{ TELLING THE FLESH }

{ TELLING THE FLESH }

*McGill-Queen's/Associated Medical Services Studies in the History of Medicine, Health, and Society*

SERIES EDITORS: S.O. FREEDMAN AND J.T.H. CONNOR

Volumes in this series have financial support from Associated Medical Services, Inc. (AMS). Associated Medical Services Inc. was established in 1936 by Dr Jason Hannah as a pioneer prepaid not-for-profit health care organization in Ontario. With the advent of medicare, AMS became a charitable organization supporting innovations in academic medicine and health services, specifically the history of medicine and health care, as well as innovations in health professional education and bioethics.

# Telling the Flesh

*Life Writing, Citizenship, and the Body in
the Letters to Samuel Auguste Tissot*

SONJA BOON

McGill-Queen's University Press
Montreal & Kingston • London • Chicago

ISBN 978-0-7735-4576-2 (cloth)
ISBN 978-0-7735-4639-4 (paper)
ISBN 978-0-7735-9740-2 (ePDF)
ISBN 978-0-7735-9741-9 (ePUB)

Legal deposit third quarter 2015
Bibliothèque nationale du Québec

Printed in Canada on acid-free paper that is 100% ancient forest free
(100% post-consumer recycled), processed chlorine free

This book has been published with the help of a grant from the Canadian Federation
for the Humanities and Social Sciences, through the Awards to Scholarly Publications
Program, using funds provided by the Social Sciences and Humanities Research
Council of Canada. Funding has also been received from Memorial University of
Newfoundland's Publications Subvention Program.

McGill-Queen's University Press acknowledges the support of the Canada Council
for the Arts for our publishing program. We also acknowledge the financial support
of the Government of Canada through the Canada Book Fund for our publishing
activities.

LIBRARY AND ARCHIVES CANADA CATALOGUING IN PUBLICATION

Boon, Sonja, 1969–, author
Telling the flesh : life writing, citizenship, and the body in the letters to Samuel
Auguste Tissot / Sonja Boon.

(McGill-Queen's/Associated Medical Services studies in the history of
medicine, health, and society ; 44)
Includes bibliographical references and index.
Issued in print and electronic formats.
ISBN 978-0-7735-4576-2 (bound). – ISBN 978-0-7735-4639-4 (paperback). –
ISBN 978-0-7735-9740-2 (pdf). – ISBN 978-0-7735-9741-9 (epub)

1. Physician and patient – Europe – History – 18th century.   2. Patients' writings –
History and criticism.   3. Sick – Europe – Psychology – History – 18th century.
4. Human body – Social aspects – Europe – History – 18th century.   5. Human
body – Politicals aspects – Europe – History – 18th century.   6. Citizenship – Political
aspects – Europe – History – 18th century.   7. Medicine –  Europe – History – 18th
century.   8. Tissot, S. A. D. (Samuel Auguste David), 1728–1797.   I. Title.
II. Series: McGill-Queen's/Associated Medical Services studies in the history of
medicine, health, and society ; 44

R726.5.B68 2015      610.9409'033      C2015-902654-7
                                       C2015-902655-5

Set in 10/13 Sabon with Scala Sans
Book design & typesetting by Garet Markvoort, zijn digital

# { CONTENTS }

CONTENTS

{ ACKNOWLEDGMENTS }

This book represents over four years of researching, thinking, writing, and sharing, and could not have been completed without the help of many.

First of all, I thank the Social Sciences and Humanities Research Council of Canada for their generous support of this project, which enabled me not only to work extensively with the archival materials and to share my research at conferences in Canada and abroad, but also to support the work and training of graduate students. I am also grateful to the staff at the Bibliothèque cantonale et universitaire de Lausanne (BCUL), in particular Mme Danielle Mincio and M. Daniel Gombau, for their welcome, helpfulness, and quiet efficiency. The BCUL is a most marvelous place to work, and this is due in no small part to the staff. My thanks, too, to the anonymous readers of this manuscript. I benefited enormously, not only from their enthusiastic response to this work, but also from their thoughtful comments, critiques, and suggestions, which have strengthened my writing and thinking. Thanks also to Joanne Muzak, for careful and thoughtful copyediting. Your eyes saw what mine could not and this book is the better for it. To Kyla Madden, senior editor at McGill-Queen's University Press, my deepest gratitude for believing in this project right from the beginning and for your commitment to it through the many years of researching and writing. Your assistance and support have been invaluable.

I am grateful to the seven graduate students who contributed their energies to this project in numerous ways: Jess Khouri, Sarah McQuarrie, Erin Mobley, Kira Petersson Martin, Ilaria Pivi, Gina Snooks, and Zaren Healey White. I am also indebted to my undergraduate and graduate seminar students in feminist theory, feminist methodologies, and life writing, with whom I have had rich and productive discussions about bodies, embodiment, theories, histories, and citizenship. Thank you for your stimulating conversations, probing questions, and passion for learning. We have journeyed far together, and your thinking has enriched mine.

I thank, too, the lunching ladies – Marica Cassis, Jennifer Selby, and Amanda Bittner – for conversations, laughter, and moral support; Joan Butler for her sense of humour and her moose sausage, and for being an absolute administrative rock; Craig Maynes for help with an errant bit of Latin; Scott and Melody Morton-Ninomiya for a well-timed holiday and a dining room table, the combination of which allowed me to revise three chapters in my very own local "writing retreat." To Jocelyn Thorpe, my thinking and writing partner in crime: thanks for your inspiration, your generous and positive outlook, your unflagging energy, and your deep commitment to living and working with integrity, grace, and passion.

My thanks go, too, to the editors of the *Bulletin of the John Rylands Library* and *Limina*, as well as to the University of Toronto Press, publisher of the edited volume, *The Secrets of Generation: Reproduction in the Long Eighteenth Century* (eds. Ray Stephanson and Darren Wagner) for their permission to draw on material included in other publications. These publications are: "Gender, Class and Epistolary Suffering: Narrating the Bodily Self in Women's Medical Consultation Letters to Samuel Auguste Tissot," *Bulletin of the John Rylands University Library* 90, no. 2 (2014): 143–61; "Maternalising the (Female) Breast: A Comparison of Marie-Angélique Anel Le Rebours' *Avis aux mères qui veulent nourrir leurs enfans* (1767) and La Leche League International's *The Womanly Art of Breastfeeding* (1963)," *Limina: A Journal of Historical and Cultural Studies* 15 (2009): 1–16, http://www.archive.limina. arts.uwa.edu.au/past_volumes/15/boon; and "Mothers and Others: The Politics of Lactation in Medical Consulting Letters Addressed to Samuel Auguste Tissot," in *The Secrets of Generation: Reproduction in the Long Eighteenth Century*, edited by Raymond Stephanson and Darren Wagner, 258–77 (Toronto: University of Toronto Press, 2015).

And finally, to my family – Búi Petersen, Stefan Boon-Petersen, and Tóbin Boon-Petersen – who have lived with all the fireworks that accompany the research and writing of a book: my thanks for your hugs, your encouragement, your patience, your goofiness, your smiles, and your late-night brownie baking. I couldn't have done this without you.

{ TELLING THE FLESH }

{ TELLING THE FLESH }

{ INTRODUCTION }

# Bodies and Stories

When we tell or write about our own lives, our stories establish our
identities as both content – I am the person who did these things – and
as act – I am someone with a story to tell. And we do something even
more fundamental – we establish ourselves as persons: I am someone,
someone who has lived a valuable life, a value affirmed precisely by any
life story's implicit claim that it is worth telling and hearing.

Paul John Eakin, *The Ethics of Life Writing*

At a fundamental level, this book is about stories, the stories our bodies
tell and the stories we tell about our bodies. It is about the stories we
tell ourselves and those that we tell others. And it is about the ways that
we integrate such stories into broader political narratives about citizenship and belonging. Finally, it is about the limits of storytelling; that is,
it is about those stories that cannot easily be told and also, about those
stories that cannot be told at all. At a meta-level this book asks us to
consider why we tell stories and what purposes stories serve. It asks us
who has the right to tell stories, and it asks us who doesn't. It asks us to
consider the role of the body in our storytelling and finally, it asks us how
stories of the body – fleshy and enfleshed narratives – come to matter.

At its heart, this book is, itself, a story: the story of suffering individuals who took pen to paper in an attempt to articulate their bodily
woes to Samuel Auguste Tissot, the most famous doctor in Enlightenment Europe. Consultation letters, as these missives are generally
termed today, are an important but, until recently, relatively overlooked
source of insight into embodied autobiographical subjectivity. Yet, consultation by correspondence – the art of writing one's bodily story and
sharing it with one's doctor – was a mainstay of the eighteenth-century
medical encounter; indeed, in many instances, consultation took place
entirely by letter. Written by individual patients as well as by primary

physicians, family members, and church authorities, these narratives offer a unique window into the nature of corporeal experience and cultural understandings of embodiment during an era when the medical encounter was largely limited to external examination. The extensive corpus of letters addressed to Tissot – the focus of this particular study – is matched by similarly rich collections of letters addressed to numerous other doctors around Europe, among them Sir Hans Sloane, Etienne-François Geoffroy, William Cullen, and others.[1]

Consultation by correspondence, what Philip Rieder has termed a "lay medical culture,"[2] made medical encounters in absentia possible, enabling individuals in far flung locations to maintain contact with leading physicians during this period.[3] But it also did something more: it provided the opportunity for individuals to conceive their psychic and somatic sufferings in textual form. In the process, these individuals created textual selves, articulating bodily autobiographies, if you will, identities deeply shaped by bodily experience. However, this is not just a story about bodies and medicine. Rather, this book is a story about the ways in which these suffering individuals came to understand their bodies as sites of political engagement; that is, it is a story about how people claimed their bodies' stories as sites for the articulation of embodied citizenship.

This book is, ultimately, a story about bodily stories. We tell stories to make sense of our world, to give voice to our thoughts, and, perhaps, because we feel that the story needs to be heard. We tell stories that have never been told, and we tell stories that have always been told. We tell stories, as writer and filmmaker Nora Ephron wrote in her memoir, *Heartburn*, so that we can shape them as we please.[4] We tell them to protect ourselves and to make sense of our lives. We tell them, Ephron writes, so that they are *our* stories, so that we can claim (and retain) ownership over them. And in this final statement, Ephron gestures towards the political domain of storytelling. By claiming authorship – by putting our name to our story – we claim the right to be heard.[5]

Two well-known eighteenth-century bodily stories might illustrate these points. In 1725, the French court musician and composer Marin Marais published his fifth book of *Pièces de viole*. Included among the many and varied movements is the "Tableau de l'opération de la taille," from his *Suite in E minor*. The "Tableau," a programmatic composition, not only exploits the voice of the viola da gamba, Marais's chosen musical instrument, but also deploys these musical gestures in an introspective examination of the depths of human fear and pain as they might have been experienced during the course of a surgery to remove a bladder stone. Nobody really knows if Marais actually underwent this operation. What is known is that bladder surgery was relatively common at that time.[6] In this sense, its program would have been recognizable to both performer and audience: fear, inevitability, shivering, incisions, pain – *so very much pain* – blood, resignation, rest.

As contemporary listeners well removed from such corporeal experiences, we are drawn into a foreign musical world, joining Marais as he recalls the rising bed, the drops of blood, and the patient's shriek followed by an almost ominous silence, and finally, a return to bed. The musical composition embodies, in a very literal way, the abject horror of this experience. We shudder as we listen, even as we find ourselves incapable of blocking the sounds from our senses. But at the end of the opening "Tableau," as the work transitions to the much more lively movement that follows, we are left with many questions. Why would Marais have chosen to put such an experience to music? What was the purpose of making this body experience visible in musical form? Why formalize this bodily story? Why publish it, in the process ensuring not only its wider dissemination but also, its posterity?

I find myself asking similar questions about famed British novelist and playwright Fanny Burney's carefully detailed and dramatically complex narration of her mastectomy, an operation she underwent in 1811, almost a full century after Marais published his "Tableau." This letter, addressed to her sister and written over a period of several months following the event itself, is housed in its own special folio, annotated, in Burney's hand: "Breast operation / Respect this / & beware not to injure it!!!"[7] Why was it so important for Burney – known to be an inveterate scribbler – not only to record this experience in narrative form, but to ensure its safekeeping? Why did she insist on sharing these details with others?

There are elements of voyeurism in both Fanny Burney's and Marin Marais's works. Reading Burney's narrative is excruciating. As creatures of sensibility, we feel her helplessness. We feel her bodily sorrow. We feel her fear. And we feel, too, her power as she responds to her doctor's query: "*Qui me tiendra ce sein?*" "Who will hold this breast for me?"[8] This almost obscenely intimate gesture sets up Burney's moment of grace, an astonishing display of strength and a powerful act of corporeal witness: Who will hold this breast for me? "*C'est moi, Monsieur.*"[9] "I will."

The return of the "I" at this point in the narrative is transformative. This is no longer an anatomy lesson enacted on a docile body; no, this is an active subject in full control of her own bodily narrative. Perhaps, then, it is the idea of bodily memory and corporeal agency that we are meant to take away from Burney's epistolary remembrance. Perhaps we are meant to reflect on Fanny's strength of character as she held her diseased breast out to her doctor in the presence of so many other men, all voyeurs in this staging of surgical skill. Perhaps she meant to turn their rapt attention away from the surgeon and toward the patient. As a reader, I, too, am called to bear witness. Not to surgical skill, but to the willpower, courage, and strength that it took to undergo this operation and later, to the brutal honesty, inner fortitude, and literary prowess that enabled Burney to produce this narrative.

Unlike Burney, Marais does not overtly include an "I" in his work. He writes from the perspective of the terrified patient, but it is not clear that this patient is Marais himself. Part of this is likely due to the nature of the genre itself. Marais was not writing an intimate letter to his sister; he was writing a musical work, a narrative that would come into its own only in the act of performance. Marais's "I," therefore, emerges in the communion between musician and score, and then, in the ephemeral spontaneity that unites performers and audience. The temporal nature of this work brings an immediacy that printed word or visual image alone lack. It is this very immediacy that evokes the "I"; in performance, the musical text becomes an autobiographical text, manifest and embodied through the bodily gestures of the performer. How might this have played itself out in the context of eighteenth-century bodily experience? Would performers have recognized their own bodily experiences, and would those experiences have transposed themselves onto and through the musical text? Would they, too, have borne witness to psychic strength in the face of somatic frailty?

In some ways, both of these works follow the tradition of the anatomy lesson paintings so common in the Dutch Golden Age. Constructed through a sort of doubled gaze – intended, that is, for at least two audiences, both the immediate audience of medical professionals actively working on the body *and* the audience of readers and viewers who later encounter these visual and textual narratives – they offer voyeuristic insight not only into the body and its workings but also into bodily identity, the subjectivities that emanate from bodily being.

Marais's "Tableau" and Burney's letter, one published in 1725 and the other written in 1812, bookend my study chronologically. As powerful narratives of bodily selves, they also ground it conceptually, critically, and creatively. Both Marais and Burney were masters of their respective crafts. They knew how to shape a narrative: how to build to a high point and how to release us and return us to ourselves. These are not mere autobiographical recollections; these are carefully structured and considered evocations of corporeal suffering and distress. As time capsules, both works bring us into the bodily thought worlds of the eighteenth and early nineteenth centuries, revealing worlds that might otherwise remain hidden. What might we learn from them as we consider the meanings and politics of bodies past? What stories do they tell? What can we learn from them about the relationships between lived bodies and textual bodies? What do they say about matters of life and death, story and experience, private and public, personal and political?

Stories are our way of living in the world. Stories allow us to imagine our world in new ways. When we tell stories, we insert our voices into the grand narratives of humanity itself, adding them to a collective history of storytelling that stretches back through centuries and forward through the voices of those to come. Scheherazade wove a seductive spell with her stories, in the process saving not only her life, but the lives of all the women who might otherwise have followed her. La Fontaine offered moral lessons through his, teaching the values of patience, virtue, and industriousness. In the nineteenth century, the Grimm brothers gathered oral stories of beautiful mermaids, winsome char girls, evil stepmothers, and handsome princes, all of whom were later made famous by Walt Disney. And oral stories, today, form the basis of Canada's Truth and Reconciliation Commission. As Thomas King reminds us, "Stories are wondrous things. And they are dangerous."[10] Stories, in a word, matter.

There are about 1,300 stories in the Fonds Tissot, a rich archive of material related to the life and work of Samuel Auguste Tissot housed in the Bibliothèque cantonale et universitaire de Lausanne, Switzerland. These stories offer insights into the ways that eighteenth-century individuals experienced and understood their bodies. They tell us how bodies spoke and they tell us how individuals transformed bodily experience into textual identity. But they also tell us more: they tell us how individuals understood their bodily selves in relation to broader political discourses of belonging and citizenship.


## SAMUEL AUGUSTE TISSOT


Such was the renown of the Swiss physician Samuel Auguste Tissot that, in the weeks leading up to his death, the Lausanne Council withdrew permission for an anticipated social event: "The medical condition of

Professor and Doctor Tissot, who lives in the Maison Fraisse, across from the Hôtel de ville does not allow the possibility of proceeding with the Regiment Officers' Ball, which was scheduled to take place in the Salle des Deux Cents. As such, we have rescinded the permission we previously accorded for this event."[11]

Samuel Auguste Tissot (20 March 1728 – 13 June 1797) was one of the most famous physicians in Enlightenment Europe. A native of Switzerland, he undertook medical training in Montpellier before taking up his first position – as *médecin des pauvres* (doctor responsible for the poor) in the Canton of Berne – upon his return. He later stated that it was suffering of the poor that inspired him to write the *Avis au peuple sur sa santé*:

> Unfeignedly affected with the unhappy Situation of the poor Sick in Country Places in Switzerland, where they are lost from a Scarcity of the best Assistance, and from a fatal Superfluity of the worst, my sole Purpose in writing this Treatise has been to serve, and to comfort them. I had intended it only for a small Extent of Country, with a moderate Number of Inhabitants; and was greatly surprized to find, that within five or six Months after its Publication, it was become one of the most extensively published Books in Europe; and one of those Treatises, on a scientific Subject, which has been perused by the greatest Number of Readers of all Ranks and Conditions.[12]

Apart from short stints in France and Italy, Tissot maintained his professional practice in Switzerland. His home, across the street from Lausanne's Hôtel de ville and today marked by a tiny plaque to commemorate his historical influence, became a site of pilgrimage, as individuals from across Europe travelled to seek out his counsel. Lausanne itself came to be known as a centre for medical tourism.[13] In 1797, Tissot was still actively writing. Death interrupted the revisions of his final work, *De la médecine civile, ou de la Police de la Médecine*, a treatise that might be read as a summation of his medical, philosophical, and political beliefs through the lens of the law.[14]

Tissot's professional career spanned almost the entire second half of the eighteenth century. His fame derived largely from his writing and publishing activities. The *Avis au peuple sur sa santé*, a practical guide designed for the populace at large rather than for the medical elite, was an instant bestseller. Its influence was such that it was in constant publication for over a century. Translated into at least sixteen languages, it ran to 144 editions and reprints between 1761 and 1884.[15] The impact of the *Avis* lay in its approach. Written in plain language in the vernacular, it addressed the most common ailments of the time, offering both insight into their origins and practical remedies for their cure. It was, at its heart, a book designed specifically for the use of laypeople.

While the *Avis* might have catapulted Tissot to international fame, it was not his only influential publication. Indeed, the *Avis* was not read in isolation. Together with three of Tissot's other books – *L'Onanisme*, *Essai sur les maladies des gens du monde*, and *De la santé des gens de lettres* – the *Avis* was part of a constellation of works in the area of public health. These works addressed not only the applied nature of health as a practice (the *Avis*), but also linked health to questions of morality and citizenship. The other three works explicitly link certain categories of individuals not only with the potential for individualized bodily disorder, but further, with the potential for broader social disorder. In other words, in these works Tissot was not merely interested in matters of physiological concern; rather, as the *médecin-philosophe* that he was, he drew overt connections between physiology and morality.

This is evident in all of these publications, each of which insists on the obligations of individuals to take responsibility for their health. Consider, for example, Tissot's exhortations to girls and women, as found both in *De la santé des gens de lettres* and in an English translation of his *Essai sur les maladies des gens du monde*. Here Tissot observed that girls who read too many novels at a young age would later be poor nurses to their children; women who chose not to breastfeed, meanwhile, could suffer "a species of palsy in the uterus, which follows the loss of the milk and renders them insensible to the pleasure, and unfit for the purposes of generation."[16] For Tissot, women's health was intrinsically related not only to their reproductive capacities, but also to their reproductive obligations. So, too, was Tissot equally concerned about the social responsibilities of men. As Antoinette Emch-Dériaz observes of his *Traité des nerfs et de leurs maladies*, a four-volume work that first appeared between 1778 and 1780, "[Tissot] had little patience with male hypochondriacs whose selfishness and whims were responsible for their troubles. He explicitly noted: 'since we owe everything to God, we ought to do what pleases Him most, which is that each human being have a useful vocation and carry it out.' To fail in this duty was to betray our human nature willed by God. Nature took revenge through poor health."[17]

The *Avis* included a helpful section on medical epistolarity. In this section, Tissot acknowledged that medical epistolarity was a common feature of eighteenth-century medical practice. But he also reminded readers that consultation itself was a complex process, one rendered even more complex in the face of faulty or inadequate information: "Great consideration and Experience are necessary to form a right Judgment of the State of a Patient, whom the Physician has not personally seen; even though he should receive the best Information it is possible to give him, at a Distance from the Patient. But this Difficulty is greatly augmented, or rather changed into an Impossibility, when his Information is not exact and sufficient."[18] In order to facilitate consultation by correspondence, Tissot included a list of questions that prospective patients needed to be prepared to answer. For the most part, these questions are not unexpected and include queries about specific bodily symptoms, including pulse, temperature, breathing, aches and pains, and bowel movements. A series of questions specific to women includes such areas of medical interest as menstruation, pregnancy, and breastfeeding.

Some lay correspondents were clearly attentive to Tissot's instructions. Mademoiselle de Zerbst, for example, offers a detailed recitation of her bodily concerns: "Everything that warms [a body] does not suit me at all. Wine is so contrary to me that I won't drink it; it gives me anxiety, dizziness and an unpleasant feeling. I often have migraines, but only in the temples, especially on the left side. I eat very little, but I sleep a lot. My sleep would be good but for the fact that it has, for some time, been interrupted by choking fits which affect me much more often at night than in the daytime. Before the measles, I was as strong as an ox, but no longer."[19] In one short paragraph, Mademoiselle de Zerbst offers a wealth of insight into questions of diet, digestion, bodily experience, and medical history, all of which are integral to successful diagnosis and cure. The rest of this two-page letter is similarly detailed. In tiny, cramped handwriting, Mademoiselle de Zerbst discusses a range of bodily sufferings, from flushed skin to palpitations, fevers accompanied by delirium, choking fits, sore throat, chest pains, chills, and a bodily weakness so profound that she was only barely able to speak. Indeed, the letter, as a whole, is entirely focused on matters of bodily suffering, its detailed descriptions responding to several of the questions Tissot put forward.

If evidence from the letters is any indication, the *Avis* transformed the everyday experience of illness and health. Numerous correspondents reference direct instances when the *Avis* helped them. Madame de Bombelles, Marquise de Louvois, for example, credits the *Avis* not only for her own health, but also for that of her son.[20] A surgeon named Rouvière, meanwhile, asserts that it was Tissot's work that supported him during a thirty-three-year sojourn on St Pierre, a remote French island off the coast of North America: "It was while on these islands, where, forced to practice my art, I found myself very taken by reading your good book, and I can assure you that I followed its recommendations with utmost exactitude on every occasion."[21]

As Michael Stolberg has observed, one of the effects of the *Avis* and Tissot's other publications was to create a system of bodily surveillance,[22] a point to which I will return in the course of this book. Through reading these writings, individuals came to understand their bodily experiences as a series of measurable signs and symptoms that could give insight not only into their physical health, but also into their moral beings. Tissot's words, built on a culture already rich in bodily signs and behaviours – as evidenced, for example, by the elite practice of *honnêteté*, or in various bodily rituals associated with Christian religious practice – were a natural extension of these processes. For those who contacted Tissot, bodily signs were not just symptoms to be catalogued and read for the purpose of medical diagnosis and treatment for improved health; rather, they came to be understood as markers of moral identity, elements integral to their self-conscious iterations of selves and subjectivities in a deeply political and hierarchical world.

## SOURCES

The letters that form the basis of this work are housed in the Fonds Tissot at the Bibliothèque cantonale et universitaire de Lausanne, Switzerland, a rich archival collection of materials related to the life and writings of Samuel Auguste Tissot. The Fonds Tissot as a whole includes not only consultation letters, but also a range of other documents related to Tissot's intimate and professional lives, among them personal letters sent to and received from family and friends; professional correspondence with colleagues around Europe; manuscripts of later published work; and a range of unpublished essays on a variety of topics. The medical letters addressed to Tissot number approximately 1,300 in total.[23] Sent by over 1,000 different correspondents, they concern the health of some 1,250 individuals.[24] They originate from all parts of Europe (and beyond) and detail histories that traverse the globe. While a majority of correspondents write from Switzerland and France, letters also emanate from such countries as England, Germany, Italy, The Netherlands, Poland, Greece, Russia, and North America. Correspondents detail experiences as far afield as the Cape of Good Hope in what is now South Africa; and the island of St Pierre, today still a French territory, off the coast of the island of Newfoundland, Canada.[25] The vast majority of the letters were written in French; however, the collection also includes English, German, Italian, Latin, and Dutch documents. As a group, they span almost the entire second half of the eighteenth century, from 1761 – the year that saw the publication of Tissot's *Avis* – to 1797, the year of Tissot's death.

While, as Micheline Louis-Courvoisier and Alexandre Mauron indicate, a true "sociological profile" of the correspondents is impossible to develop, it can be surmised that the vast majority of the letters were written by socially and economically privileged individuals: in addition to being literate, they had the economic capacity to write to Tissot and to pay his consultation fee.[26] Some correspondents make mention of their professions – this is particularly the case for military men, priests, lawyers, and nuns – while others mark their social status through their aristocratic titles. A small minority of the letters concerns the health of impoverished individuals,[27] among them servants and residents of small communities. However, as Louis-Courvoisier and Mauron point out, "Generally speaking, patients and physicians mentioned in these documents seem to belong to the same social world."[28] The relative social homogeneity of this collection of documents is a limiting factor to this study. The very nature of this collection means that questions of non-elite and non-European embodiment, subjectivity, and politics remain almost completely inaccessible to me as a researcher. Nevertheless, while the correspondents occupied a very narrow stratum of elite society, the letters themselves are highly diverse in both form and content.

The documents in this collection fall under two main types: letters and medical consultations (medical consultations and memoirs authored by medical professionals as well as by suffering individuals or others in their immediate family or community).[29] Letters are generally introductory documents and might be understood as calling cards that serve to situate the correspondent in relation to Tissot. J. Pierre Gay, writing from the French city of Lyon, for example, nevertheless positions himself as one of Tissot's Swiss compatriots, writing, "I address you with confidence, persuaded that you would wish to lend your good counsel to a languishing unfortunate individual who, having been born in the Gex region in a village (Sauverny) which borders Switzerland via Chavannes, another Swiss village only one *lieue* from Coppet, is almost your compatriot."[30] This introductory document serves to frame a formal consultation that provides insight into Gay's medical situation. Interestingly, Gay's package is further framed by a third document. Written by a curate in Chalex – "in the Gex region" – this document lends credence to Gay's earlier assertions while also, by sole virtue of the fact that it is authored by a curate, presumably attesting to Gay's moral fortitude.[31] Medical consultations, meanwhile, are documents focused entirely on the concerns that directed individuals to Tissot in the first place. Detailing bodily, emotional, and personal histories that sometimes stretch across several decades, consultations – written not only by medical professionals, but also by suffering individuals, their family members, and their friends – can be understood as the "flesh" of the medical encounter. However, it is important to recognize that many documents in this collection cannot be so neatly categorized. In numerous instances, for example, letter and consultation fold into a single document, with the correspondent in question moving fluidly between social "grease" and bodily suffering.

A majority of individuals write only once or twice; however, a few pen several letters, detailing a medical relationship that spans many months or even years. In addition to this, as Micheline Louis-Courvoisier and Séverine Pilloud have discussed, mediation is a significant factor in this correspondence.[32] Letters were written not only by suffering individuals, but also by their family members, friends, and physicians. In some instances, the details of a particular case are described and discussed by a range of individuals, thus offering Tissot and the contemporary reader what Pardo-Tomás and Martinez-Vidal understand as a "polyphony of voices."[33] The letters concerning the health of Mademoiselle Disque – authored by three different doctors over a three-year period – are a case in point,[34] as are those written by various members of the d'Hervilly family in relation to the deteriorating health of an eight-year-old girl suffering from the problematic after-effects of inoculation.[35] I discuss both of these cases in greater detail later in the book.

Finally, in addition to an obviously extensive epistolary medical practice, Tissot maintained an in-person medical practice in Lausanne throughout his professional career. These two practices complemented one another: some correspondents referenced in-person consultations while others requested them. Dupan de Saussure, writing from Geneva, references both: an earlier encounter with Tissot in Rome as well as his desire for a consultation in Lausanne.[36] In this way, letters can be seen as thresholds that mediated between the doctor and his correspondents, filling in the space where an in-person encounter might otherwise have occurred.

In this study, I have been particularly interested in those letters by suffering individuals or their friends or family members. This is because these letters can offer insight into the ways that individuals experienced not only their encounters with the medical system but also how they imagined and understood their bodies; in other words, how they "describe and make sense of their intimate sensations."[37] Just over one-third of the consultation letters in the Fonds Tissot were written by suffering individuals.[38] This group of correspondents might be understood as laypeople, individuals who were not formally trained in the medical arts. Such individuals may well have had considerable lay knowledge in medicine, and many likely read one or more of Tissot's books, but these individuals were not professionally trained physicians. Many of those who wrote to Tissot demonstrate not only a clear awareness of Tissot's publications – notably the *Avis au peuple* – but also a relative facility with medical discourses of the time.[39] Medical treatises, popular literature, "self-help," and receipt books proliferated throughout this period.[40] Suffering individuals drew their bodily imaginings and understandings from a variety of sources, among them oral culture (including songs, storytelling, and poetry), religious belief systems, and popular literature (both medically or non-medically oriented).[41] Thus, while they were not professionals, they were clearly able to read and interpret themselves through a medical gaze.[42] The medical encounter, then, was a site of negotiation. Each party was actively involved in the construction of meaning.[43]

To be clear, my intent is not to set up a binary system that pits the voice of "naïve" or "innocent" layperson against the powerful and privileged voices of the medical profession. Such a binary would neither be useful nor representative of the complexities of doctor–patient relations at the time. Nor does it acknowledge the extensive privilege enjoyed by most of these individuals. Rather, because my interest lies in interrogating the nature of the relationships between life writing, citizenship, and the body, I am more intrigued by those letters that offer insight into the social and cultural understanding of the body and its workings; that is, in those letters that reveal the experience of the *lived* body, that entity which in the words of Iris Marion Young, is "always enculturated."[44]

The letters themselves are highly diverse. Nevertheless, the majority shares common characteristics. The documents in the Fonds Tissot often begin with a formal introduction that situates the correspondent in relation to Tissot. In addition to this, letters and consultations often include a detailed medical history. For some individuals, this history reached back to birth; for others, it incorporated only the parameters of the current condition. Letters conventionally record the various treatments prescribed by local doctors as well as individual engagement with these prescriptions and regimens. In many letters, correspondents also recounted matters of more personal concern – family and career issues, for example, or emotional responses to bodily suffering or the witnessing of bodily suffering.

However, beyond these broad similarities, diversity is the order of the day. Lay letters in particular tend to be "messy" documents that resist and defy easy analysis. They do not follow any particular method and are not necessarily structured in a logical fashion. There is no standardized use of language. Above all, they are subjective, offering insights only into the lived experiences of individual people. As Nahema Hanafi explains, these documents can be understood as incredibly rich "medical biographies."[45] As such, they appear to confirm the critiques of scholars who point to the inherent limitations of letters as source documents. Letters are, in a word, troublesome. Philippe Bossis lists a range of limitations: "singularity of the testimony, personal and subjective character, elitism of the writers, gaps and partialities in content, frequent absence of content and finally, an always flattering approach to writing."[46] Ken Plummer dismisses letters as documents of scholarly interest, noting that they "are not generally focused enough to be of analytic interest – they contain far too much material that strays from the researcher's concerns."[47] But it is that very messiness that offers the greatest potential for interrogating the questions that interest me most: it is in that unruly and sometimes chaotic cauldron of ideas and experiences located at what Hanafi terms the "midpoint between intimate writing and medical consultation" that I can trace questions of identity and subjectivity.[48] How did prospective patients respond to Tissot's admonitions, as propagated in his numerous publications? How did they interpret them in relation to their own lives and experiences? How did they navigate the complexities of social performance? And how did they understand their body experiences in relation to broader questions of citizenship? What stories did they tell?

The professional letters generally allow much less room for this sort of exploration. Ordered along much more prescriptive lines, they usually offer nothing more and nothing less than what Tissot would have needed in order to best diagnose and treat the condition the patient presented. These are, in general, neat, tidy packages that leave little to the imagination. Perhaps more importantly, they leave little room *for* the imagination. The parameters are circumscribed, including only patient medical histories, current symptoms, and attempted treatment. They focus, to a large extent, on issues of organic concern; that is, these letters understand the body not as a social or cultural entity, but rather as a material, physiological entity, and their letters reflect this. In form, too, these letters are tightly structured, leaving almost no possibility for alternative imaginings. These are the letters of professionals speaking to other professionals. Such letters are invaluable for scholars interested in the histories of diagnosis and treatment. They are, however, less relevant to my work. Nevertheless, in Chapter 6, which examines nervous disorders, epilepsy, and madness – what one might otherwise imagine as the "limits" of autobiography – I rely, by necessity, quite heavily on such sources. In the Epilogue, I question why this might be the case and the implications of this.

The lay letters are very different. While their authors do offer some of the same details included in medical letters, they articulate their stories differently and include a range of details that, at first glance, seem incidental to the larger medical concerns they are bringing to the table. These details are both corporeal and material; they relate not only to perceptions of bodily function (or dysfunction), but also to their lived social experiences. Thus letter writers might link dandruff with masturbation, for example, while omitting doctor-centred concerns such as body temperature and bowel movements.[49] Other letter writers take time to include details about their social lives and responsibilities, factors that appear much less frequently in medical narratives. Of interest, too, are patient references to political concerns: the encroachment of the French Revolution, for example, becomes an issue of concern in some of the letters sent between 1789 and 1796.[50] These letters also reveal much about elite understandings of the social contract; that is, they allow us to understand the nature of social performance and self-fashioning in a social world where who one knew was one of the most important aspects of one's identity. In short, as scholars such as Lisa W. Smith have argued, what the lay letters reveal is that embodied experiences cannot

     TELLING THE FLESH

be divorced from the social, cultural, and political; they are intrinsic to it.[51] For patients, in other words, body stories are never just about blood and guts, tissue and bone; they are about embodied citizenship – about *being* in the world.

Finally, patient-authored letters also function as active sites of critique. As mentioned previously, the majority of these writers were not passive patients, quietly awaiting a doctor's advice. Rather, they actively managed their care and the letters clearly demonstrate this.[52] If patients had complaints about local medical professionals, or about medical experiences they had undergone in the past, they made sure to let Tissot know about it. Thus, for example, the mother of the Princess de Vaudemont writes that she was overwhelmed by the sheer number of different remedies prescribed by her daughter's doctors.[53] Some, while not overtly in conflict with local physicians, did not necessarily agree with their ideas. Mademoiselle de Charitte, for example, found herself navigating professional tensions as a result of consulting both Tissot and a local doctor: "I was unable, Sir, to hide your prescription from my doctor, but I only followed your prescription (and nothing from his) as I very much respect your knowledge."[54] Others, meanwhile, were not entirely convinced by Tissot's medical vision.[55] Others, still, understood themselves – and their bodily sufferings – as active agents in the production of medical knowledge. Such individuals revelled in their ability to relate bodily experiences that lay outside of common medical understandings. Consider, for example, the words of Madame de La Millière: "Sir, having been, for the last six years, in a terrible state, and having found but little comfort from all the remedies that have prescribed to me, I am addressing myself to you with confidence, having heard much about your abilities. Because the sickness that I will recount to you is so extraordinary, I believe it is important for me to speak about the period that preceded it. This could give you some insight into the cause of my sickness, which has, up to this point, been unknown."[56] Here, Madame de La Millière not only claims full authority over her telling of her bodily narrative but also over the singular nature of her bodily suffering. Her sufferings are so unique as to have apparently confounded local doctors for six years. These narratives suggest that power moved ambiguously throughout the doctor–patient relationship, and while suffering individuals were likely to accord Tissot more authority given his international renown, they were also not averse to, on the one hand, questioning or challenging him and, on the other, asserting their own meanings. From this perspective, these letters function as affidavits that allow suffering individuals to attest to their authority over their experiences.

All of this suggests that lay letters can be understood as microcosms of the social, cultural, and political worlds their writers inhabited. Much more than mere recitations of bodily dis-ease, then, they are micro-autobiographies, fragments of the self performed and presented to the Enlightenment's most famous physician. I argue that, taken together, these letters might serve as a sort of collective autobiography, offering insight into the relationships between body and story, body and self, body and citizenship.

I should note that certain stories spoke more clearly to me than others. The voices in the Fonds Tissot all jostle for my attention and each is distinctive in its own way. Some are louder than others. Some plead. Some pontificate. Some are belligerent. Some are imperious. Some are querulous. Some blush. Many are impatient. In short, these are stories written by individuals who *want* to be heard. But some stories, it must be said, don't really jostle at all; rather, they appear content to play dead. As a result, they remain nothing more than words on a page. These factors have affected not only the way that I read the material, but also the decisions I made, the analyses I developed, and, indeed, the stories that I, myself, have written and am writing here. These clamouring voices themselves have powerfully shaped my work.

I will also state at the outset that this is not a work of medical history. Rather, my conceptual lenses are theoretical and literary. I situate these letters not solely within the context of medical history and medical epistolarity as has conventionally been the case but, rather, within the broader context of eighteenth-century epistolary practice more generally speaking. Letters proliferated throughout this period. Indeed, the eighteenth century was an era of letters – letters shaped social and self-identities, and it can be said that individuals came to understand themselves through their epistolary relationships. I suggest in this book that medical letters were an extension of an already rich epistolary practice. Furthermore, I situate these letters not as iterations of medical history – that is, as letters solely concerned with questions of illness and recovery – but rather as conscious iterations of self in a complex and shifting political landscape. This study is, in this sense, much more of a conceptual work. I draw on corporeal theories to frame and develop my arguments. Central to this reading is the entanglement of body and text – the intimate relationship between textual and corporeal selves. I use this conceptual framework to think through the possibilities and limitations of corporeal citizenship, as this notion emerges in the letters. Finally, using conceptual lenses drawn from auto/biography and life writing theories as well as feminist theory, disability studies, and fat studies, I argue that the letters to Tissot can never be seen merely as articulations of bodily suffering; rather, they must be understood as articulations of bodily *selves*, experienced and understood within a social, cultural, and political context of mid-eighteenth-century Europe.

This project reworks "the personal is political." A mantra of second wave feminist organizing in the United States, "the personal is political" gave women the courage to stand up for the things in which they believed, and to assert that the quotidian – manifest in their everyday roles and responsibilities as caregivers and homemakers – had political relevance.[57] But I take this argument in a new direction. Nothing, I would suggest, is more personal, more quotidian, than the body, that physical cadaver in which, philosophers would have it, the self resides. But the body is much more than the container for the self. It is both a site for the staging of the self, and, in its volatile unruliness, an agent of its own staging.

In Chapter 1, I explore the methodological terrain on which this study is founded. More specifically, I consider the letter and the body as sites of autobiographical self-making, looking in particular at the possibility of what I term a visceral methodology.

In Chapter 2, I take these ideas further. More specifically, I focus on the relationships between body and self as they emerge in the consultation letters to Tissot, and map out a typology of bodily subjectivity. I introduce five different epistolary selves: the quantifiable self, the storytelling self, the emotional self, the confessional self, and the resistant self, offering examples from the correspondence to support this framework.

The conceptual terrain of corporeal citizenship – the focus of Chapter 3 – is the thread that stitches this book together. What people did with their bodies, and what their bodies did for them, mattered greatly in a political environment beset by concerns about depopulation, moral depravity, and corporeal excess and organized around intricate rules of comportment and propriety. I suggest that for many of the intellectuals, political thinkers, and moralists – among them Rousseau and Tissot – the body functioned as a vital stage for the performance of virtue. Embodied virtue, virtue enacted through the bodily actions and behaviours, made possible the performance of a concept that I term corporeal citizenship, a deeply embodied – indeed, fleshy – citizenship that could be claimed only through virtuous bodily performances.

In Chapters 4, 5, and 6, I examine different manifestations of corporeal citizenship in greater detail. In these chapters, I am most interested in exploring how it was that individuals narrated and leveraged their bodily stories – from the narratives of kinship and reproduction that are the focus of Chapter 4 to questions of sexual pleasure that underpin Chapter 5, and the narratives of nervous suffering that mark Chapter 6 – in the service of corporeal citizenship. I engage in a close comparative reading of specific letters, analyzing them in the context of the larger body of letters of which they are a part.

In Chapter 4, I consider reproduction, in the broadest of terms. I start here with the question of kinship, considering how it was that individuals mobilized familial identities through medical consultation letters. Of particular interest in this chapter is a consideration of the corporeal performance of kinship – an examination of the ways that kinship manifested itself both in material functions: pregnancy, birth, infant feeding choices, parenting, but also in the form of engagement with legal understandings of kinship, such as inheritance, and ideological constructs. At issue are the social roles performed by both fathers and mothers, as well as those imputed on children. I also pay attention to claims of disrupted kinship.

Chapter 5, meanwhile, addresses the thorny issue of sexual pleasure. I consider the letters that address this issue in relation to the epistolary eroticism of libertine fiction, a popular mode of writing at the time. Central to my analysis are the twinned concepts of voyeurism and the gaze. Some individuals engage a voyeuristic lens through which to narrate their sexual histories; for others, however, the erotics of voyeurism are haunted by voyeurism's flip side: discipline and surveillance.

Chapter 6 is dedicated wholly to the question of narratives of neurological disorder. Entitled "Neurographia" in homage both to Raymond Vieussens's 1684 anatomy book *Neurographia Universalis* and to the concept of what might be termed "neuro-graphies" – or neural writings – this chapter considers the limits of storytelling. This chapter necessarily draws more on the observations of others – friends, family, and even doctors – than on the insights of suffering individuals themselves.

Finally, in the Epilogue, I ask what happens to individuals who are incapable of telling their own stories. Of particular interest here is a conversation about the ethics of storytelling and the relationships between story and citizenship. In a world that values stories, what happens to those who cannot tell stories? Are they denied access to selfhood, to humanity? Central to this chapter is a question posed first by Paul John Eakin and G. Thomas Couser, and later, referenced by literary scholar, Susanna Egan, in her 2011 work, *Burdens of Proof*: "If creating and rehearsing and developing one's own story is so crucial to self or identity, then must we assume that such people have no selves?"[58] In my particular instance, I reflect on the following question: What happens to questions of citizenship, to justice, to politics, when these terms exclude the very terms they were designed to include? My final conclusions gesture toward the possibility of what Beasley and Bacchi have referred as an "ethics of social flesh."[59] Turning my gaze out of the eighteenth century and towards the contemporary period, I consider the extent to which we might productively engage with the body – in all of its unruliness – as a site for both storytelling and citizenship.

## CHAPTER ONE

# Body Logics: Letters and Lives

I often find myself in a state which is impossible to describe; it
seems as if my whole being is in a state of constant vibration ... and
if one could compare the human body to a watch, I would say that
the movement of my lower abdomen is, up to a certain point, still
continually disturbed.

Hartmann to Tissot, 19 June 1792[1]

All I know for sure is this. I have been ill much of my life. Illness has
claimed my imagination, my brain, my body, and everything I do I see
through its feverish scrim. All I can tell you is this. Illness, medicine
itself, is the ultimate narrative; there is no truth there, as diagnoses
come in and out of vogue, as fast as yearly fashions.

Lauren Slater, *Lying: A Metaphorical Memoir*

In some respects the letters in the Fonds Tissot seem surprisingly approachable. They detail everyday experiences apparently very similar to our own: bodily signs, the confusions and fears that surround those signs, numerous visits to the doctor, medical corroboration, contradiction and conflict, and patient negotiations around medical directives. They also detail networks of family and social relations: the concerns of parents for the health of their children, husbands for their wives and wives for their husbands, friends and colleagues for their loved ones. All of this is familiar territory. Familiar, too, are the comments and worries about work and the challenges of working while suffering from some form of bodily disorder. And we might nod ruefully – and in sympathy – with the individual who has lost his prescription: "I lost M. Ackermann's prescription and, unfortunately, he himself cannot recall what he prescribed for me."[2] In a Foucauldian move, we might, after reading these letters find ourselves considering our own bodily habits, engagements, pleasures, and disorders and be sorely tempted to try our hand at writing. On the surface, then, these letters are not foreign. Rather, there is much that is comfortable. Our bodies confuse and confound us. They challenge us. They challenge our doctors. We seek numerous opinions, and, like Tissot's patients, we too could benefit from some of the good doctor's more common prescriptions: healthy food, good sleep, and exercise.

It is easy to ascribe contemporary meaning to historical descriptions of bodily disorder. But this would be a misreading. As Lauren Slater reminds us, medicine is a narrative, a story shaped by the same factors that have shaped body understandings.[3] We live in a social, cultural, and political world well removed from that of eighteenth-century Europe. Our understandings of our bodies are also, in this respect, very different. While the words themselves may be similar, the meanings may have changed, at a fundamental level.[4] Indeed, in the words of Nahema Hanafi, "[in the letters] we encounter representations of the body that appear strange to us today."[5] Furthermore, it is abundantly clear from the letters that doctors disagreed with one another, and that individual sufferers also disagreed with doctors. Bodily experience is, at its root, an *individual* experience, shaped by personal histories.

Given all of this, I am much less interested in diagnosis than I am in understanding the meanings that individuals ascribed to their sufferings. I want to know why individuals might have chosen to privilege certain bodily narratives over others. I want to poke at the bits that baffle, mystify, and confound me. In this, I am, like Robert Darnton in his now classic book, *The Great Cat Massacre and Other Episodes in French Cultural History*, drawn precisely to the ideas that make no sense, that are elusive, that resist easy analysis. As Darnton observes, "the most promising moment in research can be the most puzzling. When we run into something that seems unthinkable to us, we may have hit upon a valid point of entry into an alien mentality. And once we have puzzled through to the native's point of view, we should be able to roam about in his symbolic world. To get the joke in the case of something as unfunny as a ritual slaughter of cats is a first step toward 'getting' the culture."[6]

That said, I cannot shed my twenty-first-century self. Just as the correspondents who wrote to Tissot operated from lenses specific to their time, social location, and place, my analyses and conclusions, too, must necessarily emanate from my own social, cultural, and political positioning. Meaning making takes place at the point of encounter – at the threshold between the eighteenth and the twenty-first centuries, the moment at which the language, ideas, politics, passions, and sufferings of the past mingle with my own. Put more simply, it takes place at the smudged glass – the "area of opacity"[7] – that marks our encounter.

## IMAGINING EXPERIENCE

In the absence of a body, is a patient truly real to the doctor? What is a patient without his or her body?

Micheline Louis-Courvoisier, "Qu'est-ce qu'un malade sans son corps?"

The epigraph above, drawn from the work of the Swiss medical historian Micheline Louis-Courvoisier, encapsulates the conundrum of the scholar working in the area of medical epistolarity. While the focus of my research is the suffering body as a site of the self, I am confronted with the uncomfortable truth that I cannot access the materiality of the body; indeed, all that is left to me is the epistolary expression of that body. The body, and the individual who experienced it, no longer speaks. Where is selfhood located? Can subjectivity exist in the absence of the body? What might corporeal citizenship mean in the face of psychic rupture? These are methodological and conceptual questions that haunt this study as a whole.

In a now seminal 1985 work, Roy Porter called for medical history to change its approach, to shift its focus from the doctor to the patient.[8] Central to this conceptual shift has been an emphasis on "voice" and "experience" as sites of critical investigation.[9] Experience would appear to be a logical starting point in the case of epistolary suffering. Alun Withey, for example, points out that experience is "inherently subjective. Only an individual knows how they 'feel.'"[10] Who else but the patient, then, would be in a better position to tell their story? Key to this formulation is a claim to authenticity, an engagement with the idea that experience is a source of truth, and as such, the bedrock of the self. Even in the contemporary period, such understandings have underpinned (and, indeed, sometimes continue to underpin) social movements: identity politics, for example, relies on the foregrounding of experience as an authentic barometer for social change. The work of Barbara Duden has been foundational to the historical study of the body precisely because of its insistence on the body *as experience* – that is, the body as material grounds for the self.[11]

Such an approach stands in stark contrast to that posited by thinkers such as Judith Butler, for example, who assert the body as discursive construct, as always already within culture and as incomprehensible – indeed, entirely meaningless – outside of the social.[12] Scholars committed to a discursive and conceptual understanding of the body charge materialists with essentialism, asserting that a turn towards materiality always carries within it an insistence on bodily fixity that tends towards overdeterminacy. How, then, to reconcile two seemingly oppositional approaches to understanding that which we call "the body"? A more productive approach might be to analyze the encounter between the two – that is, to explore what happens when ideologies of the body – the body as discourse – come in contact with lived experience, or, vice versa, when lived experience butts up against discursive construction. Such an approach can elucidate each of these seemingly oppositional lenses while simultaneously opening new spaces for exploration and discovery.

At a methodological level, I draw on three distinct, but nevertheless complementary, ways of assessing the nature of embodied subjectivity. First of all, I acknowledge the work of medical historians who have, since the 1980s, worked to broaden the field of medical history. More specifically, I draw on the insights of a number of European scholars, among them Séverine Pilloud, Micheline Louis-Courvoisier, Philip Rieder, and Michael Stolberg, whose careful considerations of the body in the construction of self in relation to the Tissot correspondence have been very helpful.[13] Second, I draw on the work of scholars in the field of life writing, among them Philippe Lejeune, Paul John Eakin, G. Thomas Couser, Sidonie Smith, and Marlene Kadar, and, more specifically, on studies dedicated to the question of epistolarity, including those by Clare Brant, Dena Goodman, Marie-Claire Grassi, and others.[14] Finally, I am indebted to the insights of corporeal theorists (in the areas of feminist theory, disability studies, and fat studies, among others), including Vicki Kirby, Elizabeth Grosz, Moira Gatens, Samantha Murray, Jay Prosser, Susan Wendell, and Sara Ahmed.[15] This literature is rich and forms the basis for my own methodological and theoretical musings and explorations.

These three lenses enable me to position these letters not solely as documents of medical history, but also not entirely as life writings; instead, they become documents through which we might consider some of the broader political and social concerns of the period. This triple approach – medical history, life writing, and corporeal theories – also allows me to assert the centrality of individual subjectivity (with all its attendant complexities, contradictions, constraints, and limitations) while still acknowledging the potential of the body as an essential site of identity construction – that is, the body and its workings as both productive of the self and a key site of self-expression. Furthermore, such an approach enables me to consider illness itself – as it is manifest in the body – as agentive, as an entity that can, and often does, interfere with the individual's realization of self. As I have also argued elsewhere, suffering, in this sense, has its own subjectivity, its own meanings, and its own needs; it, too, has a self that it needs to assert.[16] The suffering body, in this framework, is an agent that acts of its own accord and on its own behalf. In the process, it can assert a self that is sometimes in contradiction with the individual to whom this body presumptively belongs.

Medical history "from below" offers the seductive possibility of imagining bodily experience from the perspective of those suffering from the complaints described in medical treatises. All of this scholarship has transformed the history of medicine, by placing what has been termed "patient experience" at the forefront of inquiry. In the intervening decades, numerous scholars have taken up this call to do scholarship from below,[17] but the project is still a daunting one. How might one approach the patient perspective? How might one tell these stories? How might one analyze the dizzying array of storytelling styles, ideas, and approaches?

Analyzing these letters is no easy task. I am indebted to the careful and thoughtful scholarship of a number of Swiss medical historians who have previously worked with the archival materials in the Fonds Tissot. Séverine Pilloud, whose doctoral research focused entirely on the medical consultation letters, has written numerous works.[18] Operating from the lens of medical history and medical anthropology, she considers the social and historical construction of the body, the histories of bodily knowledge, and the relationships between doctors and patients. Micheline Louis-Courvoisier, also drawing on the corpus of medical consultation letters in the Fonds Tissot, has written several articles that consider the doctor–patient relationship and the nature of lived bodily experience during the eighteenth century.[19] More important, however, are the methodological insights contained in her book chapter, "Qu'est-ce qu'un malade sans son corps? L'objectivation du corps vue à travers les lettres de consultations adressées au Dr Tissot (1728–1797)," where she considers critically how it is that one might *do* "bodily research."[20] Louis-Courvoisier's colleague, Vincent Barras, has written a range of articles relevant to this study. In addition to articles about Tissot and eighteenth-century medicine, he has also written about medical epistolarity, medicine and society, and the relationships between bodily experience and subjectivity.[21] Rieder, meanwhile, offers important contributions in the areas of medicalization, medical culture, and doctor–patient relations in the eighteenth century.[22] Finally, I note the contributions of scholars such as Patrick Singy, Michael Stolberg, Nahema Hanafi, Daniel Teysseire, and Antoinette Emch-Dériaz, each of whom has added to the knowledge about Tissot, medical practice, medical culture, sexuality, and patient experience during the second half of the eighteenth century.[23] All of these scholars situate their work within the framework of medical history and medical humanities. But to my knowledge, none of them has examined the links between life writing, citizenship, and the body as they emerge in this collection as a whole; that is, they have not explored the political implications of corporeal life writing.

In this book, I carry out a close textual analysis of the letters, engaging with what Catherine Belsey has articulated as the interactions between reader and text.[24] Such relationships are founded on an understanding that meaning emerges not just from the reader, but also from the encounter itself. The text, in other words, is not passive; rather, it "participates in the process of signification."[25] So, too, are the readers – both the eighteenth-century readers and their contemporary counterparts – active participants in the process of meaning making. This analytical approach mirrors the tenets of what Philippe Lejeune has referred to as the "autobiographical pact"[26] – the relationship of trust between author and reader, a relationship based on the implicit understanding that the named author is also the "I" – and complements critical understandings of and engagements with epistolarity.

A few examples from the collection can illustrate the autobiographical pact. Thomas Cranfurd, writing in 1774, establishes his pact by first positioning Tissot as the corporeal authority.[27] Through this lens, Cranfurd then situates himself as both English and, as a consequence, melancholy. He cements his "I" by offering a detailed assessment of his situation, complete with dates and carefully articulated bodily experiences (including masturbation). These details lend credence to his authorial "I"; they enable the reader to believe not only his account, but also his autobiographical integrity. So, too, does Madame Morozzo, writing from Turin in 1773, consciously situate her autobiographical pact.[28] Morozzo, writing on behalf of a girl whom she loves as her own, asserts a self whose authority derives not only from her emotional commitment to this child, but also to her clear corporeal commitment to Tissot's principles of health. She observes that she has read part of his *Avis* and that she is swayed by the international reputation he enjoys as a result of the successful regimens he proposes in the *Avis*. In this way, Madame Morozzo cements her position as both a caring maternal figure and responsible medical citizen. Again, as with Cranfurd, she offers just enough select details in order to assure her reader that she is telling the truth. Finally, the Comte d'Halgouet, writing in 1776, offers a quantitatively detailed reading: on the recommendation of one Dr Lorry, he spent fifty days at Spa, during which time he took the waters forty times.[29] During that same period, he saw his doctor twelve to fifteen times, during which the doctor palpated his body. This recitation of numbers and names enables Halgouet to assert his autobiographical truth. Self-making and authorization, as these examples suggest, occurred at the point at which bodily disorders, lived experience, and social expectations met.

In my study, I have identified three areas of corporeal and conceptual interest that align themselves most clearly with questions of citizenship and belonging: kinship and reproduction (marriage, pregnancy, labour, childbirth, lactation, and family, generally but not solely associated with the female body); sexual pleasure (generally, but again not solely, associated with the male body); and neurological conditions (from epilepsy to the more loosely defined "nervous" diseases that affected large numbers of the eighteenth-century elite). These three areas form the cornerstones of Tissot's political thought. They also mark points of performative possibility for the correspondents; that is to say, kinship, pleasure, and neurological concerns offer opportunities for individuals to stage selves that both confirm and resist the narratives of belonging put forward by Tissot. Nevertheless, it is important to note that while these three areas – kinship, pleasure, and nerves – function as distinct topics in Tissot's oeuvre, there are points of resonance among them. The pleasure-seeking body must also be seen in conjunction with both the reproductive and neurologically disturbed bodies. The same is true of the reproductive body, whose sexed and gendered situation necessarily links it to the imagined nervous body. It is, therefore, imperative to acknowledge that while the dictates of structure demand neat compartmentalization, such compartmentalization is, at a fundamental level, an artifice that can, if not carefully addressed, undermine the essential fluidity of corporeal understandings as they emerge in the letters.

About one-third of the letters in the collection deal directly with these three concerns, and while I consider the collection as a whole, it is these letters that form the basis of this study. This is, therefore, not a comprehensive study of the collection as a whole. Indeed, this work has already been done.[30] Instead, it is a more conceptual study that examines the role of the body and bodily suffering in the articulation of civic identity and the production of moral virtue. In this, I am indebted to the work of other scholars who have focused on the role of the body in the political sphere, mostly notably scholars such as Antoine de Baecque, Dorinda Outram, and Nicole Fermon, among others, each of whom has linked the body and bodily performance to broader political ideals and understandings.[31] I develop the conceptual parameters of corporeal citizenship more fully in Chapter 3.

## MEDICAL EPISTOLARITY

Considerable work exists on eighteenth-century medical epistolarity. Drawing on patient correspondence addressed to such medical luminaries as Hans Sloane, Etienne-François Geoffroy, Samuel Auguste Tissot, and Thomas Sydenham, among others, this rich body of scholarly activity has offered insight into geographically diverse histories: France, England, Wales, Scotland, Germany, Switzerland, across the whole breadth of the early modern period, from the sixteenth right through to the eighteenth centuries. A spate of new book-length studies on early modern doctor–patient relationships has emerged since 2011.[32] Doctor–patient relationships have also been the focus of numerous articles.[33] Other scholars have focused their attentions on the experiences of psychic and somatic suffering in intimate correspondence.[34] This scholarship has addressed numerous issues relevant to my study, among them the nature and logistics of consultation by correspondence, the relationships between doctors and patients, the medical marketplace, and the social experience of illness.[35] Scholars have also examined questions of bodily experience, medical theories, diagnosis and treatment, the professional and commercial status of medical practitioners and medical practice, questions of patient agency, the role of place or geography, and the effects of intersecting identity categories such as gender, race, and class.[36]

Medical consultation letters, in particular, have proven fruitful territory for methodological enquiry.[37] This body of work reveals that letters are unique and valuable sites of information precisely because they allow for a close engagement with questions of individual subjectivity. While a broad consideration of large bodies of letters, like that produced by Robert Weston, can elucidate general practice, a close and focused engagement on small collections or on specific elements within particular letter collections can enable the examination of the subjective and intimate experience of the body. Thus, Michael Stolberg's studies on masturbation, menstruation, and menopause have been particularly illuminating as, for example, has Alisha Rankin's examination of the Duchess of Rochlitz's experience of the medical encounter.[38]

Reading this source material entirely from the perspective of medical history has allowed for a detailed exploration of the nature of complaints, treatments, and relationships, and has offered insight into the nature of medical practice and patient experience, but it has not sufficiently considered the broader social and political implications – questions of identity, subjectivity, citizenship, belonging, and exclusion – of such epistolary converse. Nor has it fully considered the political implications of the suffering body itself, the stories that suffering bodies might tell about the individuals to whom they belong. Finally, such studies often engage with the figure of the "patient," an entity wholly defined in and through his or her encounter with the practice of medicine. Robert Weston, for example, offers a complex reading of practitioner motivations, but nevertheless situates the patient as a monolithic entity motivated by a single impulse: "For the patient, recovery of normal health, however he or she might perceive it, was the objective in seeking the advice of a healer," a point with which Séverine Pilloud concurs.[39] While this is a logical starting point, such a positioning ignores the fact that individuals were not necessarily, first and foremost, patients. Rather, they were, as Philip Rieder points out, individuals who happened to be suffering: "One of the main characteristics of what can be considered a 'patient history' is that the figure studied extends beyond the 'doctor's patient' or user of medical services … The 'patient' discussed … is not only the client of any given healer, but the individual as he or she deals with health-related issues."[40]

A focus on the correspondent as "patient" has significant methodological consequences. Micheline Louis-Courvoisier suggests that this approach has placed power over the bodily meaning in the hands of the medical establishment rather than in the hands of the suffering individual, an act of appropriation that undermines the possibility of individual bodily agency: "dispossessed of his body, the suffering individual sees himself stripped of his power in the therapeutic relationship."[41] Other scholars, meanwhile, stress the communal nature of bodily suffering.

Louis-Courvoisier and Pilloud, for example, argue that it is important to recognize that bodily suffering occurred in community,[42] a point also stressed by other scholars. A focus on a monolithic "patient" limits analysis to the physiology of the suffering body; an emphasis on the individual in community suggests that illness was social and, further, opens up the possibility of considering embodied citizenship.

The correspondents who wrote to Tissot identify themselves in numerous ways. One common approach was to focus on kinship ties, and thus to situate themselves as fathers, mothers, husbands, wives, sons, daughters, sisters, brothers, aunts, or uncles. Monsieur Lasseire, for example, positions himself as an exemplary father and husband. As he writes, "Monsieur Professor Tissot of Lausanne would like the medical history of my youngest son, from the time of his birth, as well as the prescribed treatment and the health circumstances of his mother. He has the right to this, because he is the happy instrument that was used to recover the health of this previously unfortunate child."[43] In this way, Lasseire responds both to his responsibilities to his family and to Tissot as the acknowledged guardian of his family's health. But Lasseire's paternal and spousal concerns reach even further. Reading through the lens of the father, we learn that Lasseire fears for his family: "During her last pregnancy – with this child – [my wife] was … very shy and suffered from nervous disorder; she was vehemently inclined to anger, almost to rage. I don't know if her nervous debility was the reason, or if her extreme anger caused her nervous debility; only the doctor can judge. I despaired of keeping a single child from her [body]; I feared that I would lose them all due to convulsions, of which the large majority of my children have died. Only three remain hale and hearty. The youngest, the subject of this letter, has, since birth, been a candidate for death."[44] In this letter, kinship inspires emotional commitment, but also intergenerational suffering and responsibility.

Kinship, it is worth noting, is not solely understood though blood ties. In one short missive, Madame de La Fosse Joly positions herself as a close family friend concerned with the health of a young child. In the process, her letter not only lends further credence to a letter previously sent by the child's mother, but also introduces La Fosse Joly's emotional obligations to her friend. She begins, "I saw the letter you wrote to Madame Poselle in which you indicated that you had not received the consultation that she sent you three months ago. I have the utmost regret; the convulsive child is very dear to his mother, who is my best friend, and I fear that this delay will only increase her misfortune. It would be a great consolation to her, Sir, if you could find some remedies and if you could communicate these to her."[45] Later in the letter, she communicates her own observations about the child's bodily experiences and, drawing on her friendship, links these with the mother's nervous sufferings.

Where relevant, correspondents make reference to career or profession, locating their identities as soldiers, nuns, students, merchants, priests, teachers, watchmakers, or actors. In some instances, as in the case of one Monsieur de Germigny, a military man suffering from rheumatism, these careers have been compromised by illness.[46] In addition to this, correspondents often indirectly reference their social status, positioning themselves as countess, duchess, or marquis.

It is also worth considering points made by Ulinka Rublack, who insists on the active role of illness itself in shaping not only individual identity and subjectivity, but also social understandings: "Illness … opened up a narrative space that individuals could use to explain their disorders in terms of disordered relationships rather than just disordered physiology. The movement of body and soul led to narratives that referred to experiences of violence and justice and called for changes in power structures or at least underlined the persistence of memories of collective suffering."[47] Bodies, in this sense, were sites of collective memory, stages upon which were played out longstanding complaints that went beyond the concerns of the individual to embrace the broader concerns of the community as a whole. Bodies and sufferings – and the narratives that flowed from them – were, therefore, political.

In January 1784, a man named Gringet wrote Tissot a four-page letter detailing his bodily history: "Persuaded that most maladies are poorly understood and poorly treated, because ill people neglect or are unable to offer the necessary details, I will undoubtedly fall to the opposite extreme and will exhaust you, Sir, with a verbosity which I hope that you, with your indulgence and your commitment to listening to complaints, will excuse."[48] Gringet's letter fits Hanafi's "medical biography" model perfectly. Much more than a recitation of bodily sufferings and medical treatments, it offers insight into the meanings he associates with bodily histories and experiences.

Both of Gringet's parents died young: his mother at thirty-three and his father at fifty. However, he suggests that these premature deaths were "accidental rather than hereditary."[49] He then goes on to explain this history in greater detail:

   TELLING THE FLESH

My mother, very negligent of anything that could conserve her health, to the point of sleeping in a room that had been bleached with lime that same day, was married at the age of 16, had 10 children (of which I am the eldest) without counting the miscarriages and haemorrhages, [and being] very sensitive to domestic troubles, could have been thrown into consumption by all of these events. My father, after having abused his youth, married my mother at the age of 30 and gave himself over to liquors, to the point of drinking full bottles during the final years of his life ... I recall that I was thin, sad, sensitive and timid, enjoying reading, painting and music. Immoderate sexual pleasures at the age of 14 with a servant further increased my thinness and my olive complexion. I was unable to escape the contagion of the clandestine and destructive tastes of college, but your *Onanism* corrected me from the age of 20.[50]

From this excerpt, it is clear that Gringet situates his understanding of health firmly within the context of corporeal responsibility. His understanding of bodily experience is founded not only on principles of health as a medical or scientific concept, but also links health with morality, emotion, and sensibility. Health, in this equation, emanates from a commitment to bodily moderation. His mother's health was compromised not only by reproduction – ten children and numerous miscarriages in a seventeen-year period – but also by her emotional state and her seemingly wilful blindness to health-based practices. His father's health, meanwhile, appears to have been fundamentally compromised by his commitment to a life of excess: he "abused his youth" and drank too much. Interestingly, given Gringet's insistence that heredity did not affect his parents' premature death, he himself appears to have inherited weaknesses from both parents: a sensitive, shy, and reclusive child, he nevertheless gave himself over to the pleasures of the flesh until he read Tissot's *L'Onanisme* and discovered the errors of his ways.

As the letter progresses, it becomes clear that Gringet's understanding of his body and its workings has been fundamentally shaped by his reading of Tissot's works. As he observes, "Your treatise *De la santé des gens de lettres*, Sir, having fallen into my hands, to my horror, I recognized myself in the different symptoms that you describe with such precision. I saw myself plodding towards the same tragic end that faced most of the examples that you cite."[51] Indeed, Tissot's words have, in this instance, actively *produced* Gringet's sick and suffering self. Tangling together bodily suffering and psychic trauma, Gringet imagines himself as a victim both of his passions and of an unruly and resistant body.

My approach, which moves away from the "ill or suffering patient" and towards the "individual experiencing illness" reflects the lenses used by those who wrote to Tissot. As I describe in further detail in an upcoming chapter, illness and suffering are understood by many as "hostile invasions," as threats to the psychic and somatic self. The suffering body, in such an equation, is a site of contestation. A stage upon and through which individuals can perform their identities, this body is also a space upon and through which illness and suffering can manifest their agency. In other words, the suffering body is simultaneously a site of the self *and* a challenge to the self. As I discuss in the coming pages – and, indeed, throughout this book as a whole – this notion of the ill body as an agentive entity is common to many who wrote to Tissot.

In conjunction with this, I stress the tensions between bodily experience, on the one hand, and illness, on the other. On the one hand, the lens of bodily experience enables me to examine the narratives from the individual's point of view without actively engaging a medical interpretive framework. On the other, an illness-based framing allows me to situate bodily experience within a particular social and political realm that valorized health, and that understood health as part and parcel of the conscious, embodied practices of individual citizens. Thus, these letters serve as a threshold between two very different ways of both imagining and articulating the body. Again, Louis-Courvoisier offers a useful articulation of this complexity: "[The body] is located at the crossroads of objectification and the expression of subjective feeling; it is observed as well as experienced and expressed; it is both lived and held at a distance."[52]

Finally, I am much less interested in medicine per se; rather, my focus is on how medicine and the suffering body might be engaged as vehicles, not only for broader social understandings, but also for the articulation of the self. To paraphrase Judith Butler, I am interested in how bodies come to matter,[53] both at an individual level and at a social level. What interests me most in the letters is how individuals mobilize their bodies towards broader concepts of citizenship, or social belonging. Thus, while it may well be the case that, as Weston argues, "for the patient, recovery of normal health, however he or she might perceive it, was the objective in seeking the advice of a healer,"[54] I argue that this was not always the case. Indeed, the question of bodily recovery was, for some individuals, a matter of only marginal importance.

 TELLING THE FLESH

Writing is language made material.

Christina Haas, *Writing Technologies: Studies on the Materiality of Literacy*

Laurel Richardson, in an oft-cited article ostensibly about methods and methodology, has argued that we write in order to think. Writing, she asserts, is in itself "a method of inquiry."[55] Writing, as a process, is an act of knowledge creation. In its gift, it is an act of dissemination. Such, inevitably, is the case with life writing. Central to any critical consideration of life writing is Philippe Lejeune's articulation of an autobiographical contract. According to Lejeune, autobiography can be defined as a "retrospective prose narrative written by a real person concerning his own existence, where the focus is his individual life, in particular the story of his personality."[56] Autobiography – and the autobiographical pact that governs it – are premised on the authenticity of the text, something that can be confirmed through the readers' belief in the reliability of the author/narrator/protagonist. This is a key point to consider in relation to the letters addressed to Tissot.

Lejeune's definition is satisfyingly neat and tidy while also allowing for some room for interpretation: autobiographies are stories of the self, as philosophically conceived and reflexively lived. Among those works that fit easily into this category is Rousseau's *Confessions*. Published posthumously in 1782, the *Confessions* begins with the self-conscious manifesto of a man determined to assert the singularity of his story:

> I am forming an undertaking which has no precedent, and the execution of which will have no imitator whatsoever. I wish to show my fellows a man in all the truth of nature; and this man will be myself. Myself alone. I feel my heart and I know man. I am not made like any of the ones I have seen; I dare to believe that I am not made like any that exist. If I am worth no more, at least I am different. Whether nature has done well or ill in breaking the mold in which it cast me, is something which cannot be judged until I have been read.[57]

Central to Rousseau's words are the components identified by Lejeune: this will be, Rousseau promises, the story of a real man, a journey into the innermost reaches of his psyche. In this work, Rousseau commits himself to moral integrity, brutal honesty, and the pursuit of truth. We can see in this work, too, a manifestation of Lejeune's "autobiograph-ical pact": as readers, we can be certain that the autobiographical "I" of the narrative is identical to Rousseau's "I," the "I" of the author whose name graces the cover of the book.

Subsequent scholars have, however, pointed to the limitations of Lejeune's theories. While useful in the sense that they allowed us to clas-sify conventional, published works of life writing, these theories exclude a broad range of life writings, and also, consequently, a broad range of possible identities and subjectivities. The groundbreaking work of Sidonie Smith, among others, has paid particular attention to the auto-biographical quandaries faced by those whose writings, thinkings, and language do not fit easily into the prescribed parameters of "autobiog-raphy."[58] In this respect, we might draw inspiration from the insights of Virginia Woolf, written now almost a century ago. "The book," Woolf writes, "has somehow to be adapted to the body, and at a venture one would say that women's books should be shorter, more concentrated, than those of men, and framed so that they do not need long hours of steady and uninterrupted work. For interruptions there will always be."[59] Woolf, of course, was not alone in her critique. To cite one more example, we might also draw inspiration from the work of Aboriginal poet and writer Jeannette Armstrong, who observes that language usage lies at the heart of oppression.[60] If this is the case – if language is a fun-damental site of oppression and exclusion – then autobiography must remain a contested genre, its definition shaped and reshaped by the voices it attempts to exclude.

Sidonie Smith and other scholars have heeded these calls and the ever-growing body of research that has resulted both attests to the breadth of writing that might be considered "autobiographical" and argues strongly for the inclusion of otherwise marginalized voices and experiences. This scholarship reminds us that stories of the self are not just limited to published prose narratives, but that they exist in many forms and can be found in the most curious of places.[61] The transition to the broader generic term *life writing* is part of this process, in that it acknowledges that a wide range of documents – and other materials – can be sites for the staging of the self. Indeed, in a move that displaces autobiography as genre and moves towards autobiography as theory, life writing is now less a *product* than what John Berger would call a "way of seeing."[62] Thus, Leigh Gilmore has articulated the possibility of examining the "autobiographics" of a text, while Marlene Kadar and her co-authors point to what they term "traces of autobiographical self-representation

     TELLING THE FLESH

in fragments of documents and image."[63] This commitment to "ways of seeing" has opened up new terrain in the area of ethics, identity, and subjectivity. How are selves made? What factors influence identity? How is it that individuals navigate the complexities of human relations as they craft storied selves? Paul John Eakin's *How Our Lives Become Stories: Making Selves* and his edited collection *The Ethics of Life Writing*, together with G. Thomas Couser's *Vulnerable Subjects: Ethics and Life Writing*, ask both scholars and readers to consider how relations of power shape the storied self.[64]

## LETTERS AS THRESHOLDS

> The epistolary genre can be defined as the genre of the in-between:
> between two people, between the written and the lived, between
> presence and absence, between connection and distance.
>
> Catherine Cusset, "La lettre ou l'utopie de l'amitié"[65]

Letters form one distinct genre within the complex generic and theoretical terrain of life writing. Letters offer a unique window into other lives, other stories, other ways of thinking and being. In letters, we can catch glimpses of lives lived, consider how individuals made meaning of and through their experiences, and from there, examine the social organization of their world. The letters in the Fonds Tissot offer rich and vibrant insight into the nature of lived identity during the second half of the eighteenth century.

Letters are idiosyncratic documents. While they are shaped by the conventions of epistolary practice, they are still highly personal and individual documents that do not easily conform to external dictates. For example, only a tiny minority of those who wrote to Tissot fully followed his directives for epistolary consultation, even as many more – among them the previously cited Madame Morozzo – made specific mention of having read the *Avis*. But Philippe Bossis observes that some of the very factors that challenge the utility of letters as historical documents might also be understood as essential conditions *for* a close engagement with them: "Their content should permit the drafting of a typology: narrative letter, business letter, pedagogical, love, family, diplomatic, administrative … [The letter] reveals norms, values, comportment, representations, and ways of thinking of a given environment."[66] Here, subjectivity and singularity are, in essence, reframed, forming the basis for a felicitous research encounter. Indeed, as many scholars have noted, letters offer unparalleled opportunity to "work from below." Literary scholars, too, have recognized the research potential of letters. As Clare Brant argues, "Since letters call canonicity into question, they support an argument for literature from below, like history from below. Letters are material evidence in the case for expanding our comprehension of what counts as 'literary.'"[67] It is, then, perhaps, wise to consider the words of Liz Stanley, who argues that letter writing is an "emergent practice": "They are not occasioned, structured or their content filled by researcher-determined concerns. Instead, they have their own preoccupations and conventions and indeed their own epistolary ethics."[68]

Critical scholarship has recognized that letters are not just private documents shared between individuals, but central to social, cultural, and political questions. In addition to a spate of books published since the mid-1990s, we can add a number of journal special issues dedicated to epistolarity.[69] All of this work demonstrates that I am not the only one to be fascinated by letters; my interest is shared by many, working in a range of disciplinary areas and across a broad historical terrain. All of us are interested in similar questions: What is a letter? What purpose does it serve? What stories does it tell (and which stories doesn't it tell)? Whose stories do letters tell? Can letters be understood as sites for the articulation of autobiographical subjectivity, or are they fictional itera-tions of desired and/or desirable lives? What role do letters play in the broader social and political sphere? Why do letters matter?

Rebecca Earle has noted that letters have been a prime medium for storytelling throughout history: "Nearly four millennia before Kipling composed his *Just So Stories*, Sumerian storytellers were affirming that the world's first written text was a letter."[70] This is particularly true of the eighteenth century. As many scholars observe, letters were *the* prime medium of written exchange. In the words of Elizabeth Hecken-dorn Cook, letters "saturated" eighteenth-century society.[71] From in-timate personal epistles, to epistolary novels, business letters, and political tracts, letters were ubiquitous to eighteenth-century culture. Gary Schneider observes that the eighteenth century can be understood as the "so-called 'golden age' of letter writing,"[72] a point with which Clare Brant agrees. Brant, author of a foundational work on eighteenth-century British letters, points to the diversity of letters, stressing their ability to transcend apparently immutable boundaries.[73] As numerous scholars have observed, letter writing both troubled *and* was implicated in conventional understandings of class, gender, and the divide between the public and private spheres. In its transition into the fictional realm,

   TELLING THE FLESH

letter writing also challenged generic boundaries, as it became a main-stay of novels during this period. Given the proliferation and diversity of letters, it can be difficult to articulate a common ground upon which to found a research project.

The letter – as form, material artifact, and method of meaning making – might be productively understood as a threshold concept. Thresholds, like boundaries, allow for an interrogation of the spaces between other-wise clearly defined concepts. Unlike boundaries, however, thresholds suggest openness rather than closure. As an opening, a threshold – like a window – promotes fluidity, but as an opening to the other, that fluidity must also be considered transformative. By positing letters as thresh-olds, I also gesture towards a notion of transformation: according to the *Oxford English Dictionary Online*, thresholds can be understood as beginnings, as sites of possibility and potential.[74] Thresholds are future-oriented. More importantly, perhaps, thresholds are – like windows – sites of interaction and exchange. That is, they serve both to delineate boundaries as well as to enable fluidity across those very boundaries. The threshold, literally speaking, separates inside from outside, marking the space between private and public, domestic and political.

Situated at the borderlands between truth and fiction, private and public, formal and informal, political and personal, letters act as thresh-olds upon and through which the tensions between constructed binaries could be explored and worked out. In this sense, letters mark the essen-tial tension of autobiography studies itself – they interrogate the very premises upon which autobiography is founded – in that they ask us to consider the truth of the author and the integrity of the autobiograph-ical pact.

### EPISTOLARITY AS GENRE

Understanding letters requires close attention to a number of factors: performance, authenticity, reciprocity, and materiality. Each of these factors both confirms and challenges the others. And all of them must be read through eighteenth-century understandings of class, gender, and citizenship.

As numerous critics have observed, performance is an integral aspect of letter writing. Bruce Redford, writing in 1986, notes that, "the eight-eenth-century familiar letter, like the eighteenth-century conversation, is a performance – an 'act' in the theatrical sense as well as a 'speech act' in the linguistic. Through a variety of techniques, such as masking and impersonation, the letter-writer devises substitutes for gesture, vocal inflection, and physical context."[75] Here, Redford refers not only to the act of translation required to transform the intangibility of the spoken word shared in person with the written text designed to traverse sometimes great geographical and mental distances, but also to the sense that letters, crafted in consort, required and involved the careful positioning and fashioning of self. We might consider here a letter written by Françoise Valérien de Mérande in 1783.[76] Madame Valérien de Mérande introduces herself via a close friend, Madame de Perron, whose son was treated and cured by Tissot. This careful framing allows her to use her social network to get her foot in the door.

By the same token, it is also important to consider the reverse action: as the previously cited letter by Gringet suggests, letters also inevitably *produced* identities; that is to say, it was through letters that individuals came to understand themselves and their world. This was particularly true of women. Seventeenth- and eighteenth-century moralists and thinkers imputed to women a "natural" inclination to letter writing; epistolarity was, by and large, understood as a specifically feminine project.[77] With its focus on the domestic, the private, the family and the affairs of the heart, familiar letters in particular appeared to have been well removed from public and political interests, even as their content often challenged such distinctions. Like women, letters were directly linked to the practice of civility and thus performed vital roles in the civilizing process.[78] But, as Ros Ballaster points out, essentialized notions of femininity could also be undermined through the very form that propagated them: an articulation of the letter as inherently performative allows us to acknowledge that women were able to deploy "the master's tools" in the service of alternative social and cultural scripts: "Women as writers are themselves aware of the significance attached to their presence in the … conversation and accrue power by demonstrating ethical postures in their writing."[79] Thus, Madame Carbounié de Castelgaillard apologizes for her gendered inadequacy. Writing, "If I had been under the care of a doctor, Sir, I would have sent you a rational and reasoned missive, but I hope you will have regard for the insufficiency of a woman," she effectively deploys naturalized feminine weakness in order to facilitate her encounter with Tissot.[80] Mademoiselle Morozzo, Comtesse de Valfenere, meanwhile, writes in her letter that she "cannot dissimulate."[81] Dissimulation, a hallmark of normative femininity, required a careful balancing act, for feminine modesty could

   TELLING THE FLESH

easily be misread as pretence or deceit. In using this language, Morozzo acknowledged both the gendered nature of dissimulation and her ability to navigate its conventions within the context of the medical epistolary relationship.

As the introductory letters in the Fonds Tissot make clear, letters and letter writing performed the work of sociability. As "instrument[s] of politeness," in the words of Clare Brant,[82] they facilitated social interactions and smoothed over any potential rough edges. Letters, Marie-Claire Grassi argues, promoted the very values the highest echelons of society held dear and that they already actively promoted through the art of conversation: *bienséance, honnêteté*, and *l'art de plaire*.[83] But Brant, Grassi, and others are also careful to point out that letters were much more than mere "instruments of politeness." Letters served vital social, cultural, and political functions in eighteenth-century Europe. Caroline Bland and Máire Cross argue that letters, as genre, are "crucial to politics."[84] Drawing on a definition of politics articulated by Nancy Fraser, which understands politics not in the narrow sense of state governance but rather "as the study of power in all its forms and relations in all spheres of life,"[85] Bland and Cross assert that "precisely *because* of their immediacy and their strength of feeling, letters offer initial expressions of political ideas in their inception or first-hand accounts of events as they unfold."[86]

This point is well taken, particularly when one considers another intrinsic aspect of letter: audience. Letters are, to state the obvious, dialogical; they are written with an audience – a specific audience – in mind.[87] As Amanda Gilroy and W.M. Verhoeven point out, "There are always (at least) two sides to any correspondence, two subjectivities telling and reading potentially different stories, two voices testifying differently in an 'event or utterance' through which self and other define and redefine each other."[88] To quote Mikhail Bakhtin, letters are always "half someone else's."[89] Unlike diaries or journals, letters are meant to travel: like Marais's musical text, they become meaningful *only* through the encounter between self and other. What this suggests is that "the *I* of epistolary discourse always situates himself vis-à-vis another; his locus, his 'address,' is always relative to that of his addressee. To write a letter is to map one's coordinates – temporal, spatial, emotional, intellectual – in order to tell someone else where one is located in a particular time and how far one has traveled since the last writing."[90] Both sender and receiver are shaped through and by the letter that unites them.

The idea of exchange – the implied assumption that a letter is not a single iteration thrust into a black void, but the beginning or continuation of a longer conversation – is also foundational to understanding a final point about letters and letter writing: the materiality of letters. Letters are physical artifacts, and the meanings they make are as much about their materiality as they are about their content. What do I mean by this? Letters are material manifestations of embodied identity. A letter shows the hand of its author. It shows the words that are tentatively written and those that are written with confidence. It shows the words that have been crossed out. It shows when a new pen is taken up. And through its structure, its penmanship, its language usage, and its spelling, it can reveal class, sex, and educational background. Other more intimate details are also revealed in letters: handwriting can offer proof of bodily weakness, with frail, or unsteady signatures serving to confirm the authors' accounts of their corporeal experiences. We might consider here a letter written to Tissot on behalf of a man named Kueffer.[91] The first two pages of the letter appear to be a consultation written in the third person. On the reverse, Kueffer attests to its veracity in his own hand – "I have nothing to add to the details of my malady that Monsieur de Coliny outlined in the two pages of handwriting that precede this one" – and signs his name with an unsteady hand. Tears, too, are sometimes visible on eighteenth-century letters, evidence of emotional intensity permanently marked on the physical copy.

Furthermore, as physical entities, letters travel. Unlike conversations, shared oral exchanges undertaken through individuals in close physical proximity, letters are fundamentally shaped by concepts of space and time. Letter writers had little or no control over the letters once they sent them away. As the plots of numerous epistolary novels of the period reveal, letters could be delayed, go missing, or even end up in the wrong hands. Manuscript collections, too, attest to this lived experience of what might be termed epistolary uncertainty. In the words of Sarah Haggarty, missing or delayed letters could leave correspondents "stranded in silence,"[92] forced to make meaning through and from their experience of lack. Haggarty notes that "even accidental delays … were decoded, and rendered intentional by their initial sender. As one is waiting for the letter that has not arrived, silence, the effect of delay, is made to speak."[93]

Delayed, lost, and misdirected letters also affected both sender and recipient's understandings of chronology, a point that is often lost in hindsight. While letters may have been composed with a certain order of events in mind, this order could easily be undermined by the vagaries of the postal system and the activities of state censors. This specific aspect of epistolarity may have held considerable relevance for those patients writing to Tissot about particularly intimate bodily problems. The letters of some onanists, for example, speak to a sense of helpless desperation as they struggle to present morally worthy identities even as they seek succour for their ailments.[94] This desperation is amplified in successive letters, as they continued to wait anxiously for responses that were either delayed or did not arrive. Thus, a young man named Thomassin, whose case I explore in detail in Chapter 5, began his second letter to Tissot as follows: "Last year, during the month of May, I had the honour of addressing to you a long consultation on a frightful subject that has tormented me for a long time. I have had the misfortune of being deprived of your response."[95] The space between sender and recipient – that space traversed by the letter – might be imagined as a sort of no-man's land that exists beyond the control of either. Anything is possible in that space and letter writers have imagined it in different ways. As such, it becomes important to consider how this epistolary uncertainty shaped the stories and identities of individual letter writers, and, it must be said, the epistolary legacies they have left behind for twenty-first-century scholars.[96] All of this suggests that letters are not, as might be superficially assumed, transparent and easily decodable documents. While they may, in their content, reflect an immediacy of lived experience, they are also marked by the conscious choices of their authors: the silences of conscious omission, for example, stand in stark contrast to what is actually written. Indeed, the vagaries of correspondence, from content to form to materiality, require us to consider letters in a much more complex way.

The conceptual motif of the threshold can, in this sense, be very useful. As thresholds, letters do boundary work, asking us to consider carefully and critically preconceived notions of fact and fiction, self and other, private and public, personal and political. Temma Berg articulates this tension as follows: "epistolary novels and published correspondences are no longer simply sites for private revelation. Instead, they realign the borders between private and public, complicate our notions of what Michel Foucault called 'the author function,' create spaces in which heterogeneous discourses – the sentimental romance, the Gothic, the domestic novel of manners, the autobiographical memoir, the political tract, the philosophical treatise, etc. – circulate indiscriminately, and dismantle any simple distinction between the real and the imaginary."[97]

The notion of an autobiographical pact, with its implicit notion of a social contract uniting author and audience, is thus a useful starting point, but it does not go far enough. Enter, then, scholars in epistolary studies. In her 1982 work, *Epistolarity: Approaches to a Form*, Janet Gurkin Altman put forward the idea of an epistolary pact. Like the autobiographical pact, this pact is fundamentally relational; however, its relationality lies not in the contract between author and reader. Rather, it is based on the dialogic nature of the letter genre itself. According to Altman, the epistolary pact can be understood as "the call for a response from a specific reader within the correspondent's world."[98] This definition, while acknowledging the symbiotic relationship between author and reader, writer and audience that marked Lejeune's autobiographical pact, nevertheless moves the focus away from questions of truth or reliability and towards the relationship itself: letters, she suggests, are overt calls for responses. In other words, the impetus is not on the author to prove the reliability of the narrative; rather, as Thomassin's previously cited letter suggests, it is on the recipient to respond to the call.

Letters – and the epistolary pact – are, at their heart, about what Liz Stanley, Andrea Salter, and Helen Dampier articulate as "reciprocity and exchange."[99] Indeed, David Barton and Nigel Hall insist that letter writing must be understood as a "social practice."[100] As such, it must be examined within a broader context that takes into account not just the text of the letters themselves, but also the personal and social contexts in which such letters emerged.[101] As Susan Foley points out, "Letter writers are not isolated individuals engaged in a solitary pursuit but participants in an epistolary culture."[102] For those who wrote to Tissot, that culture was not only the culture of eighteenth-century epistolarity broadly speaking, but also the ever growing and expanding culture of medical epistolarity. Such letters are, therefore, powerfully shaped by the expectations of the cultures in which they emerged, cultural practices that then also shaped the subjectivities of the various correspondents. As Penny Russell observes,

> The "gabble" in the archive is not only – and rarely consciously – about the constitution of a self. It is a record of how that self belongs in, relates to, and seeks to understand her world. Diaries, letters, notebooks, and laundry lists are not simply intimate spaces for the formation or expression of female subjectivity, but lie at a point of interface between the subject and her world – a power-

laden domain of imagination and experience, ideology and discourse, negotiation and agency. They are direct evidence neither of the world nor of the self, but a product of continual engagement between the two, representing multiple ways of being.[103]

Reciprocity and exchange can thus also be more broadly conceptualized, opened out to acknowledge that while the letter itself can be seen as a threshold that invites responses from recipients, it also acts as a document that is always already a response to the social world. Considering letters in terms of response and exchange opens up the possibility of fluidity and polysemy, of movement rather than stasis, ideas that will become more important as this book progresses.

Stanley, Salter, and Dampier take these ideas one step further. Reciprocity, they note, is not the same as response. Unlike response, which might be seen as the expectation of a reply, reciprocity can be understood as an active commitment to sustaining and nourishing the epistolary relationship.[104] Reciprocity resides in the relationship itself; it is the foundation for what Russell refers to above as "continual engagement." The act of letter writing thus incorporates within it notions of responsibility and obligation on the part of the recipient. This is evident in the Tissot correspondence as well. In writing their letters – in opening the epistolary conversation – many correspondents fully expect a response from Tissot, a response that will conform to their expectations of reciprocity, expectations shaped not only by the social workings of their environment, but also by their understanding of Tissot as a doctor and a man. The Fonds Tissot contain numerous instances of individuals who continue to assert their expectations of reciprocity through a series of letters, even in the face of Tissot's continued silence. A young man named Barbazan, for example, desperate for a response, resorted to extreme measures. Not only did he send four letters and three consultations, but he sent the final two letters via Tissot's publisher, Grasset, in the hope that using Grasset as an intermediary would both assure that his letters would arrive at their destination and initiate a response from the good doctor.[105]

These insights are vitally important for understanding the impulses that directed patients to correspond with Tissot. Their letters, in content, style, and form, are shaped by these very elements. They, too, were navigating the complexities of identity within a highly stratified society. As self-consciously aware individuals, their goal was to elicit a response from the good doctor. Fashioning an appealing self was, therefore, of utmost importance. But they were also doing something more. They weren't only sharing bodily events or emotions. They weren't only engaged in what might be termed business transactions. Their letters required them to articulate their bodily experiences in written form, to put the body into text – to quite literally *write the body* so that another individual might understand. Einat Avrahami, writing about terminal illness, puts forward another provocative possibility: "Autobiographies of people with terminal illness ... place both their creators and their audience at the intersection of the body and interpretation in a manner that inserts an element of contiguity between the material fatality of the physical disease and the cultural construction of illness by discursive practices. The audience thus encounters explorations of the embodiments of the self through both the writer-artist's interpretation of the past and their projection of a future self onto the text."[106] In this iteration, consultation letters might be seen as autobiographical wills or testaments that record corporeal meaning, authenticity, and truth for posterity.

## THE STORYTELLING BODY

Are bodies and selves something we "have" or something we "are"?
Paul John Eakin, *How Our Lives Become Stories*

Bodies, as the narratives crafted by both Marais and Burney introduced earlier demonstrate, have stories to tell. But in a philosophical imaginary that valorizes the activities of the mind, we often forget to listen to what our bodies are actually telling us. Rather, we take our bodies for granted, assuming that they will be there for us when we need them. The growing popularity of the contemporary illness memoir, however, suggests that we do so at our peril. They tell us that our bodies are not mute or passive containers for the self; rather, they are agentive entities, actively engaged in their own projects, projects that are sometimes radically different from those that our disembodied selves imagine for us.

Virginia Woolf, in her 1929 essay, "On Being Ill," words it beautifully:

Literature does its best to maintain that its concern is with the mind; that the body is a sheet of plain glass through which the soul looks straight and clear, and, save for one or two passions

   TELLING THE FLESH

such as desire and greed, is null, negligible and non-existent. On the contrary, the very opposite is true. All day, all night the body intervenes; blunts or sharpens, colours or discolours, turns to wax in the warmth of June, hardens to tallow in the murk of February. The creature within can only gaze through the pane – smudged or rosy; it cannot separate off from the body like the sheath of a knife or the pod of a pea for a single instant; it must go through the whole unending procession of changes, heat and cold, comfort and discomfort, hunger and satisfaction, health and illness, until there comes the inevitable catastrophe; the body smashes itself to smithereens, and the soul (it is said) escapes. But of all this daily drama of the body there is no record. People write always about the doings of the mind; the thoughts that come to it; its noble plans; how it has civilised the universe. They show it ignoring the body in the philosopher's turret; or kicking the body, like an old leather football, across leagues of snow and desert in the pursuit of conquest or discovery.[107]

Woolf argues that writing from the perspective of being ill offers a completely new view of the world – a horizontal view, rather than a vertical one – one that takes the body into account and recognizes that "all day, all night the body intervenes." It is this "horizontal" view that I engage in the next chapter, in which I examine the idea of bodily subjectivity. I want to uncover how it is that bodies speak. From there, I seek to understand how it is that those stories are interpreted and understood through the lens of culture. How do individuals make meaning of their bodily workings?

Much literary scholarship on epistolarity has focused on extended letter collections by a single correspondent. The very notion of the "epistolarium," a term coined by Liz Stanley as a result of her close work with the rich Olive Schreiner correspondence, takes for granted the idea of a single author writing extensively to multiple others, among them intimate friends, professional colleagues, and acquaintances. It is, she observes, "the epistolary output of a particular person (or organizational entity) … and the wider epistolary networks of which [this] letter writing was a part."[108] Significantly, an epistolarium situates the epistolary output of a single individual or entity within the broader context of their writing, their lives, and the politics and histories that shaped their writing (and, later, that continue to shape decisions around their publications).[109] The epistolarium, then, captures not only the original letter as a gesture towards reciprocity but also our continued scholarly engagements with letters.

I want to reverse this equation. In the letters to Tissot, the epistolarium is directed not by a single author but rather towards a single recipient. Instead of 1,300 letters by a single author, the Fonds Tissot offers almost 1,000 authors writing to a single recipient. This shifts the dynamics of the epistolarium, but the principles remain the same. As a group, the letters offer insight into the nature of psychic and somatic suffering during the second half of the eighteenth century. However, by reading them not only through the lens of Tissot's body politics, but also through broader bodily understandings of the period, these letters, as an epistolarium, do something more: they offer a window into the ways that individuals articulated the political meanings of their bodily experiences.

Rethinking the epistolarium requires attention to the fragmentary nature of this particular collection. Autobiographical fragments have, in recent years, come to be seen as integral to scholarship in life writing. Russell asserts that the "gaps and gabble" of the archive "*are* the object of enquiry, the site of self-representation and evidence of the cultural narratives amongst which a sense of self may be forged."[110] Such thinking has led to a close consideration of autobiographical fragments. In addition to Marlene Kadar and Jeanne Perreault's "traces of autobiography," we might also consider Antoinette Burton's "autobiographical assemblages,"[111] Russell's "chaos" and "gabble." Stanley, too, has considered the potential of what she terms "small epistolary insights into the mundane and ordinary, and sometime also the dramatic and tragic aspects of quotidian living."[112] Traces, assemblages, gabble, and small insights – together these form the "stuff" of the self; they are the foundations of the epistolarium.

The letters in the Fonds Tissot offer individual stories, but these stories are only partial iterations of selves – bits, pieces, and hints of lives and selves. On the surface, the very fact that, as a researcher, I can build my case only on autobiographical fragments appears to preclude, or at least compromise, my ability to explore questions of subjectivity and identity. Indeed, how might this be achieved given the impossibility of a single, extended narrative voice? There is much that we, as scholars, can never know. But putting these various traces together allows me to create a web of interlocking ideas, emotions, passions, bodies, and sufferings. From this web emerges a bigger story. This story does not resemble the grand narratives that have structured the longer history of autobiography as a practice but rather comes into being through multiplicity – that is, through a tapestry of individual colours, sounds, tastes, feelings, imaginings, and worlds. Lynette McGrath has suggested that a close reading of a range of texts can allow for the development of a "collective voice."[113] It is this collective voice that I seek to engage as well. However, by invoking the idea of collective, I do not mean to suggest that this voice is monolithic. Quite the contrary. The collective voice that I seek to bring to life is polyphonic, multiple, and complex. Dense and tangled, it is a collective whose coherence emerges not only through shared experiences and understandings but also through competing and conflicting ideas and desires. In short, this collective epistolary voice reflects the complexity of eighteenth-century society itself. In many ways, then, this is a collective autobiography of embodiment.

## AUTOBIOGRAPHICAL SKINS

Language is like the skin of culture – the surface where inside touches outside and a self encounters an other.

Arun Mukherjee, Alok Mukherjee, and Barbara Godard, "Translating Minoritized Cultures: Issues of Caste, Class and Gender"

On the surface, letters may seem like disembodied artifacts, shells of bodily selves that cannot even begin to represent the embodied reality of somatic experience. Jane Magrath, however, suggests otherwise: "Letters are intimately physical documents, an observation perhaps most applicable to handwritten letters, where the blank paper becomes, when covered with words, etched by the particulars of its writer. It is not only the words themselves but also the physical process of writing that stamps each letter with corporeal traces."[114] Such corporeal traces recall also Kadar and Perrault's evocation of autobiographical traces, of hints, fragments, bits and pieces of selves.[115]

The body is, as Simone de Beauvoir has argued, "the instrument of our grasp upon the world."[116] Even as it is through our engagement with others that we come to make meaning of our lives, it is through our physical selves that we first experience our world. The point of contact might be the skin; that which separates us from others, but also that which puts us into intimate relations with others. According to Imogen Tyler, "human skin ... is the border zone upon which self and not-self is perpetually played out."[117] Through touch, our skin is the first point of contact with the world around us, even as it simultaneously functions as the envelope that encases and protects our vulnerable and fragile flesh.

Letters evoke and provoke touch: touching a letter can stand in for touching the writer. As such, they can be read, as Magrath points out as "a kind of body double … The letter does not merely describe the body; rather it becomes a kind of partial textual embodiment, eventually cradled in the hands of the reader,"[118] a document that is both shaped by suffering but that also, in its material form, highlights that suffering. As William Merrill Decker observes, "hand writing images actual body presence."[119]

Letters situate subjectivity at the threshold between self and other. Like the skin – that material surface that lies between inside and outside, interior and exterior – the letter mediates between self and other. The relationship between body and text is integral to this study. Human skin, as the work of Jay Prosser has indicated, is a site of autobiographical inscription. As a text, it is, in Prosser's words, "the body's memory of our lives."[120] This is a particularly evocative conceptualization that enables a critical reading of the embodied experience of the myriad sufferings that physically marked the body: smallpox and syphilis, for example, ravaged the skin, leaving permanent reminders of bodily – and in the case of syphilis, moral – disorders. But it also helps us to understand both the protestations of those whose sufferings left no bodily mark at all – those individuals who had to write about bodily disorder in the complete absence of physical marking – and also the corporeal confidence of others who were able to benefit from their own unmarked bodies.

Thus, even as one anonymous correspondent acknowledged that his visage "announced a picture of perfect health," his bodily convulsions told a very different story.[121] Meanwhile, another correspondent, Monsieur Gounon, offered his reproductive health as proof that his engagements with the pleasures of the flesh were not harmful.[122] Skin, therefore, is that which manifests bodily horror but also that which conceals it. So, too, might we understand epistolarity. As conscious iterations of self, letters perform identity even as they conceal it. In the words of Prosser, "Autobiography works like a skin; it is the skin the author sends out that at once conceals and reveals the self."[123] Skin and letters might thus be productively imagined as contact zones, spaces upon which, as Tyler puts it, "self and not self [are] perpetually played out."[124]

Imagining letters as a sort of autobiographical "skin" paves the way for a particularly visceral methodology, a way of seeing premised on

 TELLING THE FLESH

corporeality, touch, and the material. Indeed, Carolyn Steedman argues that letters can be understood as body parts, sites of simultaneous wounding and revelation: "the letter is part of the body which is detached; torn from the very depths of the subject."[125] A visceral methodology is one that is attentive to such woundings, that acknowledges the entanglement of the conceptual with the material and the violence that can result from this. As Aileen Douglas reminds us in her study of the eighteenth-century Scottish doctor and novelist Tobias Smollett, "if you prick a socially constructed body, it still bleeds."[126] In this book, I am interested in exploring what emerges at the point at which the material and the conceptual meet – the point of contact between social construction and blood. I want to know what happens when ideological bodies – those bodies constructed through political discourses – encounter the bleeding, leaking, dying, pus-filled, shivering, aching, bruised bodies of lived experience. How does a socially constructed body bleed, and what might we take from this bleeding? A visceral methodology – a methodology of the skin – acknowledges the inherent tension within Tissot's bodily politics: while citizenship ideals promoted certain bodily behaviours, such ideals were filtered through the material concerns of the suffering body. Blood. Pain. Pleasure. Fear. Joy. Each of these is bodily marked, bodily experienced, bodily lived.

The work of Louis-Courvoisier and Pilloud is useful in this regard. In a 2003 article, they argue for "two dimensions in bodily experience."[127] Bodily experience, they suggest, is both external and internal; it is founded on external markers and signifiers visible both to the embodied subject and to those in his or her environment, and internal markers experienced only by the individual. One can be witnessed; the other remains within the realm of the personal and subjective. In a revealing statement, Louis-Courvoisier and Pilloud argue,

> If bodily experience is, above all, subjective and individual, it is
> also partially shared within a community. To feel is most often
> to recognize, localize or identify some phenomena in relation
> to corporal maps established from biological and cultural data.
> But the body's experience always retains, in the final analysis, a
> unique character, for any experience consists in a kind of addition, new perceptions starting to resonate with ancient ones.
> Bodily experience is thus greatly conditioned by an individual's
> biography and personality. It is, in a way, something made out
> of several layers; some are common to a socio-cultural group, as

these biologico-cultural corporal maps inform the perception of a well-functioning body; others are personal, like acute pain.[128]

Louis-Courvoisier and Pilloud offer a methodological approach attentive to the encounter between interior and exterior; that is, a visceral methodology that situates itself at the skin – the point at which the lived experience of the suffering individual and the bodily messages visible to the external gaze meet. Central to this understanding is the idea of the body as the arbiter of truth: it is the body's stories that authorize the narrative truths constructed by the author.

In this sense, the body's exterior is essential to the realization of the autobiographical pact in that it must confirm the narrative truth asserted by the correspondent. After all, narrative truth hinges on bodily evidence. But how to assert the evidence of an unseen body? Correspondents who wrote to Tissot employed numerous methods: some relied on a careful recitation of bodily signs and symptoms. Others, in an attempt to shore up the veracity of their own experiences, referenced friends or colleagues who knew Tissot or who had previously consulted him. Many, like the unfortunate Gringet, referenced Tissot's publications, in the process asserting themselves not as passive bodies but rather as knowers actively involved in their bodily care. I explore these techniques in greater detail in the next chapter. In each of these cases, questions of authenticity are never far from the surface.

Authenticity assumes the possibility of truth. Indeed, the correspondents insist on the tenets of the autobiographical pact: the reader must be able to rest assured that the story they are reading is a true story, and that the "I" of the narrator is the "I" of the author. This pact is sacrosanct. Notions of what Lisa Wynne Smith has termed reliability are central to medical consultation letters. As she observes,

> In addition to gaining sympathy from friends and family, patients may have wanted to persuade the doctor of the truth of their suffering. With doctors, however, it was not just a matter of gaining commiseration; the more detailed the narrative, the more reliable it appeared. There was a tension between physicians' need for patients' stories, issues that could affect the construction of patients' stories, and physicians' knowledge that patients could exaggerate or be unreliable. While physicians could observe their patients physically during ordinary consultations, epistolary

　　TELLING THE FLESH

consultations relied solely on the story; there was a fine balance between recounting a good story that led to diagnosis and one that was too good.[129]

In the absence of a physical body – a material entity that could provide seemingly irrefutable evidence or proof of disorder – correspondents could rely only on their words to make their case. But this was a difficult line to toe. Elite correspondence during this period was, in many respects, premised on artifice; that is, letter writing was an art of dissimulation. Furthermore, in spaces where medicine was closely linked with morality, could it be the case that the revelation of the wrong truth would undermine the relationship initiated through the letter? How, then, within these conventions, to assure the recipient of one's integrity and transparency? How, then, to prove reliability?

Truth, as numerous scholars and thinkers have observed, is complex. Truth in life writing is shaped not only by questions of memory but also by relationships, and as Sidonie Smith and Kay Schaffer observe, "Since personal storytelling involves acts of remembering, or making meaning out of the past, its 'truth' cannot be read as solely or simply factual. There are different registers of truth beyond the factual: psychological, experiential, historical, cultural, communal, and potentially transformative."[130] Such are the conclusions, too, reached by Alessandro Portelli in his now seminal 1991 work, *The Death of Luigi Trastulli, and Other Stories: Form and Meaning in Oral History.*[131] A collision between "facts" and memory, truth is rife with contradictions, but nevertheless rich with story.[132]

In their 2004 work, *Human Rights and Narrated Lives: The Ethics of Recognition*, Smith and Schaffer insist that truth is not a singular or monolithic concept; rather, it is a concept bound up in multiplicity.[133] They point to the example of the South African Truth and Reconciliation Commission (TRC), an entity charged with the responsibility to determine the truth behind the atrocities committed during the apartheid regime. As part of its mandate, the TRC interrogated the very notion of truth itself. Opposed to the taken-for-granted assumptions that underpin a monolithic definition of truth, the TRC committed itself to four different forms of truth: "factual or forensic truth, personal or narrative truth, social or 'dialogue' truth and healing and restorative truth."[134] This approach highlights the polysemous nature of truth and situates it within complex relations of power.

How do those that write to Tissot navigate questions of truth and reliability? In telling their stories, what factors do they need to keep in mind? What stories can they tell? Which truths can be shared? Which truths should remain hidden? Could a truth be dangerous? Could a truth challenge reliability? Could a truth be so ugly that it would undermine the reciprocity of the epistolary pact? These questions are the focus of the next chapter, which considers the relationships between the textual body and the textual self.

     TELLING THE FLESH

## CHAPTER TWO

# Textual Bodies/Textual Selves: Illness, Identity, and Bodily Subjectivity

I must confess, Sir, that I have not yet given up coffee. Because I have felt much better over the last while, I have even taken more than usual, and this, together with my inability to give up Spanish tobacco, is perhaps one of the causes of my current relapse.

Gualtien to Tissot, undated[1]

From the patients' perspective, sickness is rarely understood as the effect of a coherent disease – rather, sickness is related to meaning. Meaning is construed by the bodily sensation of the patient, his or her past, and sometimes with the counsel of the practitioner. In a sense, the interpretation of the patient and that of the practitioner need not meet: the practitioner offers counsel, but the understanding is more generally in the patient's hands.

Philip Rieder, "Patients and Words: A Lay Medical Culture?"

In his 1771 *"tableau de mes souffrances,"* the Chevalier de Soran imagines his sufferings as a hostile threat, "the enemy waging war against me."[2] Illness advances and retreats. It torments, poisons, and undermines him. It imprisons him in his body and in his home. And even after twenty years of attempting to repel its advances, it is always ready to attack. Illness has rendered his body helpless, fundamentally weakened by the continued onslaught. "Finally, Sir," he concludes, "I place the interests of my health into your hands."[3] He is unable to do any more.

The Chevalier de Soran's letter is, perhaps, a particularly dramatic rendering of his struggle with illness. However, a closer look at the language deployed by the hundreds of individuals who wrote to Tissot suggests that the sentiments he held were hardly unique. Correspondents were unfortunate "victims,"[4] "tormented" and "attacked" by their sufferings,[5] and subject to "terrifying" sicknesses.[6] In their descriptions of bodies under siege, these correspondents imagined illness as a dangerous and mysterious external contagion whose incursions threatened the self. Illness was understood by many to have agency over a passive and docile body held hostage by its infirmities.

In this chapter, I consider the relationships between illness and bodily subjectivity. At issue is the textual body, the body that emerges when corporeal experience encounters language. Equally important in this chapter is the relationship between the textual body and the textual self. While scholars of epistolarity have, as mentioned previously, persuasively argued that letter writers quite literally wrote themselves into existence, there has, as yet, been less engagement with the idea of the bodily self. And yet, as Susanna Egan has commented, "the word 'corpus' refers both to the human body and to a body of work."[7] This suggests that there is a foundational relationship between lived corporeal experience and textual experience, what Egan refers to as the relationship between lived identity and textual identity. I am interested in exploring how it is that individuals experienced, imagined, and then wrote their bodily experiences, how they made textual meaning out of bodily events and experiences. My central question here is deceptively simple but conceptually complex: What happens when body becomes word? Tumbling out of this question are many more. What does the body say? How does it speak? How do we know what it is saying, and, perhaps more importantly, who has the authority to determine what it is saying?

How did eighteenth-century individuals choose to organize their bodily stories? What did they do with the information they received when they entered into conversation with their bodies? What do they do with the toothaches, the sinuses, the headaches? How did they understand the blood? The pus? The sudden rashes? The aches? The pains? The swellings? The fevers, rashes, and chills? How did they make meaning out of their corporeal experiences? Of particular interest is the relationship between bodily identity and illness. I am very curious, in this chapter, to know how it is that individuals framed the various *incommodités*, or discomforts, that affected their everyday lives. I apply insights from the previous chapter to demonstrate that all bodies have narratives and, further, that individuals actively created narratives about their bodies. These narratives are shaped by geography, history, culture, society, and politics. They are shaped, too, by class, gender, sex, sexuality, and race.

    TELLING THE FLESH

I call these narratives body logics – textual iterations of how individuals understood their suffering bodies within the context of their social and cultural worlds. I demonstrate that body logics were not monolithic; rather, individuals struggled to find language to adequately relate the stories of their bodies and drew on themes both inside and outside medicine to frame their narratives. Furthermore, I observe that even medical logics were diverse: much to the evident frustration of numerous individuals, physicians – and even some of the most recognized physicians in Europe – quibbled about the meanings of illness. Bodily meaning, I argue, was elusive and always subject to interpretation. In this chapter, I am interested in the body both as a discursive construction and as "the site of experience, memory, [and] subjectivity."[8] Indeed, it seems clear to me in reading the letters addressed to Tissot that correspondents navigated competing understandings of the body, and that their own textual representations of bodily selves were shaped not only by experience but also by their situatedness within relations of power.

Bodily experiences have a deep impact on questions of subjectivity. Elizabeth Grosz has argued that "corporeality can be seen as the material condition of subjectivity."[9] Vicki Kirby takes this further, suggesting that we *are* our bodies, that subjectivity is always already embodied. In a provocative passage, she asks us to consider the relationship between corporeality and thought: "Not many would dispute the presence of a biological reality that is quite different from culture and that we imperfectly try to comprehend. But surely if we were without our skin and we could witness the body's otherwise invisible processes as we chat to each other, read a presentation aloud, type away at our computers, or negotiate an intense exchange with someone we care about, we might be forced to acknowledge that perhaps the meat of the body *is* thinking material."[10] The literary work of Susan Sontag and Virginia Woolf bears witness to these insights, situating the body and its projects at the centre of human experience and subjectivity.[11]

I begin by situating bodily experience within broader eighteenth-century understandings of sickness and health. I then offer a typology of five different narrative approaches to bodily subjectivity. This sets the stage for the rest of the chapter, in which I examine the ways that individuals negotiated these understandings within their own textual representations of self. This work serves to underpin the deeper negotiations around citizenship, bodies, and subjectivity that are the focus of the upcoming chapters.

I am a phenomenon of nature and this is what has made it impossible
for the physicians of this country to understand me.

Charier to Tissot, 10 June 1771[12]

Medical historians have observed that bodily suffering was an inevitable aspect of eighteenth-century lived experience. As Robert Weston points out, "By today's standards early modern Europe was a place where illness was prevalent, infant mortality huge, and overall, life expectancy was short. The frequency with which church bells reminded the populace of death must have been all too regular. The healthy state was certainly not something that could be assumed. The biblical notion of a man's life-span being three-score years and 10 was at odds with an actual life expectancy of around 26 years ... With epidemics ever likely to break out, death could strike at any time."[13] David M. Vess, meanwhile, offers a particularly visceral reading of the situation: "Diseases bred freely in polluted streams and in refuse-clogged roads and narrow, puddled streets. Diphtheria, measles, smallpox, and scarlet fever were killers known in every town ... Every winter and spring, epidemic pneumonias and *la grippe* appeared. Typhoid fever, dysentery, and malaria repeatedly ravaged France during the eighteenth century ... Lice and the itch were endemic, affecting practically everyone ... Venereal disease was prevalent."[14] Roy Porter puts it succinctly: "Illness and death loomed large in people's minds."[15]

These realities are reflected in the letters. Correspondents detail both short- and longer-term sufferings, from mild aches and pains to long bouts with fevers, diarrhoea, and unexplained vaginal bleeding.[16] They also mention the effects of weather, personal habits, and social encounters, among others.[17] One correspondent even details the detrimental health effects of a period of social unrest on an American slaveholding plantation: "the grief I experienced as a result of the loss of my home, which was caused by a slave revolt, contributed significantly to my slow recovery."[18] But what purpose did suffering play in their lives? How did they imagine illness? How, indeed, did they imagine health?

Weston observes that illness is an integral actor in the practice of medicine.[19] But it is equally clear that illness, as a concept, moved well beyond the medical realm. Suzanne Fleischman has argued that "diseases are ultimately constructs – of medical diagnostics in the first instance and ultimately of language,"[20] a point with which American psychologist and memoirist Lauren Slater, cited previously, would concur. Illness was a complex category of experience that shaped not only the practice of medicine, but also individual subjectivity and social relations. A closer examination reveals that eighteenth-century engagements with illness ran the gamut – from limitation right through to liberation. While the experience of illness and suffering would appear to have limited bodily agency, it also paved the way for new forms of social relationships. Illness and suffering facilitated desirable social networks, enabled individuals to express their sensibility and their commitment to bodily knowledges, and offered the possibility of liberating the psychic self. Indeed, illness and suffering were often highly productive sites of self-realization.

Eighteenth-century dictionaries explicitly link sickness and health. According to the 1694 edition of the *Dictionnaire de l'Académie française*, *maladie*, or sickness, is understood as a form of disordered, indisposed, or altered health.[21] Interestingly, however, illness is also linked with moral or mental concerns. The passions, for example, are understood as illnesses of the spirit. Homesickness, too, fits into this category; it is a disease of the spirit. So, too, is excessive desire similarly understood: the 1762 edition of the *Dictionnaire* states, "Malady also signifies, in a figurative sense, the immoderate affection that one has for something."[22] These definitions suggest that illness can be understood as psychic or somatic disorder or imbalance, a deviation from an undefined norm. As a disorder or indisposition, sickness is not fixed; rather, it is an indeterminate state that hovers between health, on the one hand, and death, on the other. This idea is reflected in the extended definition included in the *Encyclopédie*, which presents malady as a transitional state between life and death:

Illness can be regarded as a state between life and death: in the first of these two states, some functions always continue to operate, no matter how imperfect they might be; at the very least, those functions which are primarily attached to the state of life. This is what distinguishes the state of malady from the state of death ... But to the extent to which these different functions operate with difficulty, and that these functions have either been altered as a result of excess or through no fault of their own, or that they stop functioning altogether, this is what separates illness from health.[23]

Illness, here, is presented as a threshold state that troubles both life *and* death. While bodily function distinguishes the state of illness from that of death, the impairment of function makes it equally impossible to claim health. Indeed, illness is understood as a *threat* to health: "a vicious disposition, an impediment of the body or of one of its organs, which causes an injury to the exercise of one or more functions of a healthy life, or even stops it from functioning altogether, except for the beating of the heart."[24]

Health, by contrast, is understood as an ideal state of balance and equilibrium. An individual who is in good health can be said to possess a strong constitution, and, as a result is not subject to illness.[25] According to the *Encyclopédie*, health is a state of bodily perfection: "We can consequently define it: natural accord, the reasonable arrangement of the parts of the living body, from which it follows that the exercise of all its functions is done, or can be done in a sustainable manner, with ease, freedom, and to the extent which each of its organs is susceptible, according to its purpose, and relative to the actual situation, to the different needs, age, sex, temperament of the individual who is in this position, and to the climate in which he lives."[26]

But health was, as previously noted, elusive. A good constitution was a great starting point, but if the letters to Tissot are any indication, it was not enough to ensure a life free from mental or bodily disorder. Consider, for example, the case of the Count d'Adhémar, a man "born of healthy, strong and temperate parents who did not suffer from gout."[27] One might think that this felicitous bodily lineage would have set the count up for a life free from bodily suffering. However, this was not to be: his fifteen-page consultation details muscular and arthritic sufferings to which he has been subject.

Further, it is equally clear that the understandings that mark dictionary, encyclopedia, and medical definitions of health and illness do not account for the complexities of individual lived experience, complexities that rendered illness as enabling as it was disabling. The work of Jane Magrath highlights the contradictory nature of bodily suffering. Magrath, who considers English bluestocking correspondence, notes that Elizabeth Carter and Elizabeth Montagu were "not only victims of their bodies but also agents because of them."[28] So, too, were many of those who wrote to Tissot both victims of psychic and somatic disorders that profoundly limited their lives and agents of their own bodily subjectivities. Thus, while illness was disabling, it was also enabling; there were benefits to be derived from claiming and performing a sick identity. Alun Withey observes that psychic and somatic suffering, once translated into textual form, could be "tactically" deployed: "the increasing use of the written word and, in particular, the letter brought forth new opportunities for the construction of suffering ... [Literacy] offered opportunities to elaborate on the personal 'feelings' of illness, and even to construct an individual sickness 'persona.'"[29] The very fact that discussions of sickness and suffering were not confined to medical letters but proliferated throughout the letters of this period is evocative of the role of bodily malaise in the construction of the self.[30]

The body, as a corporeal tableau, served as a backdrop for embodied epistolary performances. As a site of suffering, it was the source for the textual inscription of the suffering self. This textual inscription served further to situate the epistolary self variously as a medical knower and as a moral individual. In a particularly remarkable letter complete with footnotes and references to a range of medical texts, a correspondent uses his own bodily suffering to present himself as a medical knower and, further, as a knower, to claim corporeal citizenship.[31] Bodily suffering, then, *enabled*, rather than disabled his performance of self.

We might consider, too, correspondent Jean Frédéric Borel's self-conscious assertions that he has read some of Tissot's works:

> It has been some time since I had the good fortune of reading
> your books of Medicine and Surgery, in which I noted that
> Monsieur Tissot showed great generosity and charity towards hu-
> manity, as well as a strong knowledge and experience in Medicine
> and Surgery, and intelligence, good sense and strong faith. All of
> these good qualities – together with all the others that I attribute
> with reason to Monsieur Tissot – give me great confidence in you,
> and allow me to take the liberty of asking you to allow me to
> consult you with regard to one or more of the maladies which I
> have suffered over the last several years. For this reason, I wrote
> about the state I am currently in, following the requests laid out
> in your Books.[32]

Borel's approach is mirrored by numerous correspondents. Not only does such a claim enable him to position himself favourably vis-à-vis the doctor, but it also serves a larger purpose. By engaging with Tissot's published writings, correspondents like Borel lay authorial claim to the realm of medicine, inserting themselves overtly into the grand medical debates of this period.

The possibility of basking in the reflected glow of Tissot's enlightened virtue was no small enticement. As patients of one of the most famous physicians in eighteenth-century Europe, individuals could anticipate the establishment of mutual bonds of devotion and responsibility that would cement their social position within their local communities; after all, a response from a man of Tissot's international stature was something to be treasured, something to be shared in polite company. As Cherot du Marois, writing in 1786, observed, "The frequent reading of your books, in which the Science of a True Healer reveals itself just as much as your love for humanity, has always made me want to enjoy the pleasure of knowing you personally. If I have not had the pleasure of this, at least permit me the satisfaction of conversing with you at least once in my life; your advice with regard to my condition will calm me infinitely more than a full faculty of doctors, such as those that I see on a daily basis."[33]

But such relationships, carefully established and nurtured, also laid the groundwork for further encounters: from these initial letters, correspondents established reciprocal obligations upon which they could call in the future. Thus, for example, Madame Rigoley, Marquise d'Agrain, begins her letter to Tissot by reminding him that he had previously treated her daughter. The success of that treatment – her daughter's full recovery from her ailment – underpins her current letter, which concerns the corporeal infirmity of her daughter's presumptive spouse.[34] So, too, does Madame Gounon Laborde similarly situate her authority to contact Tissot: "It is to your salutary prescriptions, Sir, that M. Gounon of Agen, my Father, and I owe the recovery of my sister and brother. Today, it is for my husband that I dare to implore the happy secret that all of Europe recognizes for the rarest and most extraordinary cures; and the humanity of your soul is so well known that I can address myself to you with the utmost confidence."[35] In each of these cases, bodily impairment serves as the primary impetus for the presentation of morally responsible self, a self fully committed not only to the principles of health espoused by Tissot, but also to the health of the family, the basis for civic happiness.

Psychic and somatic suffering also facilitated social relations at a broader level. Intimate correspondence between close friends and family frequently hinged on issues of bodily suffering. Indeed, Roy and Dorothy Porter observe that during the eighteenth century, the "golden age of diaries and letter-writing ... health is prominent in both."[36] Consider, for example the letters exchanged by Tissot's compatriot, col-



TELLING THE FLESH

league, and later patient, Suzanne Curchod Necker and her close friend, Antoine-Léonard Thomas.[37] Illness – and the sufferings of Madame Necker in particular – are front and centre in this correspondence. Furthermore, the letters exchanged by Elizabeth Carter and Elizabeth Montagu also offer evidence to support Magrath's claim that bodily suffering "may facilitate the creation of an epistolary intellectual community."[38] In such epistolary spaces, the suffering body *is* the suffering self; the two are so deeply intertwined that they cannot be separated.

In addition to this, sickness brought suffering individuals into close proximity with other suffering individuals. The growth of spa culture during this period is one example of this process.[39] Spas were spaces of healing, but they were also highly desirable spaces of sociability.[40] The work of Séverine Pilloud and others stresses the growing practice of medical tourism, in which suffering individuals with the means to do so would journey to distant locations where they could spend weeks, months, and even years under the direct care of a noted physician. While Tissot's local practice in Lausanne was a beacon that drew individuals from around Europe (to the extent that the city was incapable of housing all of them),[41] it was not the only one. Spa culture and medical tourism created far flung social networks united through shared experiences of psychic and somatic suffering, networks that were then extended and enriched through epistolary exchanges. In the process, malady, while disabling in that it limited the bodily capacity to perform to one's fullest ability, also came to be seen as intrinsic to elite identity, a point effectively made by George Cheyne in his 1733 publication, *The English Malady*,[42] and later, by Tissot, in his own published works.[43] Bodily suffering brought people together, creating imagined communities founded on the shared experience of bodily disorder.

Social networking is also evident in the Tissot correspondence itself. As Pilloud and Louis-Courvoisier have observed, numerous individuals relied on third-party mediators to send their letters to Tissot.[44] Such mediators then acted as "calling cards" that allowed for a seamless introduction between doctor and presumptive patient. Thus, the Major and Lieutenant de Bouju, writing in 1773, acknowledged the role of the Countess de Lannion in bringing his case to Tissot's attention, writing, "Permit me, Sir, to personally offer you my sincere thanks for the attention that you gave to the consultations that the Countess de Lannion undertook on my behalf."[45] Social networking served a number of functions. Not only did it allow otherwise anonymous individuals to assert a right to claim medical treatment from Tissot, but it also cemented their own social standing. It was into this environment that Tissot's prospective patients wanted to place themselves. As patients of the good doctor, they would be able to bask in the glow of reflected glory, in the process also further extending the reach and influence of Tissot's medical beneficence.

Also interesting in this regard is the position of the mediator vis-à-vis Tissot. Consider, for example, the words of one Luternau, writing from Venlo in support of an acquaintance:

> It was with much difficulty, Sir, that I was able to persuade Madame Konauw to make a final effort to recover her health, which has been lost to her for a long time. The number of medicines she has tried and the minimal benefit she has received from them have made her believe that she has little chance of recovery from her sufferings, but having noticed that she appears to be somewhat better since her arrival here, I felt that you and Nature, Sir, could render to society a woman who, by her sweetness and by the generosity of her conversation, is a gift to it. I encouraged her to write to you … I beg you to respond as soon as the multitude of your responsibilities will allow this. I am impatient to know what you think and I would believe myself infinitely happy to be the primary cause of her recovery.[46]

Here, Luternau, basking in the light of Tissot's medical expertise, imagines himself almost as a vicarious healer, a man who enabled, at least at a basic level, Madame Konauw's cure.

The suffering body itself could also function as a calling card. Medical successes – either in the form of cure or the significant alleviation of symptoms – were understood as proof positive of a given healer's abilities. Like published books or medical treatises, these recovering patients were also *ouvrages* – literally "works" – whose improved health signalled a doctor's moral and intellectual goodness. Bouju, cited above, made a point of noting his improved health while simultaneously imploring the doctor to continue to treat him: "I ask your favour, Sir, to complete you work, so well begun."[47] Bouju's healthy body here takes on the contours of Tissot's published works; in its recovery, this suffering body – a living tableau – quite literally performs the work of intellectual and moral autobiography. We can take this even one step further. It is clear that, for those who wrote to Tissot, Tissot's corporeal virtue is unquestioned; indeed, his commitment to humanity assures his position as a virtuous citizen. Such a positioning is, however, much more ambiguous for the patients who sought his counsel. After all, their abilities to realize corporeal virtue had been compromised by illness and suffering. Thus, Tissot's unsullied virtuous presence became all the more vital to their social positioning: it is through their recourse to Tissot's enlightenment that suffering individuals were themselves able to achieve virtue. As Thomassin points out in a 1775 letter, "You will return a citizen to the state and a man to humanity."[48]

As medical works in progress, suffering individuals under Tissot's care could further reflect and refract Tissot's glory. Thus, just as the art of portraiture offered insight into the moral and intellectual qualities of elite individuals – and just as the Chevalier de Soran is able to offer a "*tableau de mes souffrances*," an autobiographical narrative of bodily suffering – so too were Tissot's books and patients seen as "*tableaux*." They were, quite literally, self-portraits that, in the absence of Tissot's physical presence, nevertheless revealed, in bodily form, the moral and intellectual essence of the man himself. It is against this imagined persona that the individuals who wrote to Tissot measured themselves, against this narration of self that they constructed their own narratives.

Finally, in a somewhat contradictory move, sickness and suffering allowed otherwise bodily compromised individuals to present morally uncorrupted selves. For these individuals, casting blame on the seemingly wilfully disordered body could direct attention away from the threatening possibilities of a disordered self. Instead, by claiming that bodily unruliness was separate from the psychic self, some individuals were able to assert unsullied, unblemished – indeed, pure – moral selves. Taking such an approach requires a particularly intricate presentation of self. As Magrath suggests in the case of depression, "the body is not being blamed for hindering the self; rather, the self ... is being liberated, freed because the burden can be laid upon the body."[49] This was, however, a risky venture. While it was possible to articulate a morally virtuous self by laying the burden on an unruly body, the equation could very easily be reversed: an unruly body could be read as evidence of an equally unruly moral self. This was the quandary faced by Thomassin, a young man who contacted Tissot in 1775. In his letter, Thomassin insisted that he was morally virtuous. Bodily evidence, however – in the form of nocturnal emissions – convinced his father that he was engaged in immoral sexual behaviour: "My father, more knowledgeable than I about the wickedness of schoolboys, suspected masturbation as a cause of my problems. He tormented me cruelly in order to make me confess to a habit that I did not have … He spied on my activities and, being unable to find me at fault, he decided to check my sheets. Here he found evidence of a delight in which I only passively took part … and he confronted me … pious and devotional books on the topic were placed in my hands."[50] I examine this narrative in greater detail in Chapter 5.

All of this demonstrates that while illness was, indeed, a central feature of the medical relationship during this period, the concept of illness as experience must itself first be fully interrogated. Illness had multiple meanings and served multiple purposes and it is important to consider this. How, then, might we as researchers approach these narratives? What tools might allow me to better understand and situate the subjectivities that individual correspondents were putting forward? In the second half of this chapter, I develop what I have termed a typology of bodily subjectivity, which explores in detail the many possible selves that emerge in the Tissot correspondence.

## MANY BODIES/MANY SELVES: A TYPOLOGY OF BODILY SUBJECTIVITY

> It seems to the embodied individual as if the body itself speaks.
> Michael Stolberg, *Experiencing Illness and the*
> *Sick Body in Early Modern Europe*

The letters to Tissot can be read through a lens that acknowledges a multiplicity of subjectivities. These subjectivities – or selves – can be productively organized into five types: the quantifiable self, the storytelling self, the emotional self, the confessional self, and the resistant self. This typology of bodily suffering takes for granted the notion of the letter as a site for the conscious staging of a self. It understands the letter not only as a dialogic genre couched within the assumption of reciprocity, but as a vehicle carefully designed to ensure a positive response from Tissot; in other words, the presumptive response inheres in the telling. It is important to note at the outset that while these "selves" are distinct, they also intersect with one another; correspondents draw on elements from numerous types in order to most effectively shape their narratives and, in turn, the identities they put forward to Tissot. An exploration of these different possibilities offers a useful way of conceptualizing the complexities of the relationship between body experience and body meaning as these played themselves out in the dialogic context of eighteenth-century medical epistolarity.

The quantifiable self is most obviously marked by its adherence to the principles laid out in Tissot's instructions for medical consultation letters. As noted in the Introduction, these instructions focus wholly on matters of physiological concern: they reveal the physician's interest in the codification of bodily messages for the purpose of effective medical diagnosis. Tissot's questions are little concerned with the emotional or subjective response to suffering; rather, they are interested in bodily signs, signs that could give insight into the nature of bodily suffering. While this model is characteristic of physician-authored consultations, it is not, in its most literal form, a common feature of layperson- or sufferer-authored letters. Very few of Tissot's correspondents followed this model exactly. Nevertheless, it is clear that some individuals effectively engaged this approach in their letters.

A quantifiable approach has numerous benefits: rational and objective, it is apparently free from the messiness of subjective experience. Such an approach would be of obvious use to Tissot, a doctor attempting to cure disease from a distance, but it is also appealing to a correspondent seeking a cure from a seemingly inexplicable sickness. There is something reassuring about numbers and observations. As an easily readable entity, this body might also, presumably, be equally easily cured. A close engagement with Tissot's directives offers the possibility of writing a letter – and constructing a self – through measurable data. In the process, numbers and "facts" come to define the self.

At heart, the quantifiable self is an observed self. It is a self organized by facts and disciplined by the internal gaze, a gaze that watches, measures, and records. In its commitment to details, the quantifiable self demonstrates its willing adherence to the essential principles of the medical gaze. Significantly, however, this self is also motivated by the reciprocity inherent in the letter form. The authority of the quantifiable self resides in its ability to assert the primacy of measurable data. The performance of quantification enables suffering individuals to present selves that conform convincingly to the principles that Tissot has put forward. In the process, they can lay claim to bodily citizenship.

A man named Lavergne, writing from Lyon in 1772, offers a perfect example of this approach. Lavergne's correspondence consists of several documents, including both letters and what he terms "Memoires." All were written between May and October 1772, and all the documents reference one another. In one letter dating from September 1772,

Lavergne details how he makes *chocolat de santé* – a drinking chocolate prescribed for health-related concerns. Lavergne is scrupulous in his description: "My drinking chocolate is made with 56 ounces of cocoa, 28 ounces of sugar, never vanilla. I distinguish between three different types of drinking chocolate: the first with half an ounce of cinnamon (instead of the full ounce I used in the past), the second with a quarter ounce; the third with no cinnamon at all … if I am missing something in order to consider this a true health drink [*chocolat de santé*], please let me know."[51] Lavergne also asserts his full commitment to Tissot's medical vision, stating, "Since your *Avis* arrived, I have been following your regimen exactly; [in fact] I was doing this already, using the *Avis* as my guide, but I have redoubled my efforts since these have been confirmed by you."[52]

In this letter, Lavergne constructs himself as an exemplary corporeal citizen. Clearly concerned with his health, he offers the minutiae of his regimen in order to affirm his commitment to the principles that Tissot has laid out. His questions regarding the efficacy of his recipe for drinking chocolate suggest an engagement with common regimens of the period, and with his interest in assuring the best possible outcome for his body and his health. His commentary also alludes to an understanding of Tissot as the arbiter of citizenship: Lavergne's epistolary deference acknowledges Tissot's position while simultaneously serving to assert his commitment to the principles and practices of bodily citizenship, a conceptual framework I discuss more fully in Chapter 3.

The undated "Memoire no. 3" is a case in point.[53] Four pages in length, it reads as a carefully edited examination of what Lavergne has learned about his body, and how this knowledge has challenged beliefs he might previously have held. Lavergne organizes his insights into five main groupings that focus, among others, on questions of digestion and evacuation. Like a student who has diligently studied his lessons, Lavergne carefully and effectively demonstrates his facility with the concepts he has learned, applying these to his own situation. As a performative gesture, this document offers tangible evidence in support of his earlier claims that he is following Tissot's regimen exactly. A final supplement to "Memoire no. 3" cements this reading. Here, Lavergne details two episodes of nocturnal emission. A closer examination of the politics of pleasure, the topic of Chapter 5, reveals that many correspondents who experienced nocturnal emissions wallowed in the subjective experience of moral shame. Lavergne, however, takes a dispassionate view. Separating his rational, intellectual observations from his bodily experiences, he attributes his emissions to diet and digestion: "I experienced two nocturnal emissions during the course of the month. The first came about as a result having imprudently eaten two slices of *boeuf roti* and having drunk milk before my digestion was fully complete. This beef was too strong and too succulent for me. I will not return to this case. I am in the process of perfecting my regimen."[54] This supplement is interesting from a number of perspectives. Nocturnal emissions are conventionally understood as evidence of a failure of bodily citizenship. Nevertheless, Lavergne uses these experiences as a springboard for insisting on his commitment to bodily control: he is actively working on "perfecting [his] regimen."

The second nocturnal emission is much more complex. But its narrative deployment supports Lavergne's commitment both to a dispassionate and rational reading of bodily signs and symptoms and to an understanding of bodily management and control as ideal sites not only of bodily well-being, but also, corporeal citizenship: "I suspended my use of milk in favour of *fruits fondants*, which perhaps added too much liquid to my meals and sometimes caused my chest to be too open. I remedied this situation promptly by limiting myself to a single glass of water at dinner, which I drank in 3 sips. But after 3 days, I noted a change (for the first time since my illness began) in temperature and constipation. That night, an emission. The next day, I returned to drinking as I usually did, but in order to avoid constipation, I whipped it together with ice, which returned things to order."[55]

Interesting in these examples is the extent to which Lavergne links bodily symptoms with dietary choices. In Lavergne's framing (and, indeed, in Tissot's publications), dietary choices are acts of will; that is, they can be controlled. Bodily control can – as evidenced in this three-part correspondence – lead to positive bodily outcomes. Lavergne's correspondence offers a useful example of the quantifiable self. Lavergne uses logic, reason, and observation – the central tenets of the scientific method – to articulate his bodily signs and symptoms. In the process, he also imagines and presents a self governed by the principles of reason and individual will.

A series of seven documents – four letters and three separate consultations – sent by a young man named Barbazan over a twenty-two-month period between 22 February 1772 and 12 December 1773 is also illustrative of the quantified approach.[56] It is clear from the outset that Barbazan has studied Tissot's recommendations carefully. His first consultation, a seven-page document in tiny handwriting, is meticulous –

indeed, overwhelming – in its level of detail, outlining bodily events and treatments from his birth in 1752 right through to 1772.[57] In it, Barbazan makes direct reference to thirteen specific years, outlining not only his family history, but his experiences with smallpox, measles, whooping cough, sores, poxes of various sorts, a range of fevers, fluxes and colds, back pains, and stomach problems. This consultation also details numerous attempted remedies as well as a range of other bodily symptoms. Barbazan also provides insight into geography, referencing the places where he experienced his various sufferings. Finally, the consultation includes information about his career as a sailor. The consultation as a whole is a veritable catalogue of body data, a quantifiable self imagined and experienced through a close engagement with dates, locations, numbers, and details. In many ways this document is a *tour de force* designed not only to inform and to cure but also to impress. In the case of the quantifiable self, objective observation becomes the site of subjectivity. Quantifiable selves come to see and understand themselves through the numbers and facts that they share.

### The Storytelling Self

The storytelling self, meanwhile, recognizes that numbers alone cannot capture the essence of experience. This self is buffeted by the social world – that is, produced by its environment. For the storytelling self, there is more to life than numbers. Storytelling selves offer insight into a range of experiences and concerns that move well beyond the realm of the physiological. This is not to suggest that the storytelling self *lacks* interest in so-called hard physiological data; rather, the storytelling self is more interested in the *experience* of that data than in the data itself. The storytelling self, therefore, is a self shaped by the imagination, a self that revels in metaphors, similes, and in circuitous structures. Just as a medieval city reveals itself through hidden corners, stone walls, quiet entries, and cobbled paths, so, too, does a storytelling self reveal itself. This self is never linear or direct; rather, it is always tangly.

The storytelling self was the product of the culture of sensibility.[58] According to medical historian Alun Withey, as the eighteenth century progressed, "A heroic fatalism began to underpin eighteenth-century medical correspondence, and the sick set themselves up as romantic heroes locked in a struggle with their potentially fatal symptoms."[59] Taking their cue from the protagonists of popular epistolary novels of the period, as well as from writers such as Rousseau, who was able to im-agine himself through his pathos-filled *Confessions*, many of those who write to Tissot also position themselves as suffering heroes struggling valiantly against the incursions of hostile bodily threats. Like the fabled Scheherazade, who wove spellbinding tales of adventure and passion that captivated not only her sultan, but also an enthralled eighteenth-century audience through the vehicle of the *Arabian Nights*, some of the correspondents weave complex tales of intrigue, passion, disappoint-ment, horror, joy, and dismay. Their stories circle around their various activities, their fears and concerns.

An eight-page consultation authored by B. Polianksy in 1784, for ex-ample, is an adventure story of the highest order, complete with villains, international travel, and a never-ending search for solace and comfort. A natural storyteller who clearly delights in the various intrigues that have shaped his life, Poliansky casts himself as the hero of his little tale. In his letter, Poliansky demonstrates a clear interest in matters of bodily concern; however, unlike Lavergne and Barbazan, he situates these interests within a broader social and environmental context. He is less interested in details of bodily data and much more interested in the story that emerges as a result of a consideration of his bodily sufferings. His narrative presents itself more like what would, within contempor-ary scholarship in life writing, be understood as a memoir, a form of life writing "that takes a segment of a life, not its entirety, and [focuses] on interconnected experiences."[60]

Writing from Montpellier, Poliansky shares the following:

I am 43 years old, born with a sensitive and lively character. I have maintained an active life since childhood, engaging in much mental and physical exercise, and even though I have suffered many annoyances during my life, my health did not, thanks to my strong temperament, suffer much until 1781 when, on the second of November, I was struck by an episode of paralysis. A few months prior to this, my soul had been overwhelmed by various sorrows, and I also experienced the misfortune of falling into the hands of some brigands who attacked me while travelling. I was accompanied only by two servants and was able only to weakly defend myself against a band of thieves who left me for dead. I lost a lot of blood as a result of a being struck on the head with a large chunk of wood.[61]

Polianksy sets up his narrative with a tale of danger and adventure, a story enlivened by the introduction of numerous dramatic details that propel the narrative forward while contributing little to the medical assessment of his condition.

This attention to detail marks the rest of Poliansky's narrative as well. It is clear that he revels in bringing to life the minutiae of daily experience. Indeed, as the following example, in which he recalls further bodily experiences that also preceded his original paralysis, demonstrates, Poliansky is not at all afraid of claiming autobiographical space:

> The day before my unfortunate accident, I was eating out and I felt that something was wrong with my head. This is why I chose to return home after dinner in order to rest a bit, after which I felt much better and went out for supper again. When I returned home, I slept well and, waking at my usual time, called my valet and spoke with him for a few minutes. When he left, I (having experienced no pain at all) moved to pick up something from the floor, but I had just stretched my arm from the bed when it began to tremble. I wanted to wiggle my feet, but was unable to move the whole right side of my body. Seized with fear, I wanted to call my servants, but found that I had also lost my voice. I was in this terrible situation for two hours until my servants entered. Finding me in this state, they ran to find two doctors of my friends. When the doctors arrived I saw the fear etched on their faces because, even though I had lost my voice and was paralysed in the right side of my body, I had not lost consciousness. Their … preparations to help me frightened me even more. They gave me enemas (only the third of which worked), bled me in the arm, and … finally weakened, I lost consciousness. Returning to consciousness five days later, I was still unable to speak. I began speaking on the sixth day, but indistinctly, often choosing words that were not those that I was thinking. In 14 days, I could walk with a cane and some time thereafter, without.[62]

Later in his letter, Poliansky reflects on the vagaries of geography and weather and considers their role in his ever-declining health. After a period of time spent in St Petersburg, he decided to follow the recommendations of local doctors to visit foreign countries, preferably by boat. This, they felt, would improve the situation:

     TELLING THE FLESH

I therefore embarked [on my travels] in the beginning of July.
It took 14 days to arrive in Lübeck, but as I did not suffer from
seasickness, this journey did me neither good nor bad. Ten days
later, I took another trip, embarking for Hamburg and in 23 days
I arrived in Bordeaux without experiencing any benefit to my
health. I spent three weeks in Bordeaux and it was there that I
perceived the bodily effects of a change of climate. Within a few
weeks I travelled from Russia, which is at 60 degrees, to France,
which is at 45. Because I had travelled by boat I had avoided the
heat, but in Bordeaux it was so hot and humid that I began to
sweat. I suffered from headaches and I felt a heaviness (which
compelled me to have my arm bled) and from there I ended up in
Montpellier ... I have now spent three months in Montpellier but
I feel as if my right side is weakening and I am so sensitive that
it feels as if everything harms me. The cold, the humidity and the
slightest heat – all of these loosen my nerves.[63]

Poliansky is a natural storyteller. He delights in the various intrigues
that have shaped his bodily experiences and is content to present himself as the hero of his story. Unlike some other correspondents who
limit themselves largely to a recitation of matters of physiological concern, Poliansky takes an expansive approach, carefully crafting even the
smallest details of his narrative. But while this letter is endlessly enter-
taining and, in this way, tells us much about Poliansky's character and
personality, it offers surprisingly little of interest to the man of medicine.
Few of Tissot's recommended questions are answered. In his eight-page
memoir, Polianksy offers no extensive medical history; indeed, he barely
mentions physiological signs at all except to the extent that his paralysis
(and accompanying inconveniences) are limiting his full enjoyment of
his life.

The narrative of a young seminarian named Galliotte, written in September 1773, offers another example of a storytelling self. At issue in
the letter is Galliotte's hearing, the loss of which will affect his ability
to pursue his chosen career as a priest. While Galliotte does offer some
insight into his medical history – a childhood attack of pleurisy, and a
father who experienced hearing loss – his narrative is largely experiential and descriptive: "As a schoolboy, I had my ears pulled to the point
of bleeding. I also enjoyed listening to canons, so much so that I always
stood close to them, and this is why I have attributed my deafness to

one of these two causes, even though this did not become clear to me until later."[64] Bodily awareness, for Galliotte, comes not through an observation of bodily signs and symptoms, but rather, through youthful experiences – both pleasurable and painful – that become meaningful only several years after the fact.

What might we make of these letters? How do we situate them within the complex web of medical epistolarity? What might they tell us about bodily meaning, bodily citizenship? Storytelling selves delight in the story. Interweaving emotion with experience, they use drama as a site for the articulation of the self. They remind the reader that hard data, when included, is not the sum total of the self; rather, it serves to propel the narrative forward. For such individuals, storytelling is a vehicle that emphasizes the limitations of the purely physiological gaze.

### The Emotional Self

By contrast, the emotional self is the self governed solely by the emotional experience of suffering. A product of the rise of sensibility, like the storytelling self, the emotional self asserts truth through emotional experience. Data, in this telling, is not a matter of physiological facts regarding temperature, bleeding, bowel movements, or menstrual cycles; rather, it is shaped by the workings of the heart. The emotional self emerges through the detailing of emotional intensity: fear, love, passion, excitement, and joy. For these individuals, numbers, as such, have no meaning. Instead, the meaning of suffering resides in the subjective, emotional experience of it.

Fear, as Lisa Wynne Smith has observed, is a common motivating factor in many medical consultation letters.[65] Indeed, fear appears to take on a physical presence and is imagined by many correspondents as a menacing figure that can actively intervene in the experience of bodily suffering. This emotional agitation lurks behind a Genevan man's 1767 letter regarding problems with his eyesight.[66] His fears are so strong that he calls off his wedding. While this seems like an excessive emotional response to failing eyesight, the correspondent later reveals the true source of his fears. It is not his failing eyesight that concerns him; rather, it is what he perceives to be the cause of this misfortune: "If all of these troubles had been nourished and maintained by some form of poor conduct, then this could be the case, for at the very moment at which the power of man reveals itself, so too does one find poor examples. For at least fifteen years, I have been barely able to stop nourishing that

　　　TELLING THE FLESH

terrible habit described in your book titled *Onanism*."[67] Later in the letter he reveals that solitary pleasures have not been his only vices: "It would have been hoped for my sake that I would have been taught to enjoy women with moderation rather than to corrupt myself. Sadly, this conduct has also been detrimental to my fortunes."[68] For this unnamed correspondent, failing eyesight is, ultimately, the least of his problems. Rather, his increasing blindness manifests his moral quandary, a tension nourished by his fears. For this correspondent, and others like him, autobiographical truth is equated with emotional truth. The emotions themselves are evidence of what Lisa Wynne Smith would term the reliability of the narrative.

The emotional self is also a relational self; that is, it understands itself in and through its relationships with others. In this, it most directly channels the idea of sympathy, one of the key principles of sensibility. As Wayne Wild observes, "While sensibility was necessary for refinement ... it was the feelings generated between people through sympathy that bound them together in a civilized society."[69] Such a formulation recalls not only the definition of sensibility found in the *Encyclopédie*, but also that put forward by Sophie de Grouchy late in the century.[70] Indeed, Carolyn D. Williams notes that the idea of pleasure was, itself, intimately linked with notions of benevolent charity: "The most exquisite raptures known to mankind were supposed to flow from the ability to feel for the suffering of others, and to relieve it by acts of unselfish courage and generosity."[71] Interestingly, such a positioning suggests that emotional selves were ideally situated in relation to questions of corporeal citizenship. Writing through the lens of sensibility situates subjectivity itself as a matter of broader social concern. In the process, bodily experience comes to be understood not solely as a matter of individual concern, but as relevant to social relations, more broadly speaking.

Emotional selves are often encountered in letters written by the family members of suffering individuals. Here, emotion not only asserts the truth of physiological complaint, but also bolsters the relationship between correspondent and sufferer, in the process asserting the reliability of the narrator. That is, if the narrator is so very moved by the experience of another person's suffering as to experience extreme emotion, then this not only confirms the suffering, but it also confirms the relationship itself. In a 1770 letter, for example, a father named Börking equates his daughter's epilepsy with the suffering he experiences as a father who is witness and subject to his child's experiences. Just as his child is afflicted, so too is he, as a parent, similarly suffering: "You have already shown the generosity, Sir, of granting me your counsel on behalf of this unfortunate child (which had some effect and which I include with this letter). Sir! Please have the indulgence of according me this honour. [In so doing] you will oblige her afflicted parents, granting them lasting peace, and nothing will equal their gratitude. They will do anything for you in order to procure it."[72]

Consider, too, a letter written by Dupuy *fils* on behalf of his suffering mother-in-law. "I have the honour of having a mother-in-law to whom I owe everything and whose death would bring desolation to a tightly united family who loves her dearly," he writes.[73] It is the emotional framing of love and family that shapes this letter as a whole. Interestingly, as I discuss in Chapter 4, these emotional investments are central not only to this woman's sufferings, but to her family's concerns.[74] Thus, while Dupuy *fils* gestures towards the filial ties that link Tissot to suffering humanity in order to advance his case, Börking inverts the equation, calling on Tissot's counsel, that it might confirm the love that binds his family together.

Emotion, as the work of Lisa Wynne Smith, Michael Roper, and Wayne Wild, among others, demonstrates, is a highly relevant area of critical interrogation. Roper observes, "A focus on emotional experience reminds us that the social scripts ... circulating within a culture at any given time do not, by themselves, constitute subjectivity, but that they operate in relation to more primitive emotional investments."[75] Roper's words force us to consider that while the discursive understanding of the body may allow for an interrogation of broader social dynamics, it is only a close attention to individual embodied experience as the foundation of the self that allows at all for an examination of questions of subjectivity. The telling of emotional selves can tell us much not only about the emotional experience of suffering but also about the performance of kinship during this period, a topic which I discuss in much greater depth in Chapter 4. Consider, for example, the following excerpt from a letter by a man named Maillard:

> I beg your pardon. If I take the liberty of writing to you, it is
> because I am ceding to the tenderness so natural to a father. The
> fate of my poor daughter worries me. I would like to receive some
> news and to learn what you think in general about her condition.
> The letters that I receive from Lausanne do not comfort me; on the
> contrary, they only increase my worries ... Would you permit me,
> Sir, to present myself to you; I await the grace of your generous

and beneficent character and the kindnesses that you have for me. I still flatter myself that you will do me the honour of continuing your care for my daughter; she is worthy of your pity.[76]

Here, Maillard relies on his emotional commitment to his daughter as a way of asserting his right to Tissot's attention. Furthermore, Maillard's micro-level emotional commitment to his daughter mirrors the macro-level medical and moral commitment of Tissot – the father of medicine – to humanity as a whole.

### The Confessional Self

In contrast to quantifiable, storytelling and emotional selves, confessional selves are motivated not by data – quantifiable or otherwise – but rather by the moral implications of their bodily experiences.[77] At heart, the confessional self is seeking redemption. Confessional selves use the space of the letter to articulate their bodily sins, in the process seeking absolution. Audience is of prime importance to the confessional self; after all, a penitent requires a confessor. In confessional letters, Tissot emerges as both confessor and arbiter of bodily virtue, a messiah whose expertise and essential humanity make him uniquely placed to act as a healer of both body and spirit.

Many correspondents approached Tissot with reverence, imagining him not only as a hero and benefactor of humanity, but almost, as its saviour. To Gringet, writing in 1784, Tissot is the "Oracle of medicine."[78] Olivier, a suffering onanist in Normandy, asks Tissot to be "after God … my liberator."[79] While these correspondents are careful to position their Christian God at the top of the hierarchy, it is clear that many correspondents view Tissot as both saviour and benefactor, a man who, with God's grace, has the ability to change society. In the words of one anonymous correspondent, "I base my hopes on your enlightenment and your talents; let these hopes not be in vain; in my case, let nature obey you as well as you know how to penetrate its secrets."[80] Here, the correspondent makes it clear that it is Tissot, and Tissot alone, who has the ability not only to discern the mysteries of nature but to make nature bend to his will.

Tissot, as a modern-day messiah, has recourse to almost extraordinary resources, drawing not only on the divine, but also on the natural to cure a miserable and forsaken people. As Rossary, a sufferer of onanism, pleads, "You are the benefactor of humanity; please be mine. Do not refuse your counsel to a young man whose state is deplorable."[81] Similar ideas permeate other letters as well. Monsieur Lanjuinais, writing from Moudon in 1790, for example, begins his letter this way: "Convinced that all that concerns humanity finds easy access with you, I am taking the liberty of laying claim to the precious effects of your noble desire to oblige."[82] In this formulation, Tissot is imagined as a Christ-like figure who draws unfortunate souls into the circle of his benevolent presence.

Correspondents who present confessional selves often feel the need to unburden themselves in relation to corporeal habits that are seen as problematic, questionable, or even unsavoury. Bodily excess is a common feature of many of these letters. Dietary excess, for example, might include a taste for wine, fat, or rich meats. Sexual excess, meanwhile, usually includes overindulgence in sexual activities or, more troubling to eighteenth-century mores, masturbation. Others indicate excessive engagement with parties and games, both of which lead to late nights. Finally, some reference excessive intellectual engagement. In each of these cases, excess – a result of moral disarray and lack of will – is correlated with bodily disorder.

One young man suffered from a form of hypochondria, which manifested itself in the form of light convulsions and emotional agitation:

> He believes himself to be exhausted and weakened to such an extent that he can feel nothing and persuades himself that he is on the verge of death, says his last goodbyes, and requests his final sacraments. These crises vary considerably in duration; sometimes only a couple of hours, sometimes a whole day. They return more or less frequently in relation to the extent to which this young man indulges in dissipated behaviour ... or by some slightly excessive exercise (such as horse riding), or by a long walk, or by the cold (to which he is particularly sensitive), or by the loss of seminal fluid, even if this happens naturally during the night.[83]

This young man's bodily disorder appears to be a direct result of his moral weaknesses. He masturbated actively between the ages of eleven and sixteen, at which point, after reading numerous publications, he came to learn of the dangers that could befall him. He also engaged in numerous sexual liaisons, and while his doctor does not feel that these would have compromised his health, it is nevertheless evident that the young man harbours some fears that his actions may be the cause of his bodily disorders.

A confessional self uses the space of the letter both as a way of acknowledging moral weakness – and the bodily disorder that results from it – as the first step in a journey towards redemption. In the case of the young man cited above, the doctor's assessment is clear: "It seems evident that the vapours were produced by both a physical and moral cause. We have need of enlightenment in order to destroy the first of these causes. His parents, meanwhile, will unite their attentions in order to stop the second."[84]

In recognizing Tissot as the arbiter of bodily virtue, confessional selves position him as the source of redemption; it is through Tissot's grace that they might achieve peace. A letter written by Olivier, a thirty-seven-year-old curate from Normandy offers a prime example of this process. Olivier finds himself in a deplorable state of nervous disorder, which he attributes to two causes: his own engagement with masturbation and a friend's epileptic seizures. He writes,

> I am sending you this letter by chance. If it arrives, I will consider myself fortunate; I hope to find in the regimen that I beg you to provide a solace that nothing else has yet been able to grant me … I am 37 years old. From the age of twelve, I contracted the frightful custom of masturbating almost every day (sometimes even repeating the act). This confession is humiliating. At almost the same time, I witnessed one of my peers overcome by two epileptic seizures, which made me fear this malady. This fear, which should have dissipated because it could not possibly have had the effects that I was dreading, together with my enormous [moral] crime – two subjects which occupied me – caused me to become vaporous without even really knowing it.[85]

This youthful experience of illicit pleasure juxtaposed with the extreme horror of witnessing epileptic seizures sets the tone for the next years of Olivier's life. Emotional and moral distress colour all of his experiences, from his single sexual liaison with a woman to his various experiences with medicinal remedies. He has visited numerous doctors, to no avail. Indeed, his symptoms have only increased, to the point where he embodies the spasmodic body he so feared. In a passage reminiscent of those penned by emotional selves, Olivier writes, "Along with these worries and great sorrows which I often experience, my sorrows cause me to think the darkest thoughts."[86] For Olivier, this letter serves as a sort of confessional. He confesses to the crime of masturbation, outlines

the deleterious psychic and somatic effects of his moral fall, and re-
quests absolution from Tissot, the man best placed to deliver him from
evil. "This, Sir, is my situation," Olivier concludes, "Please give me a
remedy. You will find me as docile a patient as those whom you describe
in your publications."[87] Shaped by the framework of confession and absolution that marks his religious calling and career, Olivier's letter itself
also draws much from the literary examples to which he refers, a point
I discuss in greater detail in Chapter 5.

### The Resistant Self

Finally, the correspondence reveals evidence of what might be termed a
resistant self. Most often in dialogue with the confessional self, the resistant self challenges not only the authority of numbers and other "data"
but also the conventional interpretations that might arise from them.
More significantly, it resides in bodily experiences that cannot easily be
slotted into conventional understandings. Resistant selves tell stories of
bodies that do not conform and challenge readers to find new meanings.
Instead, they share alternative body narratives and body interpretations.
Intriguingly, the resistant self resides not so much in the text as it does
in the body; it emerges from the body and it asserts the body itself as
the site of the self. Resistant selves complicate textual representations.
Indeed, in their resistance they complicate the very grounds of what is
traditionally understood to be the "self": that conscious, moral, knowing, and reflecting entity to which we conventionally grant authority.

In a lengthy letter, Martin, a twenty-one-year-old medical student,
offers Tissot the "horrifying tableau" of Claude Joseph Demeunier, a
"victim of onanism."[88] Although Demeunier's bodily sufferings appeared to be directly linked to his excessive engagement in onanist behaviours, Demeunier himself actively resists this diagnosis, seeking out a
broad range of alternative medical opinions. In his excessive behaviour,
Demeunier refuses the call of temperance and moderation. Bodily evidence, in the form of nightmares, spasms, and convulsions, too, attests
to his resistance. Indeed, if we are to take Martin at his word, Demeunier's resistance is wilful, an active engagement with bodily excess that
has fundamentally undermined his health and well-being. I examine this
case in more detail in Chapter 5.

These five "types" offer a productive way of engaging with the various
subjectivities at play in the letters. Unfortunately, most selves do not

manifest themselves in such easily packaged forms. Stories, and selves, are rarely as neat and tidy as Tissot's carefully ordered questionnaire would suggest. Nor do they comply neatly or tidily with this typology. Thus, while this schematization is seductive, and offers eminently useful lenses through which to read and understand the epistolary stories in the Fonds Tissot, it is also deceptive in its apparent simplicity. Indeed, it quickly becomes clear that the vast majority of those letters that resonate in relation to this particular study of corporeal citizenship are shaped not by a single type but rather by several types, all of which jostle for attention. As one self gained ascendancy, other selves receded into the background.

Being able to locate these elements, however, helps to situate these stories as iterations of self – and selves – within this particular historical period. This typology is also useful in that it allows me to understand how individuals might have deployed these selves in their performances of subjectivity, particularly in a textual context founded on notions of reliability, on the one hand, and reciprocity, on the other. In addition to this, it allows me to examine how the different selves can both shore up and undermine one another. Thus, the quantified self can be given credence through lived emotion: a turn to facts could forestall a diagnosis of hypochondria, for example. Meanwhile, the quantified self can draw on its emotional and storytelling counterparts in order to assert the humanity of the suffering individual – that is, to bring forward the human subject lurking within, around and beneath what could otherwise be read as a dry recitation of bodily data. Silence, too, is worthy of consideration. For example, emotional and storytelling selves can work in consort to confirm the experience of suffering even in the absence of measurable data. Thus, for example, as noted previously, while one anonymous correspondent observes that his physiognomy presents a picture of vigour and health, he nevertheless insists on his subjective experience of malaise.[89] By the same token, these selves sometimes tangled with one another; for example, the confessional or redemption-seeking self can struggle with the resistant self, while the assertions of the emotional self sometimes come into direct conflict with the measurable data that marks the quantified self. In some instances, the various selves are in balance, offering the reader the illusion of equilibrium.

It is also important to situate this typology within a broader social and cultural context. As scholars of epistolarity have noted, epistolary selves were the product of social, cultural, political, geographic, and economic jostlings. Such jostlings shaped individual identity at a fundamental level, and, from there, predetermined, to a large extent, the kinds of narratives available to them. For example, gender, as some writers point out, shaped not only how the story was told, but also, how it might be received.[90] Madame Carbounié de Castelgaillard, writing about her husband's seizures, demonstrates her awareness of discourses of gender by closing her letter to Tissot with an apology: "If I had been within reach of a doctor, I would have sent you a reasoned consultation, but I hope that you will still have regard for the insufficiency of a woman."[91] Here, Madame Carbounié de Castelgaillard gestures towards various elements of social propriety during this period: the presumptuousness of writing a consultation letter without the requisite professional medical background, but further, the presumptuousness of writing *as a woman*. By framing her letter as she does, she is able to lay claim to normative feminine propriety by stressing what was understood during her time as the naturalized "insufficiency" of her sex while still asserting her needs. Additionally, she provides some context for a doctor who might have found her summary, articulated as it was by a layperson, off-putting, thus ensuring the best possible reception for her missive. Given gender conventions of the period, such an approach was, essentially, the only option available to her as a woman of quality and propriety. As Marie-Claire Grassi observes in her discussion about eighteenth-century feminine epistolarity, "If a woman wants to be genuine, society wants her to be reserved, modest, submissive. She must, therefore, have recourse to several discourses, that of truth, that of submission … In the words of Ortigue de Vaumorière: '*Le sexe* [woman] must possess modesty.'"[92]

Narrative choices were also circumscribed by the nature of the ailments themselves. For example, it is clear from both epistolary language and epistolary content that the narrative choices available to women were very different from those available to men. So, too, might we critically interrogate the terrain of bodily experience itself. While some physiological symptoms were relatively easy to articulate and easy to share, others could be much more challenging, even morally dangerous, to reveal. Sufferings related to masturbation and lactation, for example, were deeply infused with moral overtones, making a purely objective or rational description of bodily signs challenging, even impossible, for individuals. Narratives that included bodily experiences such as these required particularly careful crafting, attentive not only to the needs of the suffering self, but also to the morally-suspect nature of their bodily sufferings.

Furthermore, in a pan-European context, epistolary selves were also shaped by language itself: while Tissot received letters in French, German, Italian, Latin, and English, many of his patients were crafting their epistolary identities in second or even third languages. This, too, affected the nature of their narrations of self. In this sense, it is important to acknowledge the abilities of individuals to navigate linguistic constructions of self. This process is made abundantly clear in a series of letters concerning the health of Madame Konauw (née Smith), writing from Venlo, a Dutch town located on what is now the border between The Netherlands and Germany.[93] Each of the three letters in this series is written by a different author, but all three are in French. Nevertheless, the third letter in the series – a letter from Madame Konauw herself – makes it clear that each of these correspondents was writing in a second language. From her letter, it is evident that Madame Konauw is aware of the formal conventions of the epistolary genre. She is also very adept at writing in French. In many respects, her letter would appear to show a far stronger grasp of formal written French than many others in this collection (including that of Madame Carbounié de Castelgaillard, cited previously). But this assumption is disrupted by her conscious decision to revert to Dutch, her primary language, when the going gets tough. She does this numerous times over the course of a four-page letter. As she explains near the end of her letter, "As I assume that you can understand all languages, I have written in Dutch everything that I could not say in French."[94] This approach performs two specific functions: it pays homage to what Madame Konauw imagines to be Tissot's obvious multilingualism, but it also, crucially, situates Madame Konauw and her bodily condition; her narrative must be read – by Tissot, by twenty-first-century readers – through the lens of bilingualism. Language, in this sense, fundamentally shapes not only her understanding of her bodily self, but also her *experience* of her bodily self.

These examples demonstrate that writing to Tissot was, therefore, no easy matter. Such a self-positioning was complex, in that these different layers of identity did not map neatly or cleanly onto one another, but in some instances challenged and contradicted one another.

This typology of epistolary subjectivity grounds my methodological approach. Situated firmly within conceptual lenses drawn from both the history of medicine and life writing theories, and drawing on the insights of feminist scholars, political theorists, and scholars in disability studies, this methodological approach enables me to consider the essentially reciprocal nature of epistolarity and to foreground it in the performance and presentation of self. It also allows me to consider actively the roles of the body, bodily experience, and bodily resistance, in the articulation of the self. In the chapter that follows, I examine in detail the notion of citizenship.

{ CHAPTER THREE }

# Corporeal Virtue and Embodied Citizenship

To ask who is to be included as a citizen is also to ask who is to be excluded from the status.

Keith Faulks, *Citizenship*

You would accomplish a great work if you could bring health to a respectable mother who is very useful to those who surround her.

Capitaine d'Arche to Tissot, 3 July 1772[1]

In 2011, a young man was denied permanent residency status in Canada. Chris Reynolds, twenty, diagnosed with both Asperger and Tourette syndromes, was deemed "medically inadmissible," his conditions potentially costing the Canadian taxpayer upwards of seven thousand dollars per year. More simply put, Reynolds was seen as an improper body, an undesirable citizen with nothing to contribute. In the words of his father, Thomas Reynolds, "The end verdict is a judgment of worthlessness."[2] Nevertheless, Immigration Canada's decision, although callous, was not necessarily surprising. As Thomas Reynolds explains in an autoethnography of theology, disability, and parenthood published just a few years before the family's application for permanent residency, when the focus is placed on disability, "features of ... personhood fully capable of making valuable contributions to the community [are] neglected."[3]

Reynolds's case revolves around the question of legal citizenship – the formal apparati of state used to determine the boundaries of belonging. Nevertheless, legal citizenship hinges on issues of ideological citizenship; it is premised on deeply embedded notions of belonging and exclusion, histories that reach back to the Ancients and that continue to inform contemporary debates. The historical record reveals that those with improper bodies – weak, disabled, deviant, or otherwise compromised bodies – have regularly been denied the full rights of citizenship. Subject to procedures such as involuntary sterilization, institutionalization, and eugenics, they have been denied authority over their own bodies. Indeed, as Reynolds observed in his 2008 book, "Based upon narrowly defined models of individual autonomy, efficiency, or productivity, certain bodily differences and impairments are perceived as liabilities that amount to deviance."[4] How unfortunately ironic, then, that ideology and law would converge on the body of his son just three years later.

Questions of bodily and embodied citizenship are central to this chapter. In it, I focus not on legal citizens, but rather on the encounter between ideologies of citizenship and the lived experience of marginalized embodiment and bodily suffering. I take for granted in this work the possibility of corporeal citizenship – that is, of a performance and practice of citizenship enacted on and through the body, a citizenship that imagines the body not only as site of its iteration but also as the source of citizenship itself. In this, I draw on a thesis put forward by Jasbir Puar in a 2012 article: "If signification and representation (what things mean) are no longer the only primary realm of the political, then bodily processes (how things feel) must be irreducibly central to any notion of the political."[5]

The case of Chris Reynolds highlights questions central to this chapter: What is a citizen? On what basis is citizenship conferred or denied? What role does the body play in such decisions? Who decides which bodies should or should not belong? What are the implications of such debates on the lived experiences of "failed" citizens? Such questions propel many of the letters addressed to Tissot. Haunting them is a further question: "Am I worthy of receiving Tissot's counsel?" In this chapter, I introduce citizenship as a key theoretical concept that structures and frames this research as a whole. Situating the concept as central to political theory, I then draw on the insights of feminist, disability studies, and fat theorists, all of whom have sought to trouble normative conceptualizations of citizenship, often through the body. In these debates, citizenship emerges both as an act – as something that one *does* – and as a status – as something that one *has*. Integral to this discussion are both the possibilities *and* limitations of citizenship. Indeed, one particular point that I emphasize is the idea of *failed* citizenship.

These discussions allow me to develop the idea of corporeal citizenship – a lens I then use to examine Tissot's published oeuvre. I suggest that Tissot's influence derived from his ability to link medicine with morality, to link bodily health with questions of citizenship and virtue.

Finally, I explore how correspondents engaged with these ideas. Drawing on a notion that might be understood as "citizenship in action," I suggest that correspondents understood their letters as acts of citizenship, spaces in which they could assert their claims to belonging. Furthermore, I argue that they imagined Tissot as an arbiter of bodily virtue – that is, as the individual best placed to evaluate their bodily citizenship. At the same time, however, correspondents also assert their own claims to corporeal virtue, claims that sometimes run counter to the principles established in Tissot's published works. In this chapter, the body emerges as a terrain of contestation. On the one hand, the body and its workings are evocative of the "Natural" – models of the rightness of nature and the organic system; on the other, they are a site of conscious staging, a carefully constructed artifice designed to present and perform virtue. For those who wrote to Tissot, bodies, as sites of citizenship, are understood as a locus for the presentation of selves as citizens, spaces on and through which individuals claim rights to belonging.

Citizenship as performance presupposes the idea of will – a conscious engagement with and staging of the self. As will become evident in this chapter and those that follow, will is not merely a matter of asserting the mind over the body. Rather, I consider the notion of will in the context of a symbiotic relationship between mind and body. Thus, just as the mind asserts its will over the body, so, too, as we shall see, does the body also assert its will over the mind. Indeed, in some instances, a reading of bodily agency is key to understanding questions of resistance. As Judith Butler reminds us, "Bodies do not always comply with the norms by which their materialization is impelled."[6]

I consider acts of will from two perspectives. First, I am interested in those acts of will performed by individuals as they assert their right to be heard (in Tissot's presence), in the process, asserting their claim to membership in the imagined community not only of medical correspondents and bodily citizens but also of eighteenth-century Europe. To get at this, I carefully consider the ways that individuals interpreted and articulated their bodily signs and symptoms, and the meanings that they ascribed to those symptoms within the broader terrain of their lives. Conscious will, in this sense, is integrally tied to the notion of epistolary performance – that is, to the construction of bodily narratives. This is particularly important given the historical and political context of these letters. As Roy Porter has observed, "In the secularised world of the Enlightenment, physical existence became the site for those aspirations of life traditionally assigned to Heaven."[7] In other words, bodies and bodily experience came to be understood as key loci for the articulation of autobiographical subjectivity during this period. Will as a question of mind over matter, psyche over soma, is the most traditional definition. Indeed, it is this definition that underpins accepted definitions of citizenship. But I also consider will from a second perspective: the notion of the body itself as "will-full."[8] Integral to this is an understanding of the body itself as an agentive entity capable of asserting its own meanings. From this perspective, I argue that the body is always concerned with its own projects, projects that are sometimes at odds with the impulses of the rational, autonomous individual. What I mean by this is that the needs and concerns of the body do not always align themselves perfectly with those of the mind. Psyche and soma are not necessarily neatly interwoven with one another; indeed, they are sometimes at cross purposes. Sometimes bodies act of their own accord. Sometimes bodies resist. Sometimes bodies appear to actively undermine a correspondent's attempts to control their narratives. Sometimes bodies have their own stories to tell and sometimes these narratives challenge the very nature of corporeal virtue itself. This second lens is integral to troubling normative understandings of citizenship. Indeed, it is the basis for a re-imagination and reconceptualization of the possibilities of citizenship. It is, ultimately, this second act of will – bodily will – that influences the conceptual questions that underpin this work as a whole.

The letters to Tissot suggest that writing itself can, and should, be understood as an act of citizenship. Letter writing, in particular, is a gesture that transforms intimate self-reflection into a conversation. The letter, as the point of encounter between the suffering individual and the audience, can be imagined as a civic performance. A process of self-reflection, the crafting of a consultation letter suggests a conscious engagement not only with the body and its workings but also with questions of bodily responsibility and obligation in relation to the notion of health as both physiological and moral ideal. Such letters initiate the idea of the suffering self as corporeal citizen. Furthermore, they introduce the notion of the suffering self as a willing object of physician's gaze – a bodily self open to public scrutiny. In the words of Suzette A. Henke, who considers the writing of trauma, "The act of life writing serves as its own testimony and, in so doing, carries through the work of reinventing the shattered self as a coherent subject capable of meaningful resistance to received ideologies and of effective agency in the world."[9] For those who wrote to Tissot, the letter is an act of reflection and observation –

an epistolary dance, if you will, directed towards the one individual best placed to measure and assess the worth of both the letter and the bodily behaviours and practices it described in relation to idealized corporeal citizenship. In this epistolary dance, the suffering body, as imagined, experienced, and lived, becomes a stage for the performance of citizenship.

There are, as I stated in the previous chapters, standard conventions to letter writing. Stories emerge in normative formats. Conventions shape how stories are told. There are also conventions to telling the flesh – that is, to telling stories about bodies. Questions of citizenship, too, have their conventions, conventions that determine not only who belongs and who is excluded but also how belonging and exclusion might be articulated and measured. But, as will become clear in this chapter and those that follow, letters are also inherently creative spaces. Even in the face of powerful conventions, individuals can – and do – shape stories to suit their own needs. In the process, they also reshape the parameters of citizenship itself.

### IMAGINING CITIZENSHIP

Being a good citizen means conforming to and performing particular types of ... identities.

Lynda Johnston and Robyn Longhurst, *Space, Place and Sex: Geographies of Sexualities*

When Aristotle declared that to be fully human was to be a political animal, he positioned citizenship as the basis for humanity. The individual alone was not inherently human; rather, it was when one was admitted fully to, and accepted, the privileges and responsibilities of citizenship, that one was, in the words of J.G.A. Pocock, "empowered to be human."[10] But what, precisely, does this mean? What are the relationships between humanity, on the one hand, and citizenship, on the other? Margrit Shildrick offers some insight: "To be a self – and more significantly a subject – with effective agency is, in every sense of the word, to be capable of exercising autonomy. Because the western logos privileges the freedom and rationality of the putatively disembodied mind as the irreducible marker of the sovereign subject, it follows that the body itself is relatively unimportant, so long as it falls within normative parameters that pose no hindrance to the implementation of self-determination."[11] Western philosophy has imagined – and indeed continues to imagine – the self as an autonomous being capable of rational thought and self-determination: "a cognitive, active, moral, intellectual and political being."[12] The human individual, in his or her incarnation as citizen-subject, is a creature of will – a being able to assert the primacy of mind over body. Citizenship is founded on similar principles.

Understandings of citizenship rest on two sometimes contradictory premises, both of which were in circulation during the eighteenth century. On the one hand, the citizen is responsible to the needs of the community as a whole; on the other, the citizen is a rights-bearing individual, possessed of privileges by virtue of membership in the polity alone. Citizenship, as both a practice and a status,[13] is thus a balancing act that "contains both individualistic and collectivist elements."[14] The tensions between rights and responsibilities can be productive in that they offer the possibility of transformation, for a reconceptualization of the parameters of citizenship itself. Thus, for Engin Isin and Patricia Wood, citizenship is "not only ... a set of legal obligations and entitlements which individuals possess by virtue of their membership in a state, but also ... the practices through which individuals and groups formulate and claim new rights or struggle to expand or maintain existing rights."[15] Imagined this way, citizenship is a dynamic and mobile concept, its borders the site of continued interactions and contestations. In the words of Kathleen Canning and Sonya Rose, "the distinctions between those who are and those who are not full citizens are recurrent matters of contestation. Not only those who have been excluded, constrained or marginalized, or who have been engaged in contestation, but also those in control of maintaining the boundaries of belonging, entitlement and participation have been politically engaged around these issues."[16] Indeed, it is worth emphasizing that citizens are not passive creatures. They are "creative agents ... [who] will always find new ways to express their citizenship."[17] This notion of a dynamic citizenship underpins my own analysis.

Eighteenth-century sources gesture towards this oscillation between self-interest and collective good, status and act. The definitions included in the 1762 edition of the *Dictionnaire de l'Académie française*, for example, draw overtly on the Ancients, and define the citizen as follows: "bourgeois, inhabitant of a city. In previous times, Roman citizens were not just those born in Rome, but those who had acquired the rights and privileges of the citizen, even if they came from another country."[18] This approach reflects the notion of status while also gesturing indirectly towards questions of obligation. By 1787, on the eve of the French Revolution, this definition had expanded to include a much more overt

   TELLING THE FLESH

statement: "zeal for the homeland," thus evoking the idea of citizenship as a collective impulse directed towards a shared common patriotic ideal.[19] This collective impulse is central to definitions found in the *Encyclopédie* as well. In a philosophical rumination that considers the citizen in relation to the inhabitant and the bourgeois, Diderot writes, "Habitation presupposes a place. Bourgeoisie presupposes a town. The character of a citizen [presupposes] a social organization in which each individual knows what is happening, loves the good, and can promise himself to aspire to the highest dignities."[20] These definitions postulate citizenship as a profoundly relational construct: citizenship is about the structure and organization of the community and about the self *within* that community. Citizens are social beings who claim their positions on the basis not just of their names but in relation to their active participation in, and for the good of, the polis as a whole.

Key to emerging eighteenth-century understandings of citizenship is the concept of *patrie*, or homeland, understood by some correspondents as a source of pride, fulfilment, and belonging. The success of the homeland is dependent on the zeal of the citizen. By the same token, the good of the citizen is realized through the success of the homeland. As I will discuss later in this chapter, the willingness of the citizen to serve and die for the homeland – Aristotle's citizen-as-warrior – is not only an indication of his engagement with the collective good but is also linked with his individual well-being. So, too, is the lactating mother, the site of beneficent generosity, imagined as a metaphor for the homeland herself, a concept I develop more fully in Chapter 4. The homeland, in this incarnation, is both that which must at all costs be protected, but also that which nurtures and nourishes. It is, in essence, an articulation of the family writ large.

### IMAGINED COMMUNITY

At its heart, citizenship is about belonging; it is about the fabric that, as Ronald Beiner explains, "draws a body of citizens together into a coherent and stably organized political community, and keeps that allegiance durable."[21] Beiner's explanation reflects Benedict Anderson's now foundational notion of imagined community as a group of individuals who may never personally know one another but nevertheless share "the image of their communion" and, in so doing, shape and affirm the boundaries of their membership.[22] The imagined community is "a source of identity, of moral and social stability, of shared meaning and mutual cooperation."[23] Put more simply, it is the fabric that keeps individual subjects together.

Anderson's model suggests the possibility of an idyllic community of individuals united in the pursuit of common goals, a community that draws its strength and sense of identity from the bonds of reciprocal obligation. But this is only half the equation. Nira Yuval-Davis observes that the notion of "community" is itself never value-neutral. Rather, communities are "ideological and material constructions, whose boundaries, structures and norms are a result of constant processes of struggles and negotiations, or more general social developments."[24] As Anderson and others have observed, imagined communities are as exclusionary as they are inclusionary. The parameters of the nation are constructed and sustained by the nation's Others, those whom it actively excludes from membership. Scratching the surface of citizenship reveals its profoundly exclusionary nature: gender, class, sex, sexuality, race, ethnicity, ability – all of these markers have been used to deny individuals and groups the rights and responsibilities of citizenship. In the words of Moira Gatens, "At different times, different kinds of beings have been excluded … often simply by virtue of their corporeal specificity."[25] Historically, exclusion has been much more profound than inclusion. While an "idealized citizenship" appears to gesture towards a promising universal, this ideal masks a reality of systemic oppression. In the context of this particular study, bodily health itself becomes a marker of belonging and exclusion, a site that determines an individual's ability to claim corporeal virtue.[26]

What, then, happens to those excluded from these very narrow parameters of citizenship? What hope do they have of claiming a place in the body politic? And on what basis can they make those claims? Randolph Hohle suggests that it might be productive to consider the relationship between what he terms idealized citizenship and symbolic citizenship.[27] He suggests that symbolic citizenship allows those who do not have easy access to membership in the polis to assert belonging through a strategic engagement with the embodied and bodily practices of idealized citizenship. Mimicking the contours of idealized citizenship can allow symbolic citizens to assert their right to membership in the imagined community. "The idea of symbolic citizenship," he writes, "highlights the discursive, performative, and embodied aspects of citizenship as well as the impact of idealized citizenship on how social movements make claims for equality."[28] Hohle's conceptualization thus imagines citizenship as a form of masquerade, a consciously staged

   TELLING THE FLESH

performance complete with carefully studied lines, gestures, costumes, and makeup. Carefully prepared, such performances offer the illusion of idealized citizenship, in the process enabling otherwise marginalized individuals to access the privileges of idealized citizenship.

Nevertheless, symbolic citizenship may not be enough. As a mimicry of idealized citizenship, it cannot expand its parameters. Instead, symbolic citizenship just further fortifies the conventions, rather than opening them up. In the process, those unable, or unwilling, to claim symbolic citizenship – men, for example, like Demeunier, the wilfully obtuse onanist introduced in the previous chapter – "are found, in some circumstances, to be deficient."[29]

Such individuals come to occupy the status of what Samantha Murray has referred to as "failed" citizens.[30] Murray observes that within a model of citizenship premised on notions of bodily will and self control, non-compliant bodies are inevitably understood as sites of excess, as resistant and threatening entities that "refuse to regulate … needs and impulses."[31] This framework situates the resistant body – in Murray's case, the fat body – as "a moral failure, a diseased body and as a site of unmanaged desire,"[32] ideas that will come to the fore in Chapters 5 and 6. Significantly, this failure of citizenship is not only personal, but social, in that it disrupts the bodily wills and citizenship strivings of those who surround the failed citizen. Failed citizens "[fray] the very (moral) fabric of society,"[33] and as such, are the *source of suffering for others*."[34] In other words, failed citizens are points of horror; not just failures to the self, they are, as Murray has observed, constituted as a threat to virtuous citizens and as an "affront" to society.[35]

The problem with a binary model is, of course, that it casts all non-normative citizen bodies as Other, in the process excluding them from the parameters of mainstream citizenship. Unable to conform, deviant and disordered bodies are rendered unintelligible within dominant discourses and, as a result, their stories are silenced. Corporeal citizenship, within such a framework, remains an impossibility. Scholars in areas as diverse as feminist, queer, disability, fat, and African American studies have pointed out that this rhetoric has significant implications not only for the lived experience of non-normative embodiment and bodies but also for the presumptive political agency of those positioned as failed citizens.[36] As I discuss later in this chapter, the horror of failed citizenship haunts many letters addressed to Tissot and individuals assert a range of possible bodily identities in an attempt to deflect the possibility of failure. As I intimated in the Introduction, failed citizenship also haunts this book as a whole: What happens to those who cannot tell their own stories?

CITIZENSHIP IN THE FLESH

> My temperament was of a dry constitution, strong and vigorous in the face of any work, because, having been in commerce since the age of five, the activity of both mind and body did not cost me a thing. I have travelled a lot and worked constantly. Otherwise, [I am] always well presented and regulated without excesses of any kind.
>
> J. Claret to Tissot, 7 April 1790[37]

> What does it mean to lay claim to one's body? And how is this connected to state practices of citizenship, (il)legality, and the problem of agency and autonomy within hegemonic processes?
>
> Mimi Sheller, *Citizenship from Below:*
> *Erotic Agency and Caribbean Freedom*

Jean-Jacques Rousseau began one of his most famous works, *The Social Contract*, with the body. "Man is born free," he wrote in a now oft-quoted commentary, "and everywhere he is in chains."[38] Citizenship, for Rousseau, rests on a bodily foundation. And while these chains might be metaphorical, the very fact that he starts not only with the body but with bodily imprisonment is telling. Later in the century, these same chains would underpin the politics of the American and French Revolutions. They would also come to represent the atrocities of the slave trade.

The body and its workings figure prominently in eighteenth-century discourses of citizenship and belonging. Bodily workings, practices, pleasures, weaknesses, instabilities, disorders, deviances, and aberrations are all imagined and understood as markers of, or barriers to, citizenship. The body's workings come to symbolize aspects of corporeal citizenship: the enslaved individual, the lactating mother, the powerful soldier, the corrupt onanist, the dissipated aristocrat, the noble peasant. In each of these cases, the body figures prominently. In this sense, the body was at the very centre of political thought during the second half of the eighteenth century.

However, even as the body provided a powerful political metaphor for citizenship, ideologies of citizenship have been premised on a curiously *dis*embodied foundation. Mainstream understandings of citizenship take disembodiment for granted. Indeed, they are premised on a notion of the body as "mere matter," as "that which has no intrinsic form or identity and which is devoid of striving, purpose, expression or meaning."[39] The citizen, in this incarnation, is an autonomous man of reason who consciously engages his critical faculties in the assertion of his humanity. The body, as an agent in its own right, has little room to manoeuvre here.

Feminist and disability scholars have pointed to the profoundly embodied nature of ideologies of citizenship. Even as the ideal privileges the presumptively disembodied autonomous man of reason, it relies on the unruly over-embodiment of its Others in order to police its parameters. As Carol Bacchi and Chris Beasley observe, "Conceptions about bodies act as a dividing line between full and lesser citizens."[40]

Given that the ideal embodied citizen, or citizen body, as numerous thinkers have since pointed out, was specific in its construction (male, rational) and, in its normalization and naturalization, universal, it is perhaps more accurate, then, to assert that idealized citizenship naturalizes normative masculine embodiment to such an extent that it is rendered wholly invisible. In the process, other bodies become overdetermined, hypervisible, and over-embodied in their alterity. Using language that is eerily similar to that found in the letters to Tissot, Vicki Kirby details a philosophical history of "somatophobia" that continues to haunt the Western philosophical imaginary:

> Perhaps commerce with the body is considered risky business because the split between mind and body, the border across which interpretations of the body might be negotiated, just cannot be secured. This fear of being discovered unwittingly behind enemy lines, caught in the suffocating embrace of that carnal envelope, menaces all conciliatory efforts … Any exchange between the mind and the body demands explanation; a minimal reassurance that incursions into the body's foreign spaces will be temporary and provisional – a "tactical" or "strategic" necessity that justifies the risk … It is as if we are held hostage *within* the body, *embod*ied, such that the site of the self, the stuff of thinking and consciousness, is an isolate made of quite different matter.[41]

Fear, horror, risk, threat – all mark this engagement. The body is threatening, menacing, overwhelming in its carnality. In its presence, the presumptively rational self cannot escape. The body is insatiable in its desires. Possessed by its overwhelming materiality, the self is held hostage, trapped, unable to flee the fleshiness of embodiment. I am reminded of Julia Kristeva's evocative imagery: "I expel *myself*, I spit *myself* out, I abject *myself* within the same motion through which 'I' claim to establish *myself* ... During that course in which 'I' become, I give birth myself amid the violence of sobs, of vomit."[42]

Fleshiness – the material incarnation of the self – has ever been a philosophical problem.[43] Ambivalence. Somatophobia. Horror. Feminist thinkers have stressed the excessive unruliness of the body in contrast to the contained order of the mind. Focusing in particular on the female body – *le sexe*, as eighteenth-century thinkers would have it – they propose alternative understandings of embodiment. Instead of asserting the material fixity of the body, they turn to fluidity and multiplicity.[44] The female body, overwhelming in its absent presence, might, as Elizabeth Grosz has put it, be understood "in a mode of seepage."[45] While feminist thinkers have often drawn on the female body as their model, their goal is to challenge the presumed stability of the so-called universal body and to put forward an alternative that has the capacity to fundamentally reimagine social relations: If not the autonomous, self-determining man of reason, then who?

This work of reimagining has deep implications for questions of citizenship. If the human is the citizen and the citizen is the human, and the human takes on bodily form in the form of the autonomous, self-determining man of reason, then what might this mean for bodies that do not fit, bodies that don't play according to the rules, bodies that refuse containment, bodies that are unruly, excessive, disobedient? What does it mean for the selves possessed by such bodies, overwhelmed, engulfed, held hostage by hostile flesh? Indeed, what might it mean for the Chevalier de Soran, whose story opened Chapter 2?

Over the course of numerous articles, Chris Beasley and Carol Bacchi argue that "bodies give substance to citizenship and ... citizenship matters for bodies."[46] Observing that the worlds of citizenship and corporeal theory rarely meet up, they propose a concept that they term "social flesh," a model of citizenship founded not on the autonomous individual but rather on fleshy intersubjectivity. This model attends not only to the materiality of the body and of intersubjective relations but also to how these relationships shape political understandings of citizenship. Integral to this framework is an understanding of the body as not only performative but as the very stuff of the social. Drawing on the work of feminist theorists of the body, they argue that "the body is not simply an outcome, it is not simply written upon, but materializes the operations of power in social life (Balsamo 1996: 3). It literally *is* what is social, since subjectivity is always embodied. Subjectivity, including political subjectivity, is fleshly, is made out of flesh."[47]

Such an approach to questions of citizenship relies necessarily on a shift from the politics of sight, or visibility, to one of touch, which, in the words of Beasley and Bacchi, "highlights how subjects are constituted by the manner in which they are touched or not touched."[48] They argue that the emphasis of citizenship should not be on the needs and concerns of individuals but rather on the encounter that shapes the relationships *between* individuals. This political ethos appears to draw much of its creative power from the foundational work of Luce Irigaray, whose "*corps-à-corps*," "two lips," and "mechanics of fluids" all rely on the disruptive potential of touch.[49] So, too, does it appear to recall the utopian potential of Hélène Cixous's "The Laugh of the Medusa": "In one another we will never be lacking."[50] Intriguingly, this approach, which stands in opposition to the autonomy and rationality of the disembodied male citizen-subject, also, in its materiality, mirrors the conceptual monstrosity of the pregnant female body, which can, as Robyn Longhurst has observed, "be seen to occupy a borderline state as [it] disturb[s] identity systems and order by not respecting border, positions and rules."[51]

Mainstream understandings of citizenship have been less than enthusiastic about the role and function of the body in citizenship discourses. Rather, mainstream approaches prize reason, self-control, and property. The body, as an agent in its own right, has little room to manoeuvre. Instead, ownership and control over the body are presented as two of the hallmarks of ideal citizens. However, as Bacchi and Beasley observe, "Conceptions about bodies act as a dividing line between full and lesser citizens."[52] Not all bodies can so easily be "ruled by reason." Many bodies resist containment. Fundamentally compromised, such bodies actively undermine any claims to corporeal virtue. Failed citizens are possessed of unruly bodies, bodies that will not, and in some case cannot, conform to the principles of moderation. Such bodies are excessive. In their actions, presentation, behaviours, these bodies are monstrous, grotesque, uncontrolled. In a word, they are excessive to the boundaries of the larger community.

During the eighteenth century, doctors occupied a unique position. At once guardians of the physiological health of the individuals in their communities, they also actively situated themselves as public intellectuals and moralists, claiming roles as "health activists" in order to "make a more perfect polity."[53] The so-called *médecin-philosophe*, or doctor-philosopher, attended not only to the needs of his patients but to the good of humanity as a whole. A reading of numerous medical treatises of the period suggests that *médecins-philosophes* styled themselves as both medical and moral arbiters, constructing professional identities that positioned them at the forefront of not only medical and scientific thought but also of moral and political thought. Tissot contributed his knowledge in the form of treatment (both in person and by correspondence) and through the publication of numerous treatises, in the process broadening his social and political influence and cachet. Physicians such as Tissot saw health as a cornerstone of good citizenship: good health was integral to the political and social health of the community as a whole. Anne C. Vila outlines the nature of the *médecin-philosophe* as follows: "the cosmology that dominated French medical thought in the latter half of the [eighteenth] century was both highly polemical and highly popular. The medical theorists who embraced this cosmology sought systematically to expand the function of their field and practice beyond the realm of the purely corporeal, and into that of the ethical, cognitive, and spiritual. Thus the philosophical medicine of the French Enlightenment was, by nature, an anthropological endeavour, promoted by theorists eager to catapult their professional specialty to the forefront of the more general effort to illuminate and improve humanity from its physical condition on up."[54]

Kathleen Wellman has demonstrated "the centrality of biological thinking" to Enlightenment thought.[55] Doctors, moralists, and intellectuals alike struggled to understand the relationships between morality and physiology, focusing their attentions specifically on the tangled intersections between body, sex, class, and gender. For all of these thinkers, one thing was clear: physiology and morality were intimately linked together. Wellman's work reveals the utilitarian agenda of eighteenth-century thought. No matter what their ideological approach, doctors, moralists, and thinkers were, at a fundamental level, interested in improving society as a whole and further concerned with the individual's capacity for realizing this vision. A morally infused physiology (or physiologically infused morality) was seen as a tool for understanding and managing social relations.

For some, like Jean-Jacques Rousseau and the physician Pierre Roussel, this entailed a careful adherence to naturalized and essentialized gender roles. Roussel's medico-philosophical system, as Vila observes, relied on a neat symbiosis between physiology and social construction: "from puberty on, from their souls to their toes, men are literally firm and resistant, thanks to their vigorously developed organs and minimum of mucus tissue; women, in contrast, remain literally the soft, vulnerable, and oversensitive beings they were as children ... Nature thereby dictates that, in their physiology and moral comportment alike, men naturally resist or overcome unwelcome irritants and obstacles, whereas women cede involuntarily to the multiple stimuli to which they are subject, because they have no more power to resist than do children."[56]

For others, like Charles Vandermonde, this involved rational reproduction, a proto-eugenics-based approach that encouraged an emphasis on what Wellman refers to as the "physical and hereditary aspects of sex."[57] Indeed, as Sean M. Quinlan observes, doctors "began commenting upon a wide array of concerns not usually associated with public health: ideal health and beauty, upper-class morals and manners, the place of women in society, child education and sexual hygiene."[58]

Wellman's "biological thinking" approach situates eighteenth-century citizenship at a profoundly corporeal level, in that it engages the embodied experiences and bodily responsibilities of those who sought to claim membership in the broader polity. Which bodies could contribute to the national good and what would such bodies look like? What would such bodies do? What corporeal responsibilities did individuals hold and how would they fulfill these responsibilities? These are just some of the questions that interested thinkers during the second half of the century.

Tissot was an intrinsic part of this medical and philosophical community and his work was clearly influenced by it. Within Tissot's thought-world, bodily maintenance, control, moderation, and surveillance provided hard evidence of individual engagement with what an anonymous author in the *Encyclopédie* referred to as the *état de nature* – the natural state of the individual. According to the anonymous author, the state of nature is an ideal state: "This *state of nature* is a *state* of perfect liberty; a *state* in which, without depending on the will of anyone else, men may do as they please, disposing of their persons and their possessions as they see fit, provided they remain within the limits of natural law. This *state* is also a *state* of equality, such that all power and jurisprudence is mutual: because it is evident that beings of the same species and the same order, who share equally the advantages of nature, and who have the same faculties, must similarly be equals among themselves, without subordination, and this *state* of equality is the foundation for the duties of humanity."[59]

Intriguing in this definition are conceptual links to the definition of health, and further, implicit and explicit references to questions of citizenship and humanity. Consider, for example, the following passage, which draws on questions of rights and responsibilities: "Although the state of nature may be a state of liberty, it is not at all a state of licence, because a man in this state has not the right to destroy himself, no more than he does to do harm to others: he must make the best use of his liberty, required of him by his own preservation. The state of nature has natural law as its rule: reason teaches all men, if they truly wish to consult it, that all being equal and independent, none should do wrong unto another in terms of his life, his health, his freedom, or his wealth."[60]

This trio of ideas – nature, health, and citizenship – shapes Tissot's medical and moral thought throughout his quartet of bestselling books. The ideal citizen, in this formulation, is one who balances freedom with responsibility and practices moderation in all things. For Tissot, this attention to the self for the good of the community manifests itself at a corporeal level. From this perspective, Tissot's medical treatises should be understood not just as manuals to treat the physical concerns of the populace, but also as moral guides designed to develop a worthy citizenry. Public health was not just about the treatment of physical disease, it was about treating both moral and physical corruption, and in this way increasing the citizenry's capacity to fulfill its social and political roles. Through the ideology of public health, individuals came to understand themselves as bodily citizens.

Tissot's perspective was situated within broader philosophical, moral, and medical conversations about the improvement of humanity. The targets of these conversations were the unthinking men of leisure, who, in the words of Michael Winston, were "victims of their own intemperance ... [who] not only condemn themselves to a life of languor, but also visit the ill effects of their libertinage on subsequent generations."[61] Distressed by what they imagined as the internal corruption of eighteenth-century society and disturbed by the lasting psychic and somatic legacies of dissipation and excess, the intellectual elite sought to transform not only bodily behaviours and practices but also moral understandings. Tissot's contribution to these debates include his belief in humanity's capacity – and responsibility – for self improvement, his understanding of the central role played by the elite in setting the tone and tenor of social change, and his insistence on bodily discipline as a moral good. In the words of Antoinette Emch-Dériaz, "Tissot associated decent health with a purposeful life and, later advocated good health as an unalienable right, as a real property which [could] enable its owner to earn a decent living."[62]

Health, for physicians like Tissot, was political. Indeed, it was integral to the realization of the social contract. After all, as Emch-Dériaz observes, for Tissot, "sickly persons depend on others, a state not far from parasitism."[63] Health, in other words, was the glue that ensured the strength of the imagined community. Indeed, according to Emch-Dériaz, Tissot's approach might be imagined along similar lines as that of the Protestant reformer John Calvin.[64] Just as Calvin's translation of the Bible into the vernacular enabled the fostering of personal spiritual relationships with the divine, so too did Tissot's approach (what she perceives as the democratization of medical science) allow for individual patients to take more personal responsibility over their health and enable them to claim more authority over their own physical experiences. Within this framework, medicine might be understood, as Tissot's compatriot Suzanne Curchod Necker has observed, as a "theology of the body."[65] Here, the physician is reimagined a moral messiah, a man of knowledge and virtue who would guide the populace out of its corporeal misery and towards the light of a strengthened republic of virtue. As noted previously, this is precisely how some individuals approached Tissot in their letters.

Tissot expressed his medical and moral vision in his quartet of influential works. Of these, the *Avis au peuple sur sa santé* was, undoubtedly, the most popular. A corporeal bible of sorts, its title – *Avis* – gestured towards both the agency and responsibility of the reader. As Emch-Dériaz explains, "The choice of title, in particular the word 'avis,' while reflecting the emerging mentality of improvement by education, also implied a possibility of choice: one can accept or reject advice, using one's own judgment to check its validity and then decide to follow up or not … More generally, the use of the word 'avis' became a declaration of the author's intent to enlighten the population and move them to action."[66] The *Avis*, together with the treatises directed towards onanists, sedentary persons, and people of fashion, was intended as a moral guide through which individuals would come to know themselves and their responsibilities better. In these works, Tissot asked readers not only to focus on their health but to consider bodily health in relation to broader moral, social, and political concerns. Thus, while these works, and the *Avis* in particular, were practical in nature, they were also designed to promote reflection and consideration. As Emch-Dériaz observes, "Tissot wanted his readers to ponder the meaning of their lives and callings, to set in proper proportion their well-being, their ambition, and their way of life."[67]

Not all of Tissot's contemporaries approved of his approach. For some, works like the *Avis* were dangerous documents that placed medical knowledge into the hands of untrained laypeople.[68] But it was precisely this gesture that was central to Tissot's medical and moral philosophy. Like Rousseau, who embraced what Nicole Fermon has referred to as a "homeopathic" approach to social reform,[69] Tissot, too, imagined that those most responsible for bodily and mental decay were also best placed to reverse these trends. This is particularly evident in his book, *Essai sur les maladies des gens du monde*, in which he pits the bodily experiences of the dissipated man of pleasure against those of the wholesome and morally sound peasant. Tissot argued that humanity's addiction to the vice of luxury led to innumerable physical ailments. Luxury was a poison that festered among the elite, and their domestic servants, in the cities and threatened the health and well-being of the noble peasants of the countryside, whose natural behaviours, diets, and physical activities represented the potential for regeneration of society as a whole.

The dangers of luxury were manifold. Addiction to luxury led to unhealthy behaviours such as overeating and poor food choices, including overindulgence in wine, chocolate, cream, and rich meats. Luxury encouraged individuals to abandon traditional lifestyles. More importantly, however, an addiction to luxury was psychologically disruptive. Manifesting itself in such dangerous passions as avarice, jealousy, anger, resentment, and an insatiable desire for material goods, it led to feelings of discontent, unreasonable competition, and disappointment. Tissot's understanding of health and illness here appears to mimic Necker's "theology of the body" in that it is founded on a concern with the physical, moral, and spiritual welfare of his patients – and of society as a whole.

For Tissot, the healthy body is that body which conforms most effectively to its natural state. This ideal was materialized in the body of the rural peasant, who lived simply, in harmony with nature and his or her community, and who used his body to the fullest extent to which it is ca-

     TELLING THE FLESH

pable. The peasant lived a sober, regular, tranquil life.[70] Little disturbed by the anxieties of city life, the peasant was oriented towards his or her community and lived in accordance with the laws of nature. Governed by firm and steady nerves, the peasant enjoyed equal perspiration, equal circulation of the blood,[71] and a calm, rational life that drew its inspiration from the rejuvenating powers of a beneficent, uncorrupted nature:

> The morning air gives to him who breathes it, a strength and spirits which he feels the remainder of the day; the exhalations from the ground, the moment the plough opens the furrow, and those of the dew intended as vegetable nourishment, are a volatile balm; and those of the flowers, which are never so lively as when the sun rises, give such as enjoy the country air, under these circumstances, a principle of life unknown to those who only breathe the air of chambers; who by their care to ventilate them, prevent it from becoming malignant, but cannot render it salutary; it sufficeth to support life, but cannot establish it.[72]

The man of pleasure, however, challenged nature at every turn. Driven by lust, ambition, luxury, desire, jealousy, and fear, he suffered from irregularity and excessive sensibility. His internal systems were fundamentally disordered, corrupted, confused, and deprived. Tissot paints this image vividly in the excerpt that follows:

> The man of fashion, disturbed by business, projects, pleasures, disappointments, and the regrets of the day, heated by food and drinks, goes to bed with trembled nerves, agitated pulse, a stomach labouring with the load and acrimony of his food, the vessels full, or juices which inflame them, indisposition, anxiety, the fever accompanies him to bed, and for a long time keeps him waking; if he closes his eyes, his slumbers are short, uneasy, agitating, troubled with frightful dreams, and sudden startings; instead of the labourer's morning briskness, he wakes with palpitations, feverish, languid, dry, his mouth out of order, his urine hot, low spirited, heavy, ill tempered, his strength impaired, his nerves irritated and lax, his blood thick and inflamed; every night reduces his health and fortifies the seed of some disease.[73]

For Tissot, illness, among the elite in particular, was the result of disordered living. That is, disordered behaviours produced the disordered body. The narrative of an unnamed prince, contained in a third-person consultation sent in 1796, would appear to lend credence to this argument. From the outset, the narrative presents the reader with the image of the dissipated aristocrat: "The Prince ... aged 24, of a delicate constitution and a decided taste for women, and thwarted by different circumstances, abandoned himself to the unfortunate habit of masturbation."[74] The narrative continues by outlining numerous episodes of *maux de nerfs*, or nervous disorder, that occurred at various times during the three-year period that preceded the consultation. Although these attacks abated somewhat in the face of serious responsibilities the young prince was forced to undertake, he soon found himself almost continually "tyrannized" by a fear of madness: "every day, this feeling becomes strong. For a few hours, he believes himself to be completely mad or at least, he is overcome by the fear, even as he is completely rational for the rest of the day."[75] Such a body, out of balance and indisposed, was inherently incapable of realizing its full citizenship potential.

Tissot's delineation between illness and health rests primarily on a class-based foundation. The rural peasant was healthy; the person of society was ill. Tissot's juxtaposition of the sick elite with the healthy poor was both an articulation of his moral stance and also an astute political strategy. Indeed, such understandings had a particularly utilitarian bent. Individuals had responsibilities and obligations to society according to their classed and gendered social positions. By diagnosing the elite as ill, and as necessarily ill because of the trappings of their social status, Tissot was able to critique what he perceived to be their wilful bodily abdication of their civic duties to the population as a whole:

> Leave me, like others, to behold with regret, that persons who, by
> their birth, station, and education, ought to give essential exam-
> ples to society, to whom they are dear, and whose health is as
> important as their influence might be powerful, are precisely those
> who give the worst, because they continually labour to destroy it,
> by following a mode of life which is directly opposite to it, and
> which is so far from increasing their pleasures, shortly deprives
> them of the very power of enjoying them, by throwing them in
> to that state which excludes all ... Can the inestimable benefit of
> health be so perfectly unknown in all orders of society, as to be
> scarcely desired, or what is worse, that languor [sic] should be as

   TELLING THE FLESH

attractive as frost to the inhabitants of the Alps, or blackness to the Negro? This thoughtless excess is scarcely credible; for sure none but a malicious satyrist can say *that it is not fashionable to be well*. What fashion is it but a fashion which renders it impossible to be happy, and to discharge our duty properly?[76]

All in all, this is a damning portrait of self-inflicted bodily disorder and decay. Was it any wonder that, as numerous philosophers argued, Europe was in such crisis?

Tissot develops similar ideas in his *De la santé des gens de lettres*.[77] Citing the Ancients, he observed that "study, though essentially necessary to the mind, is hurtful to the body."[78] He insists on a conceptual framework that imagines body and mind to be intertwined, so deeply integrated into one another that neither can exist without the other: "So close is the connexion between mind and body, that we cannot well conceive the operations of the one independent of some correspondence with the other. For as the senses are incapable of conveying the materials of thought to the soul, without the motion both of their own fibres and those of the brain, so, whilst the mind revolves these cogitations, the organs of the brain are more or less stimulated to act, stretched, and have oscillatory motions excited in them. The mind agitates the machine."[79] Elaborating on these points, he offers numerous horrific examples of individuals whose overindulgence in learning and intellectual activity had fundamentally compromised both their physical and mental well-being. Consider, for example, the following passage, in which he links his own observations with those of two other eminent Enlightenment physicians:

BOERHAAVE, who resided a long time in a city renowned for learning, has observed, that studies excite a disagreeable sensation at the upper orifice of the stomach; and that, if this be neglected by the studious, madness ensues (i). My illustrious friend POME [sic] knew a man of learning, who had made his stomach so infirm by intense application, that immediately after eating he vomited (k). I myself have seen some, who, when their minds were wearied out with constant study, being taken ill, at first lost all appetite, then were seized with a weakness of their whole bodies, and at last with dreadful paroxysms, which began with vomiting, and ended in convulsions and a total privation of their senses.[80]

Corporeally and emotionally exhausted, studious individuals must ultimately give up their intellectual preoccupations.

Tissot's prescription is unsurprising. Like the recommendations he puts forward in his other works, he stresses the benefits of exercise, fresh air, and a healthy diet – a simple lifestyle that resembles those of rural peasants, whose bodily routines assured healthy outcomes.

On the one hand, Tissot's approach can be understood as a fundamentally humanitarian project. After all, he himself observed that many people were, if not dying, then suffering terribly.[81] It is also evident, as noted previously, that many correspondents viewed his work as essentially humanitarian in nature. But his was a deeply political project, engaged with ensuring the development of not only moral upstanding individuals but of feeding morality through the body, creating corporeally virtuous citizens, individuals whose moral virtue could be read through their commitment to "health," now reimagined as a moral ideal, and of using that corporeal commitment as a basis for social change. Indeed, a careful reading of all four of these books suggests that Tissot had little patience for those who did not take bodily responsibility for themselves. As Emch-Dériaz has observed, "The message of contempt for the parasites of society was made clearer in each succeeding book."[82] What was at stake for Tissot was not just the health of the individual but the regeneration and rejuvenation of society as a whole.

### TISSOT AS CORPOREAL CITIZEN

In the formal introductions that preface many letters, correspondents pay homage to what they see as Tissot's essential moral goodness. As noted previously, correspondents imagine him as a saviour and "friend of humanity," a beneficent being whose overriding concern lies in the health of the populace as a whole. Indeed, through his public actions – his publications and his healings – he embodies the very citizenship ideal that he professes. But these same actions *also* position him as a *corporeal* citizen. That is, they offer proof of the profoundly embodied nature of citizenship itself. Interestingly, while the correspondents assert their citizenship through their *own* bodily engagements, Tissot's corporeal citizenship emerges as a result of the corporeal experiences of those whom he has treated.

As noted previously, the healthy body – a body that has recovered from its sufferings – attests to Tissot's corporeal citizenship. In its recovery, it can be understood as a bodily manifestation of Tissot's commitment to the needs of humanity as a whole. In this way, Tissot is able to assert his citizenship not only through his publications but also through his medical practice: each individual healed as a result of an encounter with Tissot offers bodily proof of Tissot's moral goodness.

The Major and Lieutenant de Bouju, for example, understands his own recovery as intrinsic to not only to his own well-being but also to Tissot's performance corporeal virtue: "I ask you respectfully, Sir, I call on your benevolence to complete your project so well begun and to regulate my life."[83] This notion of the recovering body as *oeuvre*, or work, permeates other letters as well. A woman named Marianne Grand writes the following: "I am recovered, Sir, and my first emotion, after that of joy, is of great gratitude for he who, after God, delivered me from my suffering … Here then, is twice now that you have returned me to life. You alone knew the causes of my ills and you alone, by the circumspection dictated by providence, knew how to deliver me from them."[84] Grand's language is particularly intriguing. The references to the divine – God, providence, delivery from evil – suggest a link with celestial virtue, an approach that envisions the patient as the work of the doctor just as the human might be seen as the work of God. Every body treated by Tissot offered a further testament not only of his skill but of his commitment to the needs of humanity as a whole. As his influence spread, so, too, did his commitment to virtue expand. In this way, Tissot came to be understood as the ideal corporeal citizen, a man who, through his actions, had ascended almost to the heavens.

Tissot, as the ideal corporeal citizen, was also perfectly placed to act as the arbiter of corporeal virtue. It is this understanding that underpins many letters to Tissot. Correspondents were not just seeking a cure; they were also performing selves. Such performances required attentiveness not only to questions of physiology – the conventional domain of the medical encounter – but also to questions of morality and virtue. Suffering individuals had to demonstrate that they were morally worthy of Tissot's attention and ministrations; that is, they had to demonstrate their full commitment to Tissot's citizenship ideal. Reading for corporeal citizenship enables us to make sense of passages that seem, at first glance, wholly out of place in otherwise medically oriented letters. It helps us to understand the slippage between lay letters and their medical counterparts. And it gives us a lens through which we might come to understand how individuals understood the nature of their encounters with Tissot.

I am useless to my homeland, my family, and my self.

J. Lipinski to Tissot, 20 January 1792[85]

In 1792, a Frenchman named Martin wrote to Tissot to inquire about the health of his brother, who had come to Lausanne to be treated by him. But this is not the most interesting aspect of the letter. More intriguing is this political commentary that takes up nearly half the letter:

> You are so very fortunate, Sir! A free citizen occupied, from your earliest years, with the good of humanity – you have nothing more to desire. What a contrast with our position. Only today I learned of the sad events in Paris. From this, we can only moan and hope to find ourselves in the position of those who say: *"Nos patriam fugimus"*; God willing that we still have a homeland. It is with tears in my eyes that I formulate this wish. I beg your pardon, Sir, if I stray so far from my subject, without even having the benefit of knowing you. At this moment, it is an irresistible penchant which comforts my heart since I have the honour of engaging with a philosopher such as yourself.[86]

Martin's words, written in the chaos of the French Revolution, reflect not only the melancholy that accompanies the loss of one's homeland but also the fear of the future and the tenuous promise of political and moral freedom. In making this statement, this particular individual imagines and understands himself overtly as a political actor – that is, as a member of the broader polis – and, as such, endowed with both the rights and responsibilities of his position. As a citizen, Martin is deeply concerned about the health of the French nation. But he is also entitled to the audience of other citizens. In other words, he claims his right to be heard by Tissot on the basis of their shared membership in the imagined human community united by the principles of liberty and justice. For this correspondent, these shared interests forge an invisible bond between these two men.

Very few of those who wrote to Tissot were so overt in their language. The vast majority make no overt reference to the words "citizen" or "nation" at all in their letters. What, in this sense, enables my analysis to proceed? I argue that understandings of citizenship infuse their letters in the ways that they draw on epistolary and bodily performances to imagine themselves as citizens. In telling stories of their bodies, the correspondents also told stories about themselves. Thus, citizenship emerges in the ways that they perform the various duties of their daily lives, in the kinds of issues they bring to the fore, and in their understandings of the relationships between their bodies and their social roles. For those who write to Tissot, citizenship is about their performances of fatherhood, motherhood, and questions of kinship; their engagement and understanding of questions of productive labour; their moral sensibilities as men and women of reason, moderation, and enlightenment; and their mental faculties. Citizenship also rested on their abilities to express the meanings inherent in their bodily experiences. Citizenship emerges in epistolary style and language as well as in structure. It can also be read through silences – through what is not written at all.

The letters to Tissot provide ample evidence of the global reach of Tissot's influence. Given this influence, it would be tempting to assert a neat transmission from ideology into practice, or to suggest that individual correspondents fully incorporated Tissot's vision into their bodily practices and autobiographical subjectivities. However, correspondents exercised considerable agency over their narratives. Correspondents were not passive beings subject to whims of their physicians. In their narratives, they tell stories, challenge local doctors, introduce unique bodily experiences that are not detailed in Tissot's books, and assert alternative diagnoses. Some even take Tissot himself to task. In short, the transition from ideology to practice was messy. While some conformed fully to Tissot's vision, presenting corporeally virtuous identities, others resisted this imperative. Others still experienced a slippage between moral will and bodily reality that resulted in a form of unruly citizenship. The discourse on health, responsibility, and morality was fluid. It was one that shaped their engagements with Tissot, but it was also one to which they responded to individually and through their own lenses. Thus, while it is evident that prescriptive literature, like Tissot's contributions to public health, actively sought to instil particular understandings of citizenship, and while it can also be argued that such works influenced those who read them, it is not entirely clear that the individuals who wrote to Tissot accepted these prescriptions without question.

In a normative sense, bodily citizenship relies on the assertion of the body as the product of rational processes. The ideal citizen body is carefully monitored and controlled.[87] In the letters to Tissot, such bodies are carefully managed and maintained; "moderation" is shorthand for a commitment to bodily virtue. Such bodies are also, significantly, "productive";[88] that is, they can contribute actively to the well-being of the larger community. Good citizenship is, in this sense, performative – a series of repeated acts that, taken together, give the illusion of careful bodily management. Consider, for example, the words of G. Roche, who wrote to Tissot in March 1785: "I have not eaten meat, nor have I touched women or wine during the past two months."[89] In this statement, Roche presents himself as a man who has successfully controlled his bodily passions for an extended period of time, in the process enacting corporeal virtue. Consider, too, one woman's comments about a friend who has previously been treated by Tissot: "He followed the prescribed regimen scrupulously. No wine, only vegetables, [and] he took the waters during the months of June, July, August and September, even a few times in October."[90] Like Roche, this correspondent paints a portrait of an ideal bodily citizen, a man of moderation and self-control who is wholly committed to his physical improvement. Finally, we might consider one correspondent's "*journal des mes accidens*," a detailed play-by-play of the various incidents that have befallen him between 26 April (when he last visited Tissot) and 10 July 1773 (the date of his letter).[91] A second document from the same correspondent, a man named Mathis, and dated 1 October 1773, continues this narrative, informing the reader of everything that has happened in the intervening period.[92] In their focused attention to order and detail, these documents present their author as a corporeal citizen *par excellence*.

It is clear that this model resonated with many correspondents. Regardless of their positioning on the matter, many letters reveal a preoccupation with Tissot's discourse of corporeal citizenship. This preoccupation is articulated in the form of acquiescence and approbation, but also in the form of worry or fear, and, in some instance as resistance. Correspondents engaged with questions of citizenship, situating their bodily behaviours, practices, and experiences within a moral matrix. For these correspondents, the idea of bodily citizenship acted as an anchor for the presentation of morally virtuous or morally compromised selves. What is evident in all instances is that correspondents were both aware of the dominant discourses around bodily control and health and actively situating themselves within it.

### MODERATION AND EXCESS

To consider the way that individuals navigated discourses of bodily control, it might be worth juxtaposing the cases of two very different men. The Marquis de Choisy and the Marquis de Lenoncourt were both members of the French aristocracy. The two men were, apparently, travelling together. Both wrote letters to Tissot and both included, with these letters, consultations from their local doctors. But their individual situations and perspectives could not have been more different from one another.

In his introductory letter, the Marquis de Choisy presents himself as a responsible citizen. A healthy man, he is at peace with his bodily situation. His tone is confident and free from worry.[93] This self-assessment is confirmed by his doctor – notably a doctor who has known him for seventeen years.[94] The doctor observes that while the Marquis was born with a healthy constitution and a good temperament, he has a nervous tendency and is inclined to vivid passions; however, the Marquis has moderated these innate tendencies through a sound reason and "has never engaged in excess of any kind."[95] The Marquis's life has always been well regulated and the doctor points to his diet as evidence of this: the Marquis chooses his meats carefully, eats fresh vegetables, limits his wine, and avoids overly spicy and salty foods as well as those that are excessively succulent.[96] In his bearing and behaviour, then, the Marquis de Choisy presents an ideal corporeal citizen, a man who is not only fortunate enough to possess a good constitution but who has made the most of his corporeal fortunes through a commitment to the careful regulation and management of his body, a commitment that moderates any innate bodily weaknesses he might possess. In fact, according to his doctor, the Marquis's actions demonstrate a commitment to ensuring the best possible environment for his health. These actions might thus be seen as essential to the fulfillment of the requirements of his social station. In these ways, Choisy's stance reflects the vision proposed by Tissot at the end of his treatise on the illness of people of fashion: that those who are, by fortune, best placed to be leaders should, through their bodily actions, serve as an example to those less fortunate than they.

By contrast, the Marquis de Lenoncourt's introductory letter shares none of the optimism that marks his colleague's felicitous missive. Instead, the overriding affects are fear and worry: "I have the utmost confidence in you, Sir, and in what you told me: that my illness is neither dangerous nor incurable. However, I am languishing and I await with impatience the help that I hope you can give me."[97] The Marquis continues by stating that he has been "not a single moment without suffering."[98] Chest and stomach convulsions attest to a profoundly disordered body and, at the level of emotion, the Marquis finds himself consumed by melancholy and worry. Lenoncourt's doctor appears to confirm his agitations. Unlike Choisy's doctor, who asserts his patient's moral and corporeal fortitude, Lenoncourt's places at least some of the blame for his patient's situation directly on the patient himself. While there might be a physical cause to what ails him – namely, a winter spent in a dark room that overheated during the day while being too damp at night – Lenoncourt himself shares responsibility for his condition: "born with a sanguine and lively temperament, he abandoned himself to his appetite, to foreign wines and liqueurs."[99] Furthermore, "passions of the soul and late nights"[100] also affected his health. Unlike Choisy, Lenoncourt has not lived a blameless life. Excess, rather than moderation, has marked both his bodily and his psychic existence. Lenoncourt's bodily history and current disorder appear to confirm his moral and mental disarray. Within Tissot's matrix of corporeal citizenship, Lenoncourt would be positioned as a failed citizen, a man whose apparently wilful abdication of his bodily responsibilities – or, perhaps more accurately stated, his apparently wilful abdication *to* his bodily appetites – have set the stage for disorder and disarray. In both being and action, Lenoncourt resembles not the corporeally virtuous man who takes up the mantle of bodily responsibility that accompanies his social position but, rather, the dissipated, agitated, and corporeally troubled man of excess described earlier in Tissot's book.[101]

Of course, it is not at all clear why these two men approached their bodily situations so very differently. It could just be a simple case of individual temperament. But, given the details they include and the commentary provided by their doctors, it seems entirely possible that the Marquis de Lenoncourt believed that his youthful indiscretions might have formed a troubling backdrop upon which he now attempted to make sense of his current suffering. In short, might his youthful commitment to excess have been a contributing factor to his current ailments? Corporeal virtue seems well out of reach for Lenoncourt. Lenoncourt's failed citizenship provides a counter against which Choisy's corporeal virtue might be measured. In its failure, it highlights the citizenship ideal, an ideal founded on an active commitment to the principles of moderation, balance, mindfulness, and corporeal management.

As these two examples indicate, corporeal citizenship was based on the individual's ability to fulfill the needs and requirements of their social station – to be, in the words of a Swiss man writing on behalf of a suffering colleague, "useful to society."[102] In order to do this, the individual needed to be possessed of a healthy body that conformed fully to the dictates of Nature. According to Tissot, an ideological commitment to the principles of moderation and balance was necessary in order to enable individuals to take up the practical responsibilities of their social roles. Corporeal citizenship was, therefore, as much about the practical realities of daily life as it was about ideology. As Galliotte, a novice hoping to enter the priesthood and suffering from hearing loss, observed, his "fortune" – understood in this sense not only in terms of economic security, but also in terms of his mental well-being – depended on his ability to hear.[103] If he could not recover his hearing, Galliotte would be unable to fulfill his responsibilities. But it may also be worth considering this man's chosen profession. As a novice, Galliotte was training for a life in the church. Corporeal citizenship – here understood through bodily recovery and health – was necessary not only for Galliotte's own happiness, but would also be essential to his ability to attend to the spiritual well-being of the community as a whole.

## MILITARY BODIES

We might also consider the relationship between ideology and practice in relation to the bodily concerns of soldiers, whose responsibilities lay in keeping the community and nation safe from external threat. The military body is an ideal citizen body. As Moira Gatens observes, sacrifice was a key component of the citizen. A warrior, she notes, is someone prepared to sacrifice himself for the good of the community as a whole. Thus, the citizen is not just the patriarch, the landowner, the man of reason; he is someone who is willing to give his life, to shed his blood, for a larger good.[104] The military body is also a highly disciplined body, a body carefully trained and shaped so as to withstand not only the brutalities of war but also the intense discipline required of the soldier in an army. The soldier's commitment to bodily discipline is thus part and parcel of his corporeal presentation; corporeal citizenship relies on his ability to fulfill the narratives of bodily discipline. It is through this corporeal discipline that the soldier contributes to the good of the nation as a whole.

These ideas percolate beneath the musings of an anonymous soldier who writes, "I am sixty-seven years old; I have always had a strong and vigorous temperament, having perfectly sustained the fatigues of war for many years and during very arduous campaigns."[105] There is much to consider here. In the first instance, this man presents himself overtly as a soldier, in the process asserting the primacy of the body and of bodily strength in the successful fulfillment of his duties to his homeland. But this particular soldier does not rely solely on his chosen *métier*. He is able to lay claim to corporeal virtue on the basis not only of his physical strength but also on the basis of his moral and mental fortitude. Both the psychic and the corporeal contribute to his presentation of self as an ideal corporeal citizen. In making this statement, he acknowledges the long-held understanding that citizenship is not just a matter of bearing and being; it is also a matter of will.

In the letters written by military men, active service is not only a duty for which they are responsible, but also a point of honour. Military service offered the possibility of demonstrating commitment to the values that underpinned corporeal citizenship: balance, moderation, and control, a commitment that could be read on and through the physical strength of the soldier. The successful acquitting of a soldier's duties can be read as evidence of his physical strength – consider, for example, the narrative of a man who not only "acquitted himself of all of his duties during the war" but also "succumbed to only one relatively short bout of *fièvre tierce*"[106] during this period – as well as evidence of the power of the state in action. These young, healthy male bodies were capable of sustaining the physical and mental challenges of warfare, and of withstanding the attacks of more organic "enemies." As such, these military bodies served as ideal vehicles for the display of national virtues of strength, courage, honour, and pride.[107]

### ASPIRING TO VIRTUE: COMPROMISED CITIZENSHIP

> I have not eaten meat, nor touched women or wine for the past
> two months.
>
> G. Roche to Tissot, 15 March 1785[108]

> This seizure was preceded by an abuse of sweet pastries.
>
> Joseph Camuti to Tissot, 10 February 1792[109]

As the preceding pages have made clear, membership in the imagined community of corporeal virtue was desirable but elusive. It appeared, at least on the surface, to be founded on the principles of rational thought and conscious action in the form of personal responsibility and a commitment to bodily moderation. But bodies were unruly and difficult to manage. As numerous correspondents discovered, while their will to citizenship held strong, bodily evidence appeared to suggest moral failings that risked their exclusion. For the most part, the correspondents who wrote to Tissot experienced themselves as compromised citizens; that is, while they aspired to corporeal virtue, their aspirations were being thwarted by psychic and somatic disorder. After all, it was bodily weakness that initiated their correspondence with Tissot in the first place. As compromised citizens, they understood that their experiences of psychic or somatic disorder could undermine their aspirations to ideal citizenship. Compromised citizenship, a state of striving situated between the promise of redemption in the form of ideal citizenship and the threat of failed citizenship, was necessarily ambiguous. As such, it was important for correspondents to assert their worthiness to receive Tissot's care, care that was essential to their ability to fulfill the tenets of corporeal citizenship.

In the absence of bodily health, an attentiveness to medical prescriptions became one way for individuals to manifest corporeal virtue. Such attentiveness to detail demonstrated their commitment to the principles of balance and moderation integral to Tissot's understanding of corporeal citizenship. The situation of the Vicomte de Cambis offers a case in point. Born weak and in poor health, and possessed of a poor constitution, Cambis was not well placed with regard to questions of corporeal citizenship. Bodily compromised since birth, he possessed little natural ability to fulfill the requirements of his station. Nonetheless, his doctor uses his patient's commitment to balance, moderation, and mindfulness to offer a flattering portrait of bodily virtue: "M. le Vicomte takes very few medicines; however, he observes his diet rigorously: he eats almost no meat, but does consume a lot of fish (poached or grilled); never any stock, or rather, [he eats] a veal and chicken stock seasoned with herbs and the most relevant root vegetables; rice cooked in water or prepared with this same stock; or an egg yolk. He drinks very little wine, instead flavouring his water with a small amount of Bordeaux. He engages in very little exercise but has managed to preserve his cheerful character."[110]

This quantified recitation of the vicomte's dietary habits emphasizes the performative nature of bodily citizenship. While he has suffered from bodily weakness since birth, thus throwing his claim to corporeal citizenship into jeopardy, he is able to redeem himself through a clear dedication to bodily management. At issue is not a single meal but rather a commitment to continued, repeated rituals of bodily containment and control. Furthermore, in making this statement, the vicomte's doctor assures Tissot that the vicomte's sufferings arise not from improper behaviours on his part. In other words, the vicomte is not to blame for his sufferings. This narrative allows the vicomte to sustain a position of corporeal virtue even in the face of bodily evidence to the contrary. Although compromised by his body's failings, the vicomte is nevertheless able to aspire to ideal citizenship. A man named Pictet, writing in 1767, is similarly fastidious in his dietary regulation: "However, even though I have never engaged in excess in relation to wine, I essentially forbade it; I renounced the usage of coffee with a bit of cream, which I used to drink daily, I forbade myself milk, and it was after this second privation that my colics ceased. I am also paying close attention to my nutrition: no baked goods, nor anything else that is difficult to digest. For the past two to three months I have often taken *petit lait* in the morning. In the heat of summer, I take lukewarm baths, my temperament being inclined to women."[111]

Other correspondents make reference to moderation in other areas of their lives in an effort to present virtuous selves worthy of Tissot's consideration. In their consultation on behalf of one Isnard de Reillanne, for example, two doctors offer the following statement: "Committed fully to the functions of his position as a notary, his mind is continually occupied with his business and personal affairs. Restrained in his eating habits, and even more so in his drinking habits, his most common foods (and those that most to his liking) are vegetables."[112] Isnard de Reillanne is here presented as a man of moderation in both diet and occupation, a man who appears to prefer simple pleasures and hard work. Interestingly, this virtuous framing allows the doctors to bring forward bodily concerns that appear to be the result of excess in at least one area of Isnard de Reillanne's life: "as expeditious in his meals as in his other actions, he eats too quickly and that which he swallows is, furthermore, poorly chewed given that his mouth is entirely stripped of teeth."[113]

Moderation, balance, commitment, seriousness, and simplicity form the basis for a life of corporeal virtue. Those who commit to these practices can, even in the absence of physical well-being, nevertheless present themselves as striving towards the ideal. These ideas underpin many letters. In one letter, a marquise assures Tissot that her suffering colleague, the Abbé de Chastellard, has been following Tissot's prescriptions "with the most scrupulous exactitude."[114] This type of language suggests an act of mindfulness – a conscious and sustained act of will that demonstrates a personal commitment and investment in the principles of corporeal citizenship. For each of these individuals, the assertion of corporeal citizenship relies on the presentation of a body managed by reason. Bodily unruliness is contained through the exercise of reason. In

 TELLING THE FLESH

the process, such individuals come to be understood – and importantly, come to understand themselves – as "responsible citizens carrying out their duty at various scales."[115]

Interestingly, some correspondents use the weaknesses of others to attest to their own corporeal virtue. Thus, for example, a man writing on behalf of his suffering wife observes the following: "As a girl, she already experienced the discomfort of *fleurs blanches*, a condition which has increased since her marriage, perhaps her sedentary life and the custom she has of always staying in bed for a long time are contributing factors. In relation to eating and drinking, her diet is not the most regular."[116] By delineating his wife's corporeal failures – a sedentary existence, irregular diet, and apparent laziness – and by linking these to her health problems, this correspondent demonstrates a clear awareness of the requirements of corporeal citizenship, in the process aligning himself with these principles even as his wife fails to achieve them.

More intriguing still are those who use their own weaknesses as a way of positioning themselves favourably in relation to Tissot. Such letters might be understood under a self-help rubric that situates the acknowledgment of personal failure as the first step towards transformation. Consider, for example, the words of an anonymous twenty-nine-year-old: "The individual afflicted with a chronic malady has confessed to the actions that may have occasioned it. Continual late nights during a two-year period, and hard work during this same time, long and violent hikes, [and] hunting in the marshes in both winter and summer could be the cause of the illness which has attacked me, and in particular, excessive debauchery with women."[117] This correspondent is obviously aware of the principles of corporeal citizenship. Equally clear is his awareness of his failures. Another correspondent lays blame for his bodily weaknesses on his own excessive behaviours: "In 1770 (at the age of 20), an excess of meditation and heavy study put me into a terrible state of exhaustion and languour."[118]

Finally, corporeal citizenship could also be attested through what might be termed intergenerational health; that is, one could affirm one's commitment to corporeal virtue by gesturing towards the health of one's children. As I will discuss in the next chapter, healthy children – as *ouvrages* – testified to the moral and corporeal virtue of their parents. Monsieur N.N., for example, whose case is described in a 1777 consultation, was fifty-four years old at the time of writing. Possessing a sanguine and somewhat bilious constitution, and subject to bouts of anger, he nevertheless enjoyed good health. Monsieur N.N.'s corporeal virtue demonstrated itself in numerous ways. In addition to the seriousness with which he applied himself to his work, he also lived a physically active but frugal life. Frequent horse riding, fresh air, and a moderated diet all contributed to the health he experienced in his younger years. If these behaviours were not already enough to confirm his status as an ideal corporeal citizen, his corporeal citizenship also manifested itself on a reproductive level. His doctor notes that his wife gave him "several male children, all of a strong and robust complexion."[119] The evident health and strength of these children, together with their male sex, offered yet further proof of Monsieur N.N.'s corporeal virtue. Importantly, these healthy, male children also affirm the bodily virtue of his wife. Furthermore, the existence of "numerous" children suggests that their health was no coincidence. Rather, it was the result of active parental corporeal virtue. Indeed, as I demonstrate in the next chapter, reproduction was an ideal venue for the performance of corporeal citizenship, and virility and fecundity were prime avenues of exploration.

## SELF-AUTHORSHIP AND CREATIVE AGENCY

To a large extent, the correspondents who wrote to Tissot conformed their thinking to a model of corporeal citizenship premised on rational bodily management and control, a framework in which the rational and autonomous mind asserts supremacy over the potentially unruly workings of the body in order to assure what is understood to be the most beneficial social outcome – namely, the ability of individuals to fulfill their predetermined social roles. Corporeal discipline asserts the supremacy of the mind, in the process sustaining the premises of the Cartesian *cogito*. As the examples cited earlier in this chapter demonstrate, it is clear that the correspondents mastered this language and approach. If, indeed, as Samantha Murray contends, bodily practices can be understood as "tools of self-authorship,"[120] then these letters can reveal the extent to which individuals were able to successfully parlay their experiences to fit the dictates of normative corporeal citizenship, and, in so doing, claim virtue.

However, it is also clear that the creativity with which they choose to frame their own bodily experiences suggests an engagement with a much more dynamic model of citizenship, one that is not fixed, but rather, is continually in process. Such an approach mirrors that proposed by Lauren Berlant, who argues that citizenship is "a status whose definitions are always in process. It is continually being produced out of a political, rhetorical, and economic struggle over who will count as 'the people' and how social membership will be measured and valued."[121] This model of citizenship may take the mainstream approach as its basis, but it also acknowledges that each new voice that enters the conversation subtly shifts its parameters.

A reading that stresses creative agency also suggests a need to rethink the corporeal, to move away from the model of bodily discipline promoted by Tissot and other thinkers, and towards a more polysemic model that understands bodies not as solid matter – the material representation of the rational, autonomous citizen, but rather as porous, vulnerable, and plural – thus evoking the intersubjectivity of Bacchi and Beasley's "social flesh." Such an approach can allow for the examination of a multiplicity of corporeal acts, identities, and, indeed, citizens. As Teena Gabrielson and Katelyn Parady explain, "By envisioning bodies as porous, plural and connected, a corporeal approach also acknowledges the centrality of vulnerability to the human experience."[122] In my study, this interactive or conversational model of citizenship engages the flesh – the material body – as a basis for the performance of citizenship. Bodily workings are imbued with moral meanings as individuals struggle to make sense of the role their bodies play in their subjective understandings of themselves as corporeal citizens.

The Berlant and Gabrielson/Parady arguments grant correspondents considerable agency in the crafting of their narratives. I do not want to overstate this agency. After all, it is clear that social behaviours are still profoundly influenced by the norms and conventions that govern them. However, I do think it is important to acknowledge creative agency and to consider its potential in relation to questions of corporeal subjectivity. Within this matrix, citizenship failure can still be imagined as virtue, as the cited letters have demonstrated; bodily excess can be asserted as the basis for personal transformation. At issue, in these letters, is the unruliness of a body that is sometimes wholly resistant to external control. Bodies, as I have previously argued, often have their own stories to tell, stories that can sometimes come into direct conflict with those told by the individual. These conflicts highlight a point made by Laurence J. Kirmayer: "there are at least two orders to experience: the order of the body and the order of the text."[123] This tension between the materiality of experience, on the one hand, and its productive potential, on the other, has already been explored in a previous chapter. But what I want to get at in the chapters that follow is the notion of the productive potential of bodily suffering in relation to questions of subjectivity and citizenship. What role does the suffering body play in the construction of self as citizen? Is the citizenship of the suffering self always already inherently compromised? And if so, what kinds of possibilities exist for the claiming of bodily subjectivity? What tools can individuals deploy in order to shape bodily "self-authorship" in more productive ways?

Kirmayer suggests that individuals subject to the biomedical gaze do not necessarily mirror that gaze when constructing the meaning of their experiences. Rather, they can transform it by "[putting] it to [their] own use."[124] In this, way the body might be understood not only as a site of autobiographical inscription but also a site of political inscription, a space on and through which to map alternative possibilities of self-hood and social being.[125] If bodies cannot conform to the dictates of mainstream models of citizenship, then what new stories might they tell instead? In the coming chapters, I examine in more detail the relationships between subjectivity, citizenship, and the body, considering them in relation to three distinct corporeal terrains: reproduction and kinship; sexual pleasure; and neurological and nervous disorders. In each of these instances, I highlight the mobility of the idea of corporeal citizenship, demonstrating the various ways that individuals who wrote to Tissot both engaged with and challenged its parameters.

## CHAPTER FOUR

# Constitutionally Autobiographical: Performing Kinship

We are all constitutionally autobiographical. The human genome holds the history of our lives, an ancestry that spans from primitive bacteria to ape and to nearer relatives, our social family.

Beatrice Allegranti, *Embodied Performances: Sexuality, Gender, Bodies*

"I was born of healthy parents."[1] So begins a four-page consultation letter written by the Abbé de St-Véran sometime around 1772. Such framing is not uncommon. Indeed, many letters situate illness and suffering within the context of an extensive family history. But family, for the abbot, plays a very particular role in his health: he paints the domestic sphere of the family as integral to his health and well-being. Central to this portrait of felicitous domesticity is the Abbé de St-Véran's mother, who nursed her infant son at great personal cost: she suffered from eye problems linked directly to her decision to breastfeed her children.[2] Later, at the age of eight, the abbot was sent away to school. His experience was not a positive one: "I was exiled from the paternal home in order to deliver me into the hands of bachelor schoolmasters devoid of any humanity. It is unnecessary to describe here the effect that this had on a weak and delicate child."[3] Poorly treated, the abbot succumbed to smallpox. As a result, he was forced to undergo bleeding, purging, and baths of all sorts. He subsequently contracted a tubercular disease. Rescued from certain death by his father, he returned to the family home, where he was put to bed and treated with numerous medicines. However, he returned to health only through his mother's maternal ministrations: "My mother, touched by my condition, remembered that I loved milk very much. She offered me [the opportunity] to share her breasts with one of my brothers, whom she was nursing. I accepted her kind offer and it is because of this remedy so worthy of her piety that I was returned to the state of health that I still enjoy today."[4] In this way, the abbot's mother, in a heroic act of corporeal citizenship, quite literally nursed her eight-year-old son back to health.

In his consultation, the abbot situates his family at the heart of his recovery and, indeed, central to his emotional and corporeal well-being. His health goes awry when he is "exiled" from the family home and only returns through the bodily interventions of his parents. His father, portrayed as a mythical knight, whisks him away from danger; his mother, meanwhile, a portrait of maternal goodness and generosity, gives him her milk – the perfect medicine for that which ails him. Through her actions, she foreshadows the values of the republican Marianne: her corporeal generosity – a selfless stance that undermines her own bodily well-being – assures not only her son's physical health, but also his mental and emotional health.[5] As his narrative continues, home and family continue to be integral to the abbot's health. The home, bastion of the family and source of the nation, is here imagined as a beneficent and nurturing entity that allows the abbot to recuperate from the trials and struggles of his daily life.

Beatrice Allegranti, in the epigraph that opens this chapter, offers an evocative and provocative understanding of the relationships between kinship, bodies, and autobiography. Autobiography emerges in the marrow, at the very heart of what constitutes life itself. Bodily narratives are located deep within ourselves; they are constituted from scraps of selves built from shared, intergenerational histories. For the individuals who contacted Tissot, bodily histories reached well beyond their own experiences and included the bodily narratives and histories of their forebears. So, too, did their bodily narratives extend forward into an unforeseeable future, imprinting themselves on the generations to come. Thus, nervous parents were thought to produce nervous children. *Maux de famille*, meanwhile, could affect marital prospects.

But kinship is not only read through the building blocks of biology. Corporeal autobiography brings bodily and affective experience together into a complex web shaped by social, cultural, political, and ideological imperatives.[6] As the case of the Abbé de St-Véran demonstrates, parental love and corporeal devotion could assure health. Virtuous living could assure virility, strength, and fecundity. Bodies and minds were deeply intertwined, tangled across and through generations and families. These stories were integral to their understandings of kinship and, further, to their understandings of themselves. In the letters to Tissot, bodily citizenship is not just a matter of individual lived experience; it is a matter of lineage and inheritance – a matter of genealogy. It is a story, written through generations, that can and should be further excavated.

In this chapter, I map the notion of corporeal citizenship onto questions of kinship and family. More specifically, I am interested in the following questions: How does kinship manifest itself in the letters to Tissot? How do individual correspondents use notions of kinship and family to further their bodily interests? How are ideologies of family mapped onto bodily practices and experiences? And finally, what happens to the body when kinship goes awry? The stories in the Tissot correspondence offer a complex reading of kinship, one that includes not only the narratives of mothers, fathers, and children, but that extends well beyond this to include the voices and bodies of grandparents, in-laws, siblings, and community members. These voices introduce us to performances of parental virtue, such as those described by the Abbé de St-Véran, but they also point to moments of disrupted kinship. In all instances, the eighteenth-century family, the heart of the domestic sphere and the linchpin for social and moral reform, is on full display. I begin by situating the family as a legal, ideological, and corporeal entity that can be understood along both vertical and horizontal axes. From here, I move into a discussion of maternal and paternal performances before concluding with a section on disrupted kinship.

### IMAGINING THE FAMILY

To understand kinship and its embodied manifestations in the letters to Tissot, it is important to map the shifting terrains these ideas occupied during the eighteenth century. Carol Sherman observes that the family is "the crucible of the individual's formation or destruction."[7] The eighteenth century saw a gradual shift in understandings of the family. At the beginning of the century, family was a profoundly patriarchal construct, a spaced governed by the will and word of husband and father. As James Traer observes, the husband and father "was the ruler of his own small realm, similar to the monarch in his kingdom."[8] This framework was supported both by church, in terms of moral expectations and understandings, and state, in terms of the legal frameworks, and it is reflected not only in philosophical, moral, and legal writings but also in literature of the period. Among the elite, family was understood as a means to secure lineage and inheritance. It was, in short, a business transaction. In the words of Jean Sgard, echoing Rousseau's literary hero, Saint-Preux,

"One marries … 'fortune or social status.'"[9] But the second half of the eighteenth century saw a turn towards marriages of affection and companionship.[10] Within this framework, marriage and family emerge not only as carefully arranged unions designed to secure family fortunes but also as affective spaces actively shaped by the participants.

The letters to Tissot suggest an engagement with various aspects of this spectrum of understanding. Thus, some correspondents clearly situate their concerns within the framework of the business transaction; that is, they consider the health of the family in relation to formal questions of lineage and inheritance. Other correspondents, meanwhile, articulate their kinship relations in the language of affect, situating themselves within loving, affectionate, and committed family units founded on principles of equality. Others still engage the conjugal hygiene approaches popular from mid-century.[11] In many instances, these perspectives are interwoven with one another. Thus, for example, correspondents draw on the language of affection and love to situate concerns about lineage.

At heart, family was about marriage and reproduction. Marriage, as Michael Winston points out, was the cradle of the state and a gateway to social prosperity.[12] Young women, for example, were trained and educated to their future vocations as mothers and wives. This was the expected trajectory of femininity during this period.[13] As Yvette Went-Daoust observes, "The lives of young women unfolded entirely in anticipation of marriage. This goal governed all of their education, and inevitably shaped their imaginaries."[14] But marriage, while the putative end point of many novels and fairy tales, was only relevant in relation to its much more important partner: reproduction. Carefully considered marriage was a gateway that ensured healthy reproduction, and from there, the health and well-being of family line and fortune, and the broader interests of the state as a whole.[15]

Key to this is the centrality of the child. Philippe Ariès has argued that the eighteenth century witnessed the emergence of the child as a focal point of moral and political interest.[16] Thinkers such as Rousseau, Venel, Vandermonde, and others imagined the child in relation to what Lee Edelman has referred to as "reproductive futurism."[17] That is, the child came to be understood as a site of possibility and potential, as the *only* way forward for an otherwise fundamentally diseased and corrupt society. The figure of the child is infused with promise, an entity whose health will assure the health of the social order itself. This conceptual framing permeates moral, legal, and philosophical debates throughout the second half of the eighteenth century. The child, as a symbol of hope, emerged as a being not only to be protected, but also to be nurtured, for in the child resided the potential for future moral regeneration. Such, indeed, are the imperatives behind Rousseau's *Emile*. Given this, notions of family necessarily transcended generations; one's bodily actions could have long-term social consequences. As Traer observes, "it is clear that nuclear families acknowledged and responded to the obligations and ties of the larger kinship group and to the sense of family as lineage or a chain of humans linked by blood over time."[18] "The voice of blood" is a strong one, situating extended family members in relation to one another in the search for health care and cure from Tissot.[19]

A pair of examples drawn from the correspondence to Tissot illustrates these points effectively. Madame Rigoley, Marquise d'Agrain, wrote to Tissot in relation to her daughter's prospective suitor: "You have perhaps forgotten, Sir, the good advice that you gave me with regard to the health of my daughter, and which served me well. You determined that I was raising her to be a good mother and I believe that she will be one: her growth and development have been accomplished without any of the inconveniences that concerned me. Her size and her freshness announce her good health, which was sorely tested this past winter by a most violent smallpox. All six of my children had it, [but] I treated them according to your method and all recovered."[20] Implicit in this letter are the twinned ideas that bodily health was important for the sustenance of family lines and inheritances, and therefore, that bodily disorders could impact the future family line. The correspondent presents herself as the ideal corporeal citizen. She is a mother uniquely dedicated to her children's health and well-being. Not only does she consult with appropriate authorities like Tissot to ensure their recovery from seasonal illnesses, but she is also carefully and deeply attentive to her children's future health and well-being, and, indeed, the health of generations to come. This introduction serves to situate her current concerns regarding the health of her daughter's potential husband: "[The daughter] for whom you so generously offered your medical counsel is almost 18 years old. We have found a potential suitor for her, a man whose distinguished birth and natural and acquired qualities – upon careful and scrupulous evaluation and verification – leave nothing to be desired, but there is one obstacle about which I beg you to tell me what you would do, if you were in M. d'Agrain's position, or if you were personally on the verge of getting married."[21] At issue, it seems, is a physical deformity. The marquise wants to know if it will affect future generations. As with the first part of her letter, the marquise positions herself as a virtuous mother concerned with the intergenerational health of her family. She demonstrates careful consideration, a watchful eye, and clear concern not only for her daughter – through the principles of conjugal hygiene – but for the health and strength of the family line itself. In this instance, maternal performance rests on a commitment to notions of family hygiene: as a mother, she is interested not only in her daughter's health but also in her daughter's future maternal activities.

The notion of family lineage, at an emotional or affective level, is central to a 1775 letter written by a man named Dupuy *fils*, which I first introduced in Chapter 2. Writing on behalf of his ailing mother-in-law, he comments, "I have the honour of possessing a mother-in-law to whom I owe everything and whose death would cause desolation in a tightly-knit family to whom she is very dear on many accounts. This respectable woman, aged sixty-six years, brought to the world seventeen children and has never been attacked by any sort of illness."[22] Here, the correspondent situates his mother-in-law at the head of a strong, united, and loving family; she is its emotional and psychological core. Furthermore, as mother to seventeen children, she is eminently worthy of their love and respect. Given this framing, it is perhaps unsurprising that her own vaporous sufferings appear to have come about as a result of the deaths of close family members: "It is essential to tell you, Sir, that my mother-in-law had a husband who truly loved her. She lost this beloved spouse and since this misfortune, which caused her to indulge unreservedly in grief, she has not enjoyed that robust health which she had previously. In a short period of time, she lost her father, mother, and two brothers, all of whom were dear to her (as she has the most excellent soul that I know). All of these losses have affected her morale strangely."[23] Thus, Dupuy *fils* paints two families, both of which are united by intimate bonds of love and affection, and both of which feature his mother-in-law at their heart. The living family mimics and mirrors the contours of the dead family, providing an intriguing foil through which to articulate the power of the affective family. Such longitudinal investments with notions of kinship and family were often, as we shall see, framed by concrete and pragmatic local interests and concerns about marital choice, reproductive decisions, maternal breast-feeding, and education.

Notions of family and kinship operated at ideological, legal, and corporeal levels. Thus, while moral and political imperatives situate the family as the basis for the social order and medical frameworks emphasized the need for intergenerational corporeal responsibility, legal frameworks formalized and codified these ideologies in material form. Questions of marriage, reproduction, and the family were therefore of immense importance, particularly among the elite, and these concerns underpin many letters to Tissot.

Traer situates the legal or formal understandings of marriage as follows:

> The words *sacrament* and *contract* summarize the legal definition of marriage in eighteenth-century France. For many men, marriage referred primarily to a religious act, a sacrament in which the church blessed the union of a man and a woman, declaring it indissoluble and pleasing in the sight of God. For others, jurists and those who had been involved in the process of the law, marriage meant a contract subject to the rules of royal law and the jurisdiction of royal courts. Beyond the law, marriage meant many things: an alliance of fortune and social rank, a property settlement regulating the duties and rights of the spouses and their families, a personal relationship between two individuals founded upon sentiment and free choice, cohabitation with the intent to remain together.[24]

At the level of lived bodily experience, marriage and reproduction denoted material investments in the notion of family through the passing on of titles and fortunes, on the one hand, and of moral character and bodily health, on the other. These material investments were meant to ensure the family's economic and bodily well-being across the generations.

A 1770 consultation on behalf of a man on the verge of marriage offers some insight into the complexities of the situation.[25] About ten years previously, this man had engaged in sexual relations with an unhealthy woman from whom he believes he caught gonorrhoea. She, however, denied this, claiming that she was just suffering from a particularly bad case of vaginal discharge. Nevertheless, this man experienced extensive sufferings, including burning, urinary difficulties, and bodily weakness. Over the next several years, he had been offered various remedies, including mercury. His questions to Tissot revolve around the notion of marital fitness: Can he trust that he is fully free of venereal disease and, perhaps more importantly, can he get married without fear of sharing with his wife and children "the sad fruits of his youthful errors"?[26] So, too, did another correspondent, the Marquis de Romira, reflect on his own fitness for marriage. In a desperate letter dated 28 March 1775, he writes, "I despair, Sir, to tell you that I am impotent, but such is the unfortunate reality: imagine a poor devil, thirty years of age, and on the verge of marrying a beautiful, young, and rich woman whom he adores, who becomes impotent. That is my story. Judge from this my despair and my acknowledgment for you if you are able to save me."[27] In both of these instances, bodily practices and concerns are central to larger concerns about lineage and inheritance. Indeed, the importance of kinship was not merely emotional or moral here; family, as stated previously, had legal relevance.[28]

At an ideological level, notions of family and kinship were shaped by political and philosophical debates about the role of the family in the regeneration of the nation. Rousseau and others located the cure for social and political malaise in the family, which they understood as the basic building block of the social order.[29] Citizenship, in this framing, might be understood as the ability to contribute to the greater social good through a conscious and active engagement with the bodily responsibilities of one's prescribed social roles. As Nicole Fermon observes, "It is Rousseau's contention that a reform of mores could begin only … in properly constituted family, in our earliest sociability, and that its effects would extend to the public sphere and be experienced in all forms of social interactions."[30]

Fears of depopulation, twinned with concerns about luxury and excess and moral decadence and disarray, led to renewed interest in embodied kinship.[31] Corporeal virtue offered the promise of social and political transformation, the possibility that society might be reborn, strengthened through a commitment to the politics of a body governed by an attention to "health" and family. An emphasis on sentiment and affect was central to this project of moral and ideological reform. Sentiment linked families together through bonds of affection, as the case of Dupuy *fils*, above, indicates, but it could also manifest itself in bodily form. Morally and corporeally benevolent parental performances are integral to numerous letters as individuals sought to present their cases favourably before the good doctor. Thus, a series of letters concerning the health of an eight-year-old girl apparently suffering the after-effects of inoculation reveals not only distraught parents, but a similarly troubled extended family, each of whom weighs in on the young girl's suffering. The Marquise d'Hervilly, writing in the third person, introduces the situation in the first letter, writing, "It is a father and mother, Sir, who, as a result of their grief at the unfortunate consequences that followed the inoculation of one of their children and putting their hope only in your enlightenment, beg of you not to refuse to help them. For the last four and a half months they have been consulting the best physicians in Paris, but their child is in no condition to execute their orders."[32]

The d'Hervilly's parental commitments reveal themselves in numerous ways. Notably, this consultation was written by the parents themselves, a gesture that reveals their deep investments in their child's health and well-being, and their insistence on telling the story themselves, rather than through a medical intermediary: "The statement included here was written by themselves; if they are unaware of the proper terms, it is at least certain that nothing has been forgotten."[33] While these parents may not have had the medical knowledge to write a perfectly composed letter, they can nevertheless draw on the evidence of experience in order to ensure that nothing of importance is forgotten. Central to this framing is the notion of the parent as guardian of a child's health and, in this instance, of parents so intimately involved with their child's health that they alone can reveal every relevant detail. In this way, these parents can perform moral virtue. Their virtue emerges from the care and concern that has shaped all of their interaction in relation to their child's health. At a bodily level, d'Hervilly *mère* and *père* have followed the latest medical knowledge: they had their child inoculated (a practice supported strongly by Tissot) and brought their child to the best doctors in Paris. At moral and ideological levels, they present themselves as hands-on parents who have watched over their child with diligence and care. Given this level of moral and bodily care and concern, their daughter should have been in perfect health. She should have manifested – in her body – the care her parents had bestowed on her. Her health and well-being should have provided evidence of their material, ideological, and affective investments. And yet, in her suffering, she contradicts this logical conclusion. Her bodily suffering undermines what should otherwise have been a parental legacy of virtue and goodness.

This tale of woe is then confirmed by other family voices, notably the child's grandmother and great aunt, each of whom, in updates, further situates the child within a web of love, care, and concern. This series of letters as a whole offers material evidence of the ties of affection, love, and commitment that would appear to lie at the heart of the Rousseauist family. Through this extended correspondence, the d'Hervilly family performs its own vigil. In the process, the family also seeks to secure corporeal citizenship: as a cornerstone of a renewed and revitalized citizenry, the d'Hervilly family is ideally positioned to take up its social role.

This careful positioning is particularly relevant in relation to comments made by their physician. The d'Hervilly family maintains, throughout the correspondence, that this child's condition was a consequence of her inoculation. Their doctor, however, proposed a different theory, arguing instead that the child's sufferings emanated from an entirely different cause: "M. Power said, in justification, that all of the things that happened to Mademoiselle d'Hervilly came about as a result of her ear problems, which could be regarded as a *mal de famille*."[34] In other words, blame, if it was to be accorded, lay *within* the family, not in external causes. The problem was hereditary. This extended epistolary performance of kinship, then, was of utmost importance, in that it could signal family virtue even in a space of potential bodily rupture.

This example, which emphasizes the intersections between ideology and affection, also introduces the third pillar on which notions of family were constructed: the body. Not only was the idea of inheritance relevant in relation to questions of law or custom but it was also something that could be passed on in bodily form. Thus, some letters reference the health of their extended family in order to situate the health concerns of a suffering individual. One consultation, for example, references the health of the sufferer's immediate family and that of her extended family as a way of trying to get to the bottom of her sufferings.[35] This unsigned letter was written on behalf of a sixteen-year-old girl who appears to have been in good health during her early childhood but began to suffer after an inauspicious public encounter with a soldier who was fleeing one of his superiors. According to the correspondent, this young woman was possessed of a healthy temperament. "Alert and vivacious," she had a good appetite and, apart from childhood bouts with measles and smallpox, never showed any signs of chronic illness.[36] Her immediate family, too, offers a picture of health: her parents and two brothers are healthy and strong. Furthermore, as she was nursed by her mother – another demonstration of bodily virtue – her health problems could not possibly have been the result of wet-nursing, a point to which I will return later in this chapter. Finally, while there have been some health problems in the extended family, the correspondent offers numerous reasons why these problems were not believed to be the cause of this girl's suffering. In this letter, the correspondent references family as a way of getting at a sort of genealogy of illness. In this case, however, this genealogical approach fails. The child, who should by rights have been the inheritor of bodily health and well-being and thus ideally positioned to take up her own corporeal position in a renewed polity of virtue, is suffering and the family is left with a mystery: How could such a strong bodily legacy go awry?

Within this tripartite conceptual framework – legal, ideological, and corporeal – family and kinship operated along both vertical and horizontal lines; that is, they were understood both inter- and intra-generationally. Correspondents actively positioned themselves as fathers, mothers, sisters, brothers, aunts, uncles, and even grandparents, using these accepted kinship roles as the basis both for their affective investments in the sufferings of family members and for their right, as corporeally virtuous citizens, to correspond with Tissot. Consider, for example, the case of Madame Gounon Laborde, who wrote to Tissot in May 1773 about the health of her husband, Monsieur Gounon, whom we will encounter again in Chapter 5. In her letter, Madame Gounon Laborde surrounds herself with family. Furthermore, she situates her family within the glow of Tissot's beneficent grace: "It is to your salutary ordinances that M. Gounon of Agen, my Father, owes – as do I – the recovery of my sister and my brother; today it is on behalf of my husband that I beseech the happy secret that all of Europe acknowledges for the most rare and extraordinary cures, and the humanity of your soul is so well known that I address you with the greatest confidence."[37] For Madame Gounon Laborde, family is an intimate notion that binds together the fortunes not only of her previously ailing brother and sister, but also of their father. But family also, as she points out, includes marital ties. Thus, family must be considered along both vertical and horizontal axes. Family links generations: Madame Gounon Laborde's concern for her husband articulates, at least obliquely, her interest in the generations to come, and her father's interest in the health of her siblings also mirrors this intergenerational interest. But for Madame Gounon Laborde, family also moves horizontally, tying together the fortunes of all of the siblings, each of whom will carry forward the family line.

This overview suggests that individuals understood and wrote themselves within the context of broader understandings of kinship and family. They situated themselves within a three-pronged structure that acknowledged ideological, legal, and bodily understandings of kinship and family, and also articulated the family along both vertical and horizontal axes. By drawing creatively on these frameworks, those who wrote to Tissot sought not only to claim the authority to speak on behalf of family members but also to put forward morally virtuous and corporeally blameless selves, in the process implicating themselves fully within Tissot's understandings of corporeal virtue. However, it is also important to recognize that the construction of a morally – and corporeally – virtuous self relied on prescriptive notions of gender and sex. Thus, the bodily performance of kinship was differently enacted by men and women; that is to say, men and women drew on different tropes to make their cases. In the sections that follow, I explore these ideas in more detail, considering in particular maternal and paternal performances of citizenship. I end the chapter with a consideration of ruptured kinship.

## MATERNAL PERFORMANCE: EMBODYING MOTHERHOOD

I am mother to 7 children, all in good health, thank the Lord. In 4 or 5 weeks I will give birth to my 8th.

Baby Develay (née Gonzebat) to Tissot, 21 May 1791[38]

As Nahema Hanafi has observed, women's bodies "progressively become an instrument of state power" in the course of the eighteenth century.[39] Women were key participants in Tissot's proposed medico-political reforms.[40] Like Rousseau, Tissot viewed women as prime targets for his suggested reforms and broader social vision.[41] At issue, for Tissot, was women's reproductive physiology. As Lynette McGrath explains, early modern women were breeders, their social role determined by their ability to successfully reproduce the next generation.[42] With such responsibility came considerable scrutiny, particularly in a thought world invested in the porosity of the body. In this world, Wendy Churchill points out, "the female body was considered by practitioners to be capable of manifesting, transmitting, and responding to disease and treatment in ways that the male body could not."[43] Furthermore, this unruly female body, marked by menstrual and later lactational flows, was considered to be particularly porous and thus prone to easy influence from external forces.[44] The female body was, in this sense, a potentially threatening entity, a vector for both social and moral contagion.[45] In the words of Julia Douthwaite, "Today, as [in the eighteenth century], the female body constitutes a mystery and a menace.

The dream of Enlightenment, that is, human perfectibility, was haunted by the spectre of reproduction with inferior, monstrous or sub-human beings."[46] But this body was also the incubator of the species. Through its workings it not only housed, but also nurtured, the next generation. And there was the rub: How could a body be both inherently nurturing and at the same time so potentially hostile?

But reproductive womanhood was not just about a woman's capacity to "breed." Just as doctors and natural scientists of the time focused their attentions on the biology of sexual incommensurability, so too did moralists and philosophers interrogate the conceptual idea of motherhood. Mothers, they argued, were integral to social and moral regeneration. In the words of Nicole Fermon, "Woman and women (i.e., as mothers and other care givers) play a vital role in the production of citizen-children, and that particular initial contact is the way in which a powerful antidote to corruption and decay is transmitted."[47] Indeed, as Isabelle Brouard-Arends has argued, mothers came into their own as central characters in the ideology of moral reform: "The mother does exist in the eighteenth century. Her existence is of the order of physiology, sociology, history. In this century of Enlightenment, the mother enters history: she can project herself into the future; or rather, let us use the passive voice: she is projected into a future which situates her, in relation to her child, at the heart of the central concerns of the period."[48]

Eighteenth-century understandings of motherhood and maternal performance have been extensively studied. This scholarship has focused on ideologies and politics of motherhood,[49] representations of mothers and mothering,[50] reproduction,[51] and embodied maternal practices (particularly breastfeeding).[52] From this scholarship have emerged the figures of the good mother – a selfless, generous woman whose benevolence, charity, and devotion marked both her bodily and moral engagements with her children and family – and the bad mother – "the antithesis of the good mother: selfish, unnatural, undisciplined, and externalized, and her children paid the price for her selfishness."[53]

Motherhood, as a social and political construct, emerged out of a messy cauldron of moral, medical, anatomical, scientific, and philosophical ideas that together conspired to construct an image of women as "essentially mother" – that is, as a fundamentally reproductive and maternal being.[54] As Rousseau argues in *Emile*, "Women, you say, are not always bearing children. Granted; yet that is their proper business."[55] Two centuries later, Simone de Beauvoir would take up this claim, positioning it as central to her notion of the second sex.[56] For Beauvoir, reproduction is the female's obligation to the species, an obligation to which men are not beholden.

It is clear from the letters addressed to Tissot that individual mothers situated themselves within this entangled relationship between biology and ideology. Indeed, this tangliness is central to conceptions of maternal corporeal citizenship. Within the body politics of the period, mothers had no choice but to present themselves as virtuous, both in terms of their biology and in terms of their affective relationships with their children. Epistolary spaces celebrated – indeed, venerated – the maternal as an expression of the virtuous feminine.[57] Unfortunately, it is impossible to deduce the extent to which such positionings were the product of authentic feeling or strategic alignment. The work of Elisabeth Badinter counsels the reader to be leery of taking such presentations of self at face value.[58] Nevertheless, it is equally clear, in reading the letters to Tissot, as well as other correspondence and published literary works by women authors, that women thought deeply about their maternal roles and responsibilities, and that the experience of motherhood was integral to their understandings of self.[59] Furthermore, it is equally clear that understandings of motherhood shaped the ways that women chose to mobilize themselves as corporeal citizens at a fundamental level.

At a general level, mothers had two different options available to them to articulate their corporeal virtue: they could rely entirely on the "biological data"[60] to tell their story for them, or they could situate themselves within narratives of moral virtue. A biologically oriented approach enabled mothers to present their corporeal virtue not only through the evidence of their *own* bodies (pregnancy, childbirth, breast-feeding), but also through those of their children and grandchildren. Intriguingly, some mothers chose to articulate a sort of vicarious or surrogate corporeality, revealing their own corporeal virtue through their close attentiveness to the bodily behaviours of those actively engaged in mothering activities on their behalf (for example, wet nurses). A moral approach, meanwhile, allowed women to articulate themselves as mothers by appealing to the bonds of affection and love that lay at the heart of their intimate relationships with their families. In this instance, it is important to note that affection and love were not just moral attributes; they also manifested themselves in intensely bodily ways.

For many correspondents, reproduction, at a bodily level, was a key facet of corporeal citizenship. It offered physical evidence of conformity, both with Nature and with the requirements of the social order. Indeed, as Hanafi has observed, "chastity and sterility are [understood to be]

    TELLING THE FLESH

contrary to the health of women."[61] But reproduction was a risky business during the eighteenth century. Dorothy Porter and Roy Porter call it "perhaps the highest-risk occupation of all,"[62] an idea which finds its echoes in the letters to Tissot.[63] Reproductive bodies were capricious entities. Shaped not only by the vagaries of sex but also by the realities of social and economic precarity,[64] they were unstable and unpredictable, sites of misfortune seemingly with wills of their own.[65] As Simone de Beauvoir has so evocatively captured it, "woman *is* her body as man *is* his but her body is something other than her."[66] Lynette McGrath has argued that in this situation, "the fragility and unreliability of [woman's] body must have presented a threat to a woman's sense of the self as agent even of this uniquely female act."[67]

Constructing a virtuous bodily self was difficult given this level of bodily uncertainty, and it is clear from the letters to Tissot that some women struggled as a result of difficult pregnancies, infertility, miscarriage, and stillbirth, as well as molar pregnancies, premature deliveries, and the deaths of infants and young children.[68] Madame Tollot, for example, who had given birth to seven children and experienced numerous miscarriages over a ten-year period, delivered her eighth child prematurely at seven months' gestation.[69] Two weeks later, things appeared to go completely awry: "She ran a distance of two *lieues* to see her child at his nurse, which caused her considerable fatigue. A short time later, she suffered from some sorrows, and finally experienced a violent fright, occasioned as a result of encountering a beggar in the countryside."[70] As a result, Madame Tollot's mental and physical health were profoundly compromised. Among other things, she experienced considerable agitation, her imagination was disordered, her menstruation had been completely suppressed, and her judgment was impaired.

So, too, might we consider the letter penned by Madame de Launay, who narrates the dramatic details of her 1782 pregnancy and delivery as follows:

In 1782, I became pregnant again. The multitude of accidents
that had previously befallen me led me to fear that this pregnancy
would be as disappointing as all the others. My man-midwife
was also fearful and this fear was the cause of all the mistakes
that almost ended up causing my death. During my pregnancy, I
was bled 12 times over the course of 9 months. Having arrived at
term, which he didn't think would happen, I called him as soon
as the first contractions began. Convinced that I would not be

able to deliver naturally, he decided to use the forceps after 18
hours of labour that was not progressing. After an hour of trying
fruitlessly (and injuring both the child and me in the process, to
the extent that I was significantly weakened), Mr Millot called
up Mr Baudeloque, who, ignoring both the procedure I had just
undergone and my current state, decided to let nature take its
course. But after 60 hours he judged that I no longer had the
strength to sustain this … and decided that it was time to deliver
me. Mr Millot wanted to be in charge of this procedure again.
His attempts were in vain and he left me in a miserable state. The
forceps had gone into the infant's head. I was seriously injured,
greatly weakened by the loss of all my blood, and condemned
by Mr Millot to a caesarean section. I managed to keep my head
enough to oppose this and to assert that this option should not
be attempted before M. Baudeloque had tried to deliver me. My
prayers were answered and five minutes later I was delivered of
these cruel torments.[71]

Reproduction, as these letters demonstrate, was corporeally fraught.

Given the levels and extent of maternal and infant mortality during
this period, as well as the mental and bodily sufferings experienced by
such women as Mesdames Tollot and de Launay, maternal fecundity
was understood and experienced as an accomplishment worthy of cele-
bration and veneration. Not only did successful childbearing attest to a
woman's strength of character, but it also attested to her bodily virtue:
only a woman of physical health and well-being – a woman, that is,
who embodied the ideals of corporeal citizenship – could ensure the
successful growth and development of a passel of children. The letter
from Dupuy *fils*, cited earlier in this chapter, makes this very point: a
significant part of his mother in law's corporeal virtue derives from her
fecundity: after all, she is mother to seventeen children.[72] Reproductive fecundity, in terms of either quality or quantity, was understood as
a form of active citizenship through which women, as mothers, could
populate the next generation, in the process extending their reach well
beyond the borders of their own bodies. Even stronger cases for corporeal citizenship could be made by those who were able to assert their
fecundity and the bodily successes of their children. In a social, cultural,
and political world that understood the child as the "work" of its parents (and particularly its mother), such issues as bodily strength, moral

fortitude, and, later, a useful career that contributed to the good of the nation as a whole, were ideal proofs of good corporeal citizenship.

"Good" maternal corporeal citizenship, then, extended the limits of the maternal body. As McGrath observes, "in pregnancy [a woman's] body is a container, a carrier, and the capacity to give birth to a child allows the body a sense of territorial expansion because it is able to produce an other, not the self."[73] Such commentary gains credence when considering the observations of the famed *salonnière*, Suzanne Curchod Necker.[74] In a letter she wrote to her close friend, Etienette Clavel de Brenles in the days leading up to the birth of her first and only child, Anne-Louise-Germaine, Necker wrote, "This will be the last letter that I will have the honour of addressing to you before I have doubled my self, or, rather, before I have brought to the world a new heart to love you. I sense that my child shall have the same feelings as her mother."[75]

This notion of a split subjectivity that links mothers not only to their children but also to the needs and concerns of subsequent generations is also a feature of numerous letters to Tissot. One letter, for example, links the death of a beloved child with the bodily sufferings of her mother.[76] The mother, a woman of thirty-three married at the age of fourteen, gave birth to four children, the last of whom was born nine years previously. One year before this, she had lost a daughter "who was very dear to her."[77] As a result of this loss, her whole body became flushed, and she was affected by this for two or three years. In this way, the maternal body materialized emotional distress; in its flushing, it marked the split subjectivity of a mother who could no longer access her daughter.

While reproductive fecundity would appear, at least on the surface, to offer material proof of corporeal generosity, it was not enough. After all, as the case of a mother of fourteen demonstrates, even as fecundity appears to offer evidence of maternal bodily health, it could also be the site of maternal disorder.[78] Here maternal virtuosity, marked through the fourteen successful pregnancies over a seventeen- or eighteen-year period, descends into maternal distress as the woman descends fully into nervous disorder. I develop this narrative more fully in Chapter 6.

Women could also draw on other aspects of bodily commitment. Breastfeeding offered one ideal avenue through which mothers could claim corporeal citizenship. Just as soldiers committed their bodies to the security of the nation, so too could corporeally virtuous mothers, who were left out of a militaristic discourse of sacrifice and citizenship, commit their bodies to the nourishment of the nation. Indeed, the altruistic benevolence of the lactating maternal body promised social transformation and redemption. Intriguingly, Jaucourt, in the *Encyclopédie*, imagines the homeland itself as an ideal nursing mother, a nurturing and benevolent being concerned wholly with the needs of her citizens:

> [The homeland] is a nurse who gives her milk with as much pleasure as it is received. It is a mother who cherishes all of her children, who does not distinguish amongst them any more than they distinguish amongst themselves; who would wish there to be opulence and mediocrity, but no poverty; the powerful and the less powerful, but no oppressed person; who, even in this unequal partition, preserves a sort of equality by opening to all the route to the prime positions, who does not accept any trouble in her family, except for that which she is unable to prevent – illness and death; who believes she has done nothing in giving being to her children unless she adds to this their well-being. It is a power as ancient as society, founded on nature and order, a power superior to all the powers that she establishes at her breasts … [the homeland] is a divinity that accepts offerings only in order to share them, who demands more attachment than fear, who smiles as she does good and who sighs while throwing lightning. This is the *patrie*! The love that one has for her leads to a generosity of morals, and the generosity of morals leads to the love of homeland. This love is the love of law and the love of the state, a love that appears only in democracies. It is a political virtue through which one renounces the self, the preference of the public interest more important than self-interest. It is a feeling and not a result of knowledge; even the meanest man of state can have this as much as the head of a republic.[79]

Lactation, in the form of maternal breastfeeding, operated as a potent material symbol of maternal virtue throughout the second half of the eighteenth century. Breastfeeding was seen as evidence of good motherhood, an activity that accorded the nursing mother all the benefits and privileges of corporeal citizenship. Jean-Jacques Rousseau was one of the most vocal champions of the practice. Equating bodily practice with moral virtue, he declared that "when women deign to nurse their children, then will be a reform in morals."[80] That this statement resonated within late eighteenth-century thought and action is undeniable.[81] This notion of large-scale social reform through maternal breastfeeding was

   TELLING THE FLESH

echoed in other publications, such as those by Marie-Angélique Anel Le Rebours and Roze de l'Epinoy.[82] For Rousseau, as for others, maternal nursing was evidence of altruism; that is, it was proof of corporeal generosity. This generosity, nursed at the mother's breast, would then positively impact subsequent generations.

While eighteenth-century breastfeeding ideology has been the focus of considerable discussion, much less emphasis has been placed on the lived experiences of breastfeeding mothers and breastfed children. More specifically, much less work has examined how women experienced lactation and breastfeeding, and how they understood these practices in relation to discourses of corporeal citizenship and bodily virtue.[83]

The relationship between mother, baby, and milk was a symbiotic one. They could not be disentangled from one another, and problems in one area could very easily undermine the balance of the whole. Within this matrix, breast milk itself was understood as both a beneficent, living giving entity *and* as a vector for contagion. While breast milk was undoubtedly a source of regeneration, it was also a dangerously volatile fluid with the capacity to transmit the mental, physical, and moral qualities of the nurse into the passive, accepting and blameless body of the child.[84] This symbiosis was, therefore, fraught. Fantasies of ideal motherhood imagined a beneficent, generous mother giving freely of herself for the good of her child, but the reality was much more complex. To get at this, it is important to distinguish between the autobiographical roles and functions of maternal breastfeeding on the one hand, and wet-nursing, on the other. Both of these bodily practices were engaged in the performance of corporeal citizenship. Unsurprisingly, however, these engagements differed markedly in tone and approach.

As I have argued elsewhere, breastfeeding comes up surprisingly rarely in the consultation letters, particularly given the weight given to it by doctors and moralists of the period.[85] That said, such a claim should not serve to undermine or derail a careful and close engagement with the stories of correspondents who *did* engage closely with this rhetoric – that is, the stories of those for whom these ideological positions resonated. Such letters allow the contemporary reader insight into how corporeal citizenship was imagined and experienced in the area of bodily exchange. It helps us to see how ideals of citizenship might have been transmitted, literally, through milk. These cases demonstrate that lactation was a complex site of maternal identity and citizenship performance. While maternal nursing could serve to underpin a successful performance of corporeal citizenship, this performance could easily be undermined by the vagaries of health and illness during this period. Furthermore, the politics of lactation ensured that only certain mothers could claim corporeal citizenship. Wet nurses, or mercenary mothers, were unable to assert corporeal virtue. Instead, they were relegated to the position of failed citizens, embodied beings who could claim no right to belonging.

As evidence of what Myra Hird has termed "the corporeal generosity of maternity,"[86] maternal nursing and its beneficent effects offered hard evidence of corporeal citizenship. Interestingly, such narratives are not always joyous. That is, they are not always portraits of happily nursing mothers and round, gurgling babies. However, in each of these cases, maternal nursing is framed as a bodily activity that is central not only to these mothers' understandings of themselves *as mothers* but also to their understandings of themselves as corporeal citizens.

Madame de Bombelles, Marquise de Louvois, aligns her commitment to maternal breastfeeding with Tissot's commitment to the health of humanity. In so doing, she not only gestures towards the life- and health-giving attributes of both nursing and medicine, but also situates herself in close proximity with the arbiter of corporeal virtue himself: "It was your method, Sir, that saved the life of a child born in a most terrible state at seven months' gestation. All the doctors in Paris assured me that I would be unable to raise him. [But] I nursed him with my milk [and] I bathed him in cold water, despite the rigour of the depth of winter. He will [soon] be 1-year-old. He is a superb child, both in terms of strength and weight … he is able to roll on a carpet, crawls and within a month, he will walk on his own. But I don't want to force him. I am waiting until nature commands him to support his own weight. I have just weaned him."[87] This child's health is the result of the active corporeal engagements of two "parents": his mother, who "nursed him with [her] own milk," and his "father," a doctor whose advice supported and sustained the mother's actions, even in the face of contradictory advice from local doctors. The bodily, and intellectual, health of the child, meanwhile, lends further credence to the corporeal citizenship of his "parents." As a unit, this "family" embodies corporeal virtue.

Maternal milk was not just morally beneficially; it was also materially beneficial.[88] But nursing was a contested activity during the eighteenth century. Very few women, of any social class, nursed their own children.[89] The vast majority of infants were sent to nurse, some of them remaining with their nurses for several years before returning to their homes. Unsurprisingly, given, among other things, the marginal economic situations of wet nurses, the distance that some infants had to travel, and the relative lack of wet nurses in relation to the demand, infant mortality was high. According to Nancy Senior, the vast majority of infants placed with wet nurses died.[90] Moral discourses of the time distinguished between the selfless corporeal generosity of the mother, or natural nurse, the being evoked in Jaucourt's definition of the *patrie*, and the grasping machinations of the wet nurse, or *nourrice mercénaire*, a mercenary mother whose economic self-interest undermined any claim she might make to corporeal beneficence.

The decision to draw on the services of a wet nurse was a contentious one, particularly among physicians and moralists of the period. Understood as vectors for moral and bodily contagion, wet nurses threatened the health of the public at large. Consider for example, the entry on wet-nursing in the *Encyclopédie*, which warns, "It is most important that she be free from all those sad illnesses that can be communicated to the child. We have seen too many examples of the communication of illnesses from wet nurse to child. We have seen entire villages infected with venereal disease that a few sick wet nurses have communicated by giving their children to other women to nurse."[91]

Intriguingly, it is this notion of contagion and threat on which some correspondents drew to shape their narratives. In these letters, wet-nursing emerges as a convenient prop on which families could blame the deteriorating mental or physical health of their family members. Bodily weakness, rather than inhering in a family line, thus compromising the corporeal virtue of the family as a whole, could be the result of the tainted milk of the mercenary mother, a being already marked by her profession as a failed citizen.[92] Thus, a four-year-old child suffering from a form of dementia was found to have been nursed by a woman who had not only nursed a "foreign" child but whose other charges had developed worms.[93] So, too, had a suffering priest been "poorly nursed by several wet nurses, one of whom died of consumption."[94] Another child, meanwhile, suffered from milk deemed to be "too substantial" for her.[95] A consultation written on behalf of the Countess de Jodocte in 1773 suggests that her suffering, which began at birth, might be due to the overly rich milk of her wet nurse.[96] In this iteration, the wet nurse, as the site and materialization of disrupted kinship, is figured as a source of contagion whose milk has irrevocably altered the countess's long-term health. Another man's nervous sufferings, which included suicidal tendencies and a desire to jump out a window, were similarly blamed on his wet nurse, in the form of the "excessive sorrow" that he nursed at her breast. [97] Yet another details an almost two-year history of wet-nursing misfortunes.[98] The twenty-two-month-old child, born of healthy parents, had had eight nurses, one of whom passed on venereal disease. In these examples, it is the milk of the nurse that disrupts the "natural" relationships between mothers and children. Furthermore, this bodily disruption cannot be attributed to the actions of the sufferer, whose corporeal virtue, as a result, remains intact. The nurse, meanwhile, is in this way forcibly exiled from the parameters of corporeal virtue. In these presentations of self, the wet nurse is banished to the realm of the failed citizen, a process that allows the suffering correspondent to maintain a position of corporeal virtue.

In addition to drawing on "biological data," to follow Beauvoir, women-as-mothers also situated their appeals within the language of moral virtue. Articulating their responsibilities as mothers by drawing on the moral values of love, affection, commitment, and intimacy, they position themselves as virtuous moral agents whose children are worthy of Tissot's care and attention. Thus, for example, Madame Cagnart Briod, a postmistress at Saudrupt near Bar le Duc, entreats Tissot to heal her son on the basis of her maternal virtue. After recounting his entire medical history, from his birth in 1764 to his current state (in 1791), she concludes her letter by writing, "I hope, Sir – and it is a tender and suffering Mother who begs this of you – that you will examine and reflect [on this case] with all the attention of which you are capable. You can count on the truth of my narration; we would give anything for the recovery of our son, whom we love especially because he has no faults, I can say with all honesty, and furthermore, he is a well-grounded child."[99] While this statement, with its calls to suffering, affection, attention and its references to the "good child," might be read as a performance of maternal virtue, it functions also, equally, as an implicit challenge to Tissot himself: just as Madame Cagnart Briod has put everything into her concern and care for her son, so too does she now expect that Tissot will respond with similar seriousness of purpose. Her commitment, then, serves as a foundation for the commitment that she feels she can expect in return.

Maternal love, affection, suffering, and grief could also transcend generations. One correspondent situates her own health directly in relation to her experience of maternal loss and her concerns for her

   TELLING THE FLESH

granddaughter. In this way, she extends the narratives of motherhood, invoking a chain of mothers united by common experience and purpose. She writes that her decision to write is informed by a number of factors: "The continued presence of my daughter's death, and my fear of dying and of leaving my granddaughter who, as a result, will have no other asylum but the convent."[100] This intergenerational legacy shapes her understanding of herself: at a corporeal level, she is responsible both to the memory of her daughter and to the material comfort of her granddaughter. Significantly, this intergenerational legacy will also shape her granddaughter's life: the grandmother's compromised health will limit her granddaughter's opportunities and life chances. At a corporeal level, then, this grandmother is responsible both to the memory of her daughter and the material comfort of her granddaughter.

It is also worth considering a narrative written by a man named Dollffuss, residing in Mulhausen.[101] In his letter, Dollffuss situates moral virtue as a genetic quality, something that moves through generations: "Madame is 38 years old. She was born of well-constituted parents who have never done anything be ashamed of their manners. This virtue having been transmitted to their daughter also preserved itself in her, and in 22 years of marriage, our union has always been perfect, without troubles or changes or any sort of pain. Madame had 4 children. The first two, the eldest of which is now 20, were born 15 months apart and then the other two at intervals of four years. She had these four sons with ease, having experienced neither adverse postpartum problems nor serious inconveniences."[102] Here, madame is presented as a paragon of both corporeal and moral virtue. Her lineage is strong: her parents were possessed both of good health and of a strong morality. Her children, too, provide evidence of her bodily citizenship: she is mother to four strong boys – the eldest of whom is now an adult – and suffered no bodily ill-effects. Furthermore, her reproductive history is neat and tidy: unlike many other women, she does not appear to have suffered from any miscarriages, molar pregnancies, or stillbirths.

Some letters, however, are not so neatly analyzed. These narratives are much more complex, leading to ambiguous and even ambivalent performances of motherhood. Such stories do not fit easily into dominant ideologies and understandings and, in their contradictions, they point to the limitations of those very ideologies. Consider, for example, the narrative of Madame Moreau de La Villegille, who sent three documents to Tissot in 1773.[103] Madame Moreau de La Villegille had a complex reproductive history that included four healthy children. A fifth had died of smallpox just before the age of three. She was, at the time of writing her letters, pregnant with her sixth child.

After experiencing bodily difficulties and resistance from her family, Madame Moreau de La Villegille had sent her first four children to nurse.[104] It was only after the birth of her fifth child that she plucked up the courage to assert her desire to breastfeed. She explains the situation as follows:

> I nursed only the child that I lost; I wanted to nurse the others, but with my first, I had no milk during the first days; I had no experience [and] nobody told me that it could still come in. My child was sent to nurse and this hurt me considerably. My birth was complicated, I had rheumatic fever: first in my bowels, then in my chest and finally, throughout my limbs. I was in this state for two and a half months. As for the others, I was reminded about how ill I'd been and was discouraged from fulfilling my responsibility. Finally, I took it upon myself to try to nurse my fifth child and despite everything I had been told and in spite of the fact that the child did not want to nurse for eight days, I kept at it. I followed the advice for mothers in the *Avis*. I did not swaddle my son and washed him in cold water. I was in good health and my son was very strong and very big.[105]

According to dominant ideologies, Madame Moreau de La Villegille's decision to take up the bodily responsibilities of motherhood and to enact the corporeal generosity of motherhood should have assured her son's future health. However, in an inversion of dominant logic, this child died, while the others, all of whom she had sent out to nurse, thrived. Indeed, this child's death appeared to confirm her family's resistance. But it also situated her as a failed corporeal citizen: she had put her faith, and her maternal identity, in breastfeeding, only to see it fail. What then, was a woman like Madame Moreau de La Villegille to do? How could she possibly enact corporeal virtue? After all, her one attempt to reverse her bodily legacy had resulted in failure.

And yet, it is in this very promise of maternal transformation through breastfeeding that she sought healing. Haunted by the death of a son who was healthy and strong and whose death occurred almost before she had had a chance to process the fact of his illness, Madame de

 TELLING THE FLESH

La Villegille hoped that breastfeeding her sixth child would help her recovery: "[The death of my son] is always present and fills my days with bitterness; I am also melancholy and serious. [Nevertheless] I confront with pleasure that which hurts me; I would like to nurse the child that I am carrying [and] I am convinced that this will be the best way to distract me from what I have lost. I do not dissimulate; if I do not nurse this child, I will experience true sorrow."[106] These concerns also percolate under the surface of her next letter: "I very much fear that if I must continue with these purgatives after my delivery, that my milk will be diverted and that there will not be enough for me to nurse my child. What, then, should I do, Sir, to return myself to health without denying myself the consolation of being a nurse to my child? I will not hide from you that I ardently wish to fulfill this duty, and I flatter myself that it will contribute to my recovery."[107] For Madame Moreau de La Villegille, breastfeeding, as corporeal practice, is integral to healing a wounded maternal identity. Furthermore, it is also through breastfeeding that she hopes to fully and firmly situate herself as a corporeal citizen. For Madame de La Villegille, maternal breastfeeding is about much more than infant health; in her case, it offers the promise of maternal redemption.[108]

The complexities surrounding breastfeeding and maternal performance also shape the narrative of another, in this case unnamed, woman. This mother's narrative begins in a felicitous manner. She writes that she gave birth to a large, fat baby in perfect condition.[109] In this narrative, this infant's health and size offer bodily evidence of his mother's fitness for reproduction; that is, his health stands as proof of her own bodily health. This mother's ability to bring to term a healthy, robust child bodes well for his future. There is nothing in his birth that would announce psychic or somatic weakness on her maternal part. Indeed, this delivery offers support to a reading of corporeal generosity and virtue. But this reading is quickly complicated by other factors and, as a result, this woman's performance of motherhood is not entirely unambiguous. Like the vast majority of mothers during this era, this mother chose to send her child out to nurse. Unfortunately, this decision – however common it was during this period – appears to have led to unhappy results for this woman's child. Unbeknownst to the parents, the infant's wet nurse had, as a result of an unfortunate incident, lost her milk completely. Six weeks later, when they went to see the child, they found him on the verge of death. Thinner than one could possibly imagine, he was but a mere shadow of his earlier healthy and strong self. Maternal refusal would, in this instance, appear to have had disastrous consequences.

This mother's narrative continues as follows: "We immediately found him another wet nurse who, although very good, was unable to extricate him from this situation except with much struggle and great care; we only gave him milk by degrees."[110] Interestingly, this formulation, which emphasizes the parents' close monitoring of the wet-nursing relationship, allows the non-lactating mother to take on a position of what might be termed "vicarious breastfeeding." Still actively involved in her child's growth and development, she invokes the vague but all-encompassing "*on*" – here understood as "we" – as a way of signalling her allegiance to a contemporaneous medical perspective that, as Joan Sherwood has argued, understood milk as medicine, as a life-giving drug that should be carefully dispensed under close medical scrutiny.[111] In this scenario, maternal milk is not a matter of maternal beneficence or corporeal generosity as it was for Madame Moreau de La Villegille. Rather, it is, like any prescription, a dosage that should be carefully administered. Such a framing allows this mother to assert her maternal responsibilities to her son through her commitment to an exacting regimen: "we only gave him milk by degrees." Surrogate nursing, as a medical prescription to which she, as mother, is attentive, gives credence to the authority of her later claims of emotional attachment and commitment.

This framing would suggest a desire on the part of this mother to situate her actions within the boundaries of corporeal citizenship. Her commitment to her child's bodily health is clear and unambiguous. Her responsibilities, enacted vicariously through her careful monitoring of the second wet nurse, appear to have been fulfilled. Nevertheless, this performance of motherhood is not entirely unambiguous. After all, this loving and committed mother contacts Tissot not to describe her son's health, but rather, to seek a cure for his sufferings. This boy, who almost died at the breast of his first wet nurse and was carefully nursed back to health by the second, has continued to suffer: "He fell numerous times, during the day, into a convulsive state which made us fear that we could lose him at any moment. He gained weight and grew taller, and didn't gain any strength. At the age of one and eighteen months, he had no more strength than an infant of six weeks. Finally, he nursed for three years and never grew stronger. At the age of four, he could not walk independently and at five and six he could not lift himself up when he fell."[112] The child, now a teenager, appears to have continued to develop slowly. Although he was large for his age, lively and very happy, he had no physical strength and very little intellectual ability. His current situation leaves his mother under no illusions and she is deeply concerned for his future. What will become of this young man as he enters into adulthood? How will he make his place in the world?

A Rousseauist reading would suggest that it was the mother's selfish decision to delegate her sacred duty to another woman that was the source of this young man's compromised health. After all, his health might have been saved had his mother accepted her corporeal responsibilities. But an alternative reading, one situated in relation to the construction of the letter itself, ascribes blame not to the mother but, rather, to the failings of the first wet nurse. In this reading, the mother herself is not to blame: after all, in this presentation of self, she demonstrates herself to be physically strong, capable of bringing to term a strong, healthy child. Furthermore, she shows herself to be actively committed to her child's health and well-being, not only through her careful monitoring of the second wet nurse but also through her decision to contact Tissot when clear evidence of bodily disorder emerged. Blame, if it is to be apportioned, appears to rest solely with the first, unidentified wet nurse, a woman of questionable fortitude whose bodily weakness appears to have taken root in the child. Thus, a reading of this letter from the perspective of the correspondent reveals a very personal and individual response to the question of corporeal virtue. Here, a woman who would appear to have transgressed the foundational tenets of the maternal ideal is nevertheless able to assert an alternative that relies on a form of embodied surrogacy. However, this corporeal performance can never be entirely unambiguous. This mother's son is corporeally weak, unable to take up his responsibilities in a republic of virtue.

## EMBODYING FATHERHOOD

While eighteenth-century motherhood has been the subject of considerable critical attention, the same cannot, unfortunately, be said for fatherhood. Apart from an engagement with ideologies of fatherhood, as represented in the form of the monarch, fatherhood has been the focus of limited scholarly activity.[113] And yet, as the letters in the Fonds Tissot make clear, fatherhood was a rich site of identity formation. And, like those penned by or about mothers, the letters from fathers are equally intriguing in terms of what they reveal about corporeal citizenship.

As many scholars have suggested, fathers enjoyed a privileged position in eighteenth-century society. "Most social structures put the father at the centre of power," writes Carol Sherman, "all look to him or to his representative both when they needed protection and when they want to subvert his will."[114] At legal, social, and economic levels, fathers were freely able to exercise their wills, not just with regard to their own needs but also in relation to the needs of their wives and children.[115] In this sense, fathers emerge as gatekeepers for maternal performance. We might think, here, of the role of fathers in relation to questions of maternal breastfeeding in eighteenth-century fiction and memoir.[116] Such gatekeeping was not necessarily oppressive, however. Fathers were responsible for assuring the economic and moral well-being of the family unit, and their citizenship status depended on their success in this role. Leslie Tuttle points to the notion of the "*père de famille*" as a particular ideological and political construct in eighteenth-century France:

> In early modern French usage, the term evoked more than merely fathering children or presiding over a taxable domestic unit. It connoted the responsibilities within the household, community, and commonwealth that fell to an adult man with children. The term had distinct political resonance; because a *père de famille* was held ultimately responsible for the economic and moral integrity of the household, moral and political thinkers insisted that on *pères de famille* rested the whole edifice of the social order. As the Chevalier de Jaucourt explained in the *Encyclopédie*, 'a *père de famille* cannot be evil or virtuous without consequences.' His behavior, contemporaries argued, had enormous implications for his dependents, his neighbors, and society at large.[117]

Emma Barker, in her analysis of Greuze's *L'Accordée de village*, makes the following observations: "Such a father, concerned as he was to provide for his children, was an exemplary citizen whose efforts enriched the state and provided it with new citizens to take his place."[118] Thus, as Lynn Hunt notes, just as motherhood became subject to considerable critical interrogation during the eighteenth century, so too did fatherhood emerge as a site of ideological consideration: "the ideal of the good father took shape in a variety of ways, ranging from tracts on education to paintings of sentimental family scenes. Perhaps the most influential source for new attitudes about both fathers and children was the novel. The rise of the novel and the emergence of interest in children and a more affective family went hand in hand … As sensibility and individual subjectivity, even for children, came to be more and more emphasized, the role of the father was bound to change. A stern, repressive father was incompatible with the new model of the family as emotional center for the nurturing of children and the new model of the individual as an autonomous self."[119]

This interplay between what Barker refers to as the "usurping, tyrannical" father and the "loving father figure" is evident in some of the letters directed to Tissot.[120] Male correspondents consciously articulate paternal subjectivities, situating themselves within and through the dominant discourses of fatherhood and family during this period. In many instances, fathers and mothers draw on similar gestures to make their case: reproduction and affection feature prominently. However, the tropes used to articulate these positions are very different and are defined in and through the lens of sexual incommensurability. While maternal virtue could be revealed in bodily form through fecundity and a commitment to maternal breastfeeding, paternal virtue required different bodily lexicon. Thus, for fathers, fecundity is often reimagined as virility. Lineage, too, is differently construed: while women are concerned with reproduction and the health of children, men appear to be more interested in the formal aspects of lineage – that is, in the passing on of name and title. Interestingly, however, the correspondence also offers hints of what might be termed "domestic masculinity" – a conscious construction of the masculine self not through the dominant trope of virility but, rather, through an affective commitment to home and family.

For men, bodily responsibility was framed through the relationship between biological understandings of the male body and social constructions of masculinity. Cathy McClive argues that "Ownership of a penis was not sufficient: the penis had to be seen to function correctly for its own to be declared a man in a court of law. In early modern France this meant that it had to be capable of 'erection, penetration and ejaculation.' This emphasis on the performance of reproduction accentuated the need for men as well as for women to prove that their bodies were capable of engendering, which rendered the embodiment of masculinity potentially as fragile and uncertain as that of femininity."[121] This "performance of reproduction" must also be considered in relation to the rhetoric of normative masculinity, which, as Lisa Wynne Smith explains, required men "to exert self-mastery over their bodies at all times in order to maintain their status."[122]

McClive's articulation of what might be termed "penile performativity," together with Smith's notion bodily and mental control, offer a useful conceptual lens through which to consider the performance of fatherhood. For men, paternal masculinity as corporeal virtue resided not only in the ability to produce children but, ideally, in the ability to produce strong, male children who would be best placed to take up their corporeal responsibilities.[123] Monsieur N.N., for example, introduced in the previous chapter, was "fifty-four years old and of a sanguine and somewhat bilious constitution, a quick and lively mind, and while of a generally sweet and benign temperament, also, nevertheless very subject to sudden bursts of anger."[124] His health is partially defined by his reproductive prowess: married at the age of twenty-one, he "had from his wife several male children, all of a strong complexion, and robust."[125] Here, strong male children are offered as proof not only of fecundity – he and his wife had "several" – but also, of virility. Monsieur N.N. has suffered none of the consequences that generally accompany busy, stressful lives. Instead, his proven virility, together with his "frequent horse riding, an active and tiring lifestyle, youth, the simplicity and frugality of his diet and the wholesome air" have all contributed to a general state of health and well-being and, further, to an unquestionable performance of reproductive masculinity.[126] In this instance, healthy children alone are not guarantors of corporeal citizenship; however, their presence offers material evidence of his healthy lifestyle, in the process revealing the health of the next generation.

So, too, might we consider more closely the narrative of the Comte de Ferray de Romans.[127] As a military man, he already performs virile masculinity through his profession. This impression is only strengthened in the face of his statement that he has produced twelve children, over half of whom are male. Furthermore, the vast majority of his sons have followed him into military service, thus further sustaining first impressions of virile paternal performance. Interestingly, this father cements this reading of a form of heroic masculinity by referencing his younger brother. A weak man and minister who could not manage his finances, the brother offered a perfect foil against which the count could situate his own moral and corporeal virility. The reader is left in no doubt about this man's penile performativity. As a corporeal citizen, the Comte de Ferray de Romans's membership in the republic of virtue is assured.

However, all is not well within this family, a point that I develop more fully later in this chapter.

Paternal virility was also directly implicated in the performance of masculine sociability. Consider the introduction to a 1774 letter written by a man named Reydellet on behalf of another man, whom he describes as follows: "a man aged forty years, who has eight children, a true gentleman and poor."[128] On the surface, these details seem random. Unlike the previous examples, which show clear links between the performance of fatherhood and the requirements of masculinity, this narrative is not so easily decoded. Read in combination with one another, however, these single ideas – age, family status, moral character, and economic situation – offer a picture of a morally and corporeally virtuous citizen worthy of receiving Tissot's attention and care. This man proves his worthiness at both bodily and moral levels: his bodily health can be attested to by his age and by his evident ability to produce eight living children, even in a state of poverty. Additionally, as "a true gentleman," he is clearly morally sound and socially responsible.

A lack of penile performativity, meanwhile, was significant cause for concern as it was suggestive of a troubled masculinity and a failure of corporeal citizenship. We might recall here the lamentations of the Marquis de Romira, referenced earlier in this chapter. On the verge of marriage to a beautiful and wealthy young woman, he found himself impotent and unable to realize the responsibilities of masculinity.[129] The social implications of such a situation were profound. In the words of one English correspondent, suffering from weakness that "particularly prevails in the Parts of Generation," "I would infinitely prefer death to a continuance of these sufferings for as many years to come."[130] I treat these issues in more detail in Chapter 5.

Paternal corporeal citizenship could also be assured by extra-corporeal means. In a series of four letters written over a two-month period, a Swiss pastor, Cart, writes to Tissot about his son's health.[131] In this instance, paternal concern is revealed through quantity – that is, through the careful and extended enumeration of all the details of day-to-day parental care. Paternal care, just as maternal care, is embodied in the letters themselves, each of which offers material proof of family virtue. Cart suggests as much in his first letter, where he observes that he and his wife have followed Tissot's recommendations carefully and, because the situation has not improved, he continues to write such that nobody can reproach them.[132] Each letter, then, contributes to the performance of concerned and committed parenting. Parenting, here, is imagined as a performance that can be externally judged and evaluated.[133] Fatherhood, as practice, is embodied in the materiality of the letters themselves.

Other fathers gesture towards broader concerns about inheritance and legacy. A man named Steinberg wrote to update Tissot on the health of his son, Charles: "After numerous futile attempts, it has only been since Charles has been following your remedies and your regimen, Sir, that things have improved for him, which give us hope in his perfect recovery, and I dare to abandon myself to the sweet thoughts of seeing his future secured. What a great satisfaction for you, Sir, to be able to contribute so often to the happiness of parents by prolonging the life of one who is so very dear to them ... [You can] count, Sir, on the gratitude of a man who has the very tender heart of a father for his children."[134] On the surface, Steinberg appears to articulate an emotional or affective investment in his son. While this may be true, it is equally clear that he is motivated by his commitment to the continued health of the family line. As Steinberg observes in the letter, Charles is his only son, "a son who has no brother."[135] In other words, he is the only one who can carry forward the family name. The performance of fatherhood, then, was also directly implicated in notions of inheritance.

Steinberg's letter suggests that paternal performance, like maternal performance, was also about affection, intimacy, love, and commitment. Some letters are marked by deep paternal intimacies, from the simple comments of a man named Maillard who suggests that his letter is motivated by "the tenderness of a father"[136] to much more extensive reflections on family, affection and love.[137] Consider, for example, the narrative penned by Torchon de Lihû in April 1785: "I lost my wife after few years of a most happy union; and I have consecrated myself to the education of my children. The tender attentions of a brother who I regarded as replacing me in the case of an accident, consoled me in my loss of my adored wife, and allowed me to confront death with less fear. And now, his days, too, are threatened ... What wouldn't I give to prolong them."[138] In structure and content, this narrative reveals a form of what might be termed "domestic masculinity."[139] In contrast to the performances of virility that mark the letters of military men, this letter and others like it emphasize the importance of home, family, and the domestic sphere and situate themselves and their concerns firmly within it. At the level of affect, this letter is concerned with love, devotion, commitment, tenderness, and consolation. Indeed, this devoted

     TELLING THE FLESH

father, mourning husband and worried brother cocoons himself in a web of affection.

Finally, fatherhood, as corporeal performance, was also marshalled into the service of larger medical concerns. Thus, it became part of a bigger picture of health. Consider, for example, a case recounted by a surgeon named Radaz in 1786.[140] His patient was a fifty-eight-year-old man suffering from trembling and weakness in all of his limbs. His sufferings were extensive enough that he was forced to suspend his studies and intellectual engagements. Radaz, however, can find no logical cause for his patient's sufferings. It is at this precise point that fatherhood, as penile performance, becomes integral to the narrative. Radaz writes that while these tremblings could suggest an engagement with onanism, his patient has never been debauched and has never suffered any *vice vérolique*.[141] In addition to this, Radaz does not believe that his patient has a history of masturbation. As support to these claims, Radaz turns to his patient's domestic life. This patient has been married for fifteen years and is father to two children, both of whom appear to be healthy and strong. In other words, while the signs might point to a morally and corporeally threatening conclusion, and while his virility might be questioned given the number of children he has produced, the length of this man's marriage and the health of his children confirm a different reading: this man's moral and corporeal integrity are sustained by the physical proof of healthy children.

### DISRUPTED KINSHIP: TROUBLING THE FAMILY

The performative gestures that structured the letters I have previously examined suggest that motherhood and fatherhood, as performances, were important aspects of the presentation of self. They offered individuals a way of situating themselves positively in relation to the doctor, in the process enabling a reading of a good family – and from there, good citizenship. But other correspondents were completely unable to make gestures towards good families and good citizenship. In some letters, it is clear that normative kinship structures had gone completely awry. In these letters, corporeal problems are cited as material evidence of troubled kinship. That is, bodily suffering gives voice to the emotional anguish of a family gone wrong. Such letters traverse a broad territory – from the concerns that arise as a result of reproductive failure, to emotional abuse, and to internal family struggles over inheritance and legacy.

In 1791, Madame Reverdil wrote to Tissot on behalf of an acquaintance of hers, an unmarried woman between the age of thirty and forty.[142] Possessed of strong blood and a sweet temperament, this woman's health should have been good. However, her body displayed numerous signs of disorder: among other things, she did not sweat, experienced tremblings throughout her limbs, always had cold feet (even in the heat of summer), suffered from overwhelming sadness, and had dry skin. She also suffered from fevers, irregular menstruation, and poor digestion. Madame Reverdil linked these extensive sufferings to her acquaintance's dysfunctional family life. While her acquaintance had the foundations for good health, "she is forced to live with her family, who treat her poorly."[143] One family member in particular threatened her and Reverdil observed that these episodes occured so frequently that they disrupted her health.

Another reading may also be possible: Revderdil's acquaintance was unmarried, a social condition that, some doctors believed, could cause physical problems.[144] Such a condition might, itself, also be read as a form of failed or at the very least, compromised, citizenship. Unable to locate herself within a constellation of family virtue, an unmarried woman was inevitably an outsider, not only to the concept of the family but also, and perhaps more provocatively, to the notion of corporeal citizenship.

Other disruptions, too, could cause bodily effects, particularly if they emerged in relation to challenges to normative understandings of kinship roles. For example, if motherhood as reproduction was intrinsic to women's identity-making practices and to their performance of citizenship, then failed reproduction could be experienced as a site of trauma. The Countess de Non, whose case I will examine in more detail in Chapter 6, offers a prime example of this. The Count Piossasque de Non wrote to Tissot in 1785 with concerns about a female family member's nervous afflictions – the vapours – which appear to have begun sometime around 1782.[145] According to the count, her condition was at least partially due to her way of life: the Countess de Non lived the sedentary existence common to other women of her station. However, the count points more directly to another cause: "Her health was perfect until her fifth pregnancy which was disturbed by the profound grief which she experienced as a result of having lost a child a short time previously, this sorrow having continued to afflict her during the birth brought about a sort of disturbance in her health."[146] The letter later confirms that the period of the countess's miscarriage was determined

    TELLING THE FLESH

to be the primary cause of her later vaporous condition. What makes this situation even more interesting is that the countess's reproductive failures can be said to extend beyond her miscarriage. That is, according to precepts put forward by Tissot, her sedentary life would undoubtedly have affected her reproductive health. We might here recall his warnings about girls reading novels. In addition to this, she did not nurse any of her children, thus further compromising her ability to claim virtuous motherhood.

However, this reading of corporeal failure cannot be fully sustained in that certain markers of maternal performance *are* present. After all, the countess has seven living children and her youngest child, a son, is healthy. In this way, she can, at a biological level, claim her right to corporeal citizenship. But these markers remain ambiguous because she may not have completed them fully: her miscarriage, combined with her failure to nurse any of her children and her inactive lifestyle all combine to undermine what would otherwise have been the foundation for a strong maternal performance. It is this very ambiguity, the lack of clearly defined maternal virtue, that constitutes her sufferings and, further, that contributes to a reading of disrupted kinship.

Finally, disrupted kinship can also be linked to legal and moral questions of lineage and inheritance. Consider, for example, the consultation sent by the Comte de Ferray de Romans.[147] The count, first introduced earlier in this chapter, styles himself as a retired army officer, widower, and father of twelve living children, five of whom are also in military service. Evident in this autobiographical trace is his assertion of a morally and corporeally sound self. In terms both of his family size and his career, this man is a good citizen who has contributed significantly to the good of his community. As a retired military officer, he has contributed to the security of the state; as a husband and father, meanwhile, he has presided over the birth and development of a large and strong family – twelve living children! What's more, he is able to draw on a continuing legacy: just as he served the king, so too do five of his children – almost half of his progeny and all but one of his sons – continue to serve both king and country. In short, this man and his family embody corporeal virtue.

The rationale behind this virtuous self-positioning becomes apparent later in the letter: in the correspondent's own words, his health has been fundamentally undermined by familial injustice: "It's been a year and a half since I had the misfortune of losing my mother at the age of 89 years, and she was the inheritor of my dear departed father. During my absence, others took advantage of her infirmities and her advanced age in order to have her write a new will (which contradicted two previous wills, in which she named me her inheritor) which names my only brother – younger by ten years – subdeacon and canon of this town, as her sole inheritor, and this, even though he owes a considerable sum of money and cannot manage his money."[148]

This "unjust and unexpected blow" fundamentally altered the count's health: he suffers from tightness in his upper abdomen, swelling in his legs, itchy skin, and disordered sleep.[149] Bodily health has been compromised through family hostility. Family rupture becomes the site of bodily malaise. This reading is confirmed by a diagnosis provided by Théodore Tronchin, another leading physician of the period, which was included along with the correspondent's letter: "You enjoy, Sir, good health. You had a strong chest up until the moment when a great sorrow occasioned in you a revolution and a weight, which since that time, has not dissipated … my quick response to you should stand as proof of my devotion and my zeal, both of which are due to a father of twelve children such as yourself."[150] Tronchin's response thus confirms and affirms this patient's self-positioning. It is moral malaise, in the form of family injustice, that has caused these problems. Illness, in this sense, emanates from an external rather than internal cause. It is clear that Tissot agrees, as a short notice at the top of the letter indicates: *effets du chagrin* – effects of grief.

As the examples in this chapter have shown, bodily experience was fertile ground for the performance of kinship. Notions of kinship allowed individuals to transcend the boundaries of their own bodies and enabled them to draw on the bodily experiences and signs of other bodies – those of their siblings, in-laws, and progeny – in order to make their claims. Bodily disarray, however, pushed at the limits of the idealized family. Nevertheless, it is clear that those who wrote to Tissot engaged creatively and critically with the ideologies that shaped their daily lives, in the process shaping selves that simultaneously conformed to and troubled the bodily parameters of the family.

{ CHAPTER FIVE }

# Bodily Agency and the Politics of Pleasure

> From 1751 (when I was 14) until today, I became accustomed to frequent ejaculations, especially in 1754 ... I contracted this habit so strongly that I could not go a single month without falling back into it ... It also happened, either after visiting women or while masturbating, that I held my semen in, not even stopping at the moment of ejaculation. I also engaged the services of prostitutes.
>
> Roussy to Tissot, 10 June 1774[1]

On a sunny Saturday in June, the tiny streets that wind behind the Château d'Yverdon are bustling with activity. Market vendors set up their wares and the townspeople come together to celebrate nature's bounty: fruits, vegetables, flowers, cheese, fish, and meat. It's a riot of colour, sound, and smells – an almost overwhelming sensual experience. These narrow streets have stood the test of time. The Château itself dates from the thirteenth century. Next to it is the equally impressive Temple dating from 1757, an imposing structure created from the distinctive yellow stone of the Neuchâtel region. Both stand as monuments of power: the juridical power of the state, as embodied both in the force of the Savoyard dynasty and later, the bailiffs of Berne, and the ecclesiastical power of the church, as manifest in the deep and abiding hold of Calvinism in the French cantons of Switzerland.

Yverdon-les-Bains has an impressive intellectual heritage. Jean-Jacques Rousseau sought refuge here in 1762 after fleeing France following publication of his *Emile*. Around the same time, *yverdonnois* intellectual, Fortunato Bartolomeo De Felice, together with a pan-European team of writers, embarked on the ambitious fifty-eight-volume *Encyclopédie d'Yverdon*, a massive project running from 1770 to 1780 and founded on the principles of Diderot and d'Alembert's project. And in the early nineteenth century, another thinker made his mark on the city: Johann

Heinrich Pestalozzi, renowned pedagogue and educational thinker, transformed the Château into an internationally famous school and laboratory for his pedagogical theories. The city's strategic importance can also be traced through its name: *les Bains*. With its natural hot springs and fortuitous geographic situation at the edge of Lake Neuchâtel in the pristine beauty of the Jura mountains, Yverdon-les-Bains has, for centuries been known as a centre for natural health and healing, an ideal place to recuperate from a range of illnesses and sufferings.

It was from this picturesque town – a community that boasted both the corporeally rejuvenating properties of natural hot springs as well as the intellectually stimulating projects of an active learned elite – that a young man named François Louis Gauteron wrote a series of five tortured letters to Tissot. Gauteron was an eighteen-year-old *étudiant en philosophie* when he wrote his first letter to Tissot in 1792.[2] In his first letter, he describes being "menaced by" nocturnal emissions for three years. These emissions came out of nowhere and in spite of his best efforts to follow the regimen of bodily control suggested both by Tissot and a local doctor, he found that he continued to suffer: "Often I have emissions without even waking up … I don't understand what is causing such activity during my sleep because I have eliminated all excesses. I am used to little sleep, I work in moderation, I exercise every day, and neither my reading nor my [amorous] liaisons introduce in me a single bad thought. Actually it seems that the <u>fear</u> of nocturnal emission is the cause of them, and it is enough that this idea comes to me during the night for the act to be consummated, in spite of the resistance of my mind. Sometimes I wake up in time, but this is rare."[3] Gauteron's frustration – indeed, moral discouragement – is palpable. His struggles, both moral and physical, are in vain, and in the course of the correspondence that ensues, he resigns himself to a life of insurmountable moral suffering and almost certain death: "if it is too late, if I am to languish for the rest of an unhappy life, I will place my trust in Providence, which always proportions my courage and my patience in accordance with my sufferings. Death frightens me little; I believe that my happiness will begin with death. Indeed, it is the sight of the long and painful road that I have to travel that worries me, should my malady only end then."[4] Haunted by the impossibility of realizing corporeal virtue, he reflects that he will, in this condition, be of only limited social utility: "In the state of languishing in which I find myself, I could do but little good on Earth, I see myself reduced to impotent desires that are useless to my fellow men, and which have no merit but before God, who alone can read my heart."[5]

Gauteron was not alone in his situation. Others, too, wrote to Tissot detailing not only their bodily desires but also their attempts to control them, and their moral shame. This struggle between the experience of bodily excess, on the one hand, and the felt need for bodily restraint, on the other, is a feature of many of the letters that treat questions of a sexual nature. Like Gauteron, these individuals find themselves struggling against bodily manifestations of sexual desire, which included not only involuntary ejaculation, but also such things as masturbation, "excessive" sexual engagements, and loss of virility, even as their rational and moral selves sought to assert and articulate a corporeally virtuous identity.

These tensions between bodily desire and bodily and moral restraint lie at the heart of this chapter. In it, I move from questions of kinship and reproduction to questions of sexuality. My main focus is sexual identity. I am interested in teasing out the ways in which pleasure, and particularly illicit sexual pleasure, manifests itself in medical consultation letters addressed to Samuel Auguste Tissot. What stories does bodily pleasure tell? What purpose does the articulation of pleasure serve? What role does it play in the construction of a correspondent's bodily self? And finally, in an era that venerated moderation in all things, how do individuals navigate the thorny, and inherently excessive, nature of pleasure itself? What role does the desiring body play in the development of a corporeally virtuous citizen?

Corporeal virtue is fraught here. Unlike in the previous chapter, where bodily virtue could be compromised by an array of external forces, the correspondents who contact Tissot in relation to questions of bodily pleasure find themselves struggling with, through, and against the desires of their *own* bodies. A closer examination of the excerpt from Gauteron's previously cited introductory letter, for example, is revelatory. What is interesting in this letter is the juxtaposition between psychic moderation and bodily pleasure – that is, between what Gauteron is thinking and what his body is doing. At a psychic level, Gauteron is doing what he can to live up to Tissot's corporeal ideals of balance and moderation. He has followed all the guidelines and, with his mind, he is performing virtue. In this respect, he is adhering fully to the ideal of corporeal citizenship as proposed by Tissot. But Gauteron's body refuses to cooperate, and it is clear that this is causing him significant distress.

Gauteron does not read his continuing nocturnal emissions as a sign that the body is experiencing pleasure. Rather, as another sufferer also suggests, he understands them as punishment for bodily crimes.[6] Nocturnal emissions, in Gauteron's letter, are experienced and understood as evidence of permanent disability, their presence a physical reminder of his bodily indiscretions, and, as a consequence, of his inability to conform fully to the ideas that Tissot presents. Perhaps more provocatively, such bodily unruliness might be seen as evidence of his *body's* unwillingness to conform to Tissot's model. This disconnect between performed moral virtue, on the one hand, and bodily resistance or refusal, on the other, is a characteristic of other letters as well, in which patients confess their bodily indiscretions and affirm their commitment to personal transformation and corporeal self management, only to discover that resistance is futile. The mind might be willing, but the flesh is most certainly weak.

At a conceptual level, I situate my reading within a context that oscillates between surveillance and voyeurism – that is, between the discipline of a Foucauldian gaze, on the one hand, and the autoerotic specularity of the text, on the other. I develop each of these concepts further later in this chapter. Gauteron's five lengthy letters to Tissot, together with two additional, and equally lengthy, letters he subsequently sent to a Calvinist pastor, underpin my narrative. They are, indeed, the foundation on which my analysis rests. In number, length, and detail, these letters offer a very comprehensive account of the way that one individual experienced and understood the "pleasures of the flesh." These letters also demonstrate the extent to which the psychic and somatic were implicated in one another. Finally, in their level of detail and moral tone, they offer a productive foundation upon which my analysis of the letters as a whole might rest.

### EPISTOLARY PLEASURES: *LUXE, CALME ET VOLUPTÉ*

> Là, tout n'est qu'ordre et beauté,
> Luxe, calme et volupté.
> Charles Baudelaire, "L'Invitation au voyage"

Charles Baudelaire's poem, whose now famous refrain I cite above, celebrates the sensuous mysteries of the flesh, the commingling of two bodies into one, in life, in death, on an imagined island whose contours evoke the shape of the beloved. In this sensuous idyll, everything is as it should be: *luxe, calme et volupté*. Baudelaire's words, and, indeed, the title of his poem, "L'Invitation au voyage," recall imagery integral to French eighteenth-century understandings of sensuality, pleasure, desire, and *galanterie:* the fabled island of Cythera immortalized in the work of Watteau.

The articulation of pleasure in epistolary form occurred in a social and cultural context that alternately revered the art of seduction and condemned it. Thus, among the elite, notions of citizenship demanded allegiance to the politics of pleasure, seduction, and gallantry – concepts that were integral not only to the art of conversation but also to the many linguistic intrigues, illicit liaisons, and seductive illusions and allusions that marked libertine fictions of the period. These sensual ideals were captured early in the century in Watteau's *Fêtes galantes* and the elusive sensual pleasures of the ultimately impossible *Voyage to Cythera,* and later, in the porcelain beauty of Boucher's *Odalisques* and the flirtatious sensuality of Fragonard's illicit garden encounters. We might also cast our gaze on such curiosities as James Graham's theatrically and multimedia-infused Temple of Health, home to the infamous electrified "Celestial Bed." Identified by Peter Otto as "perhaps the world's first sex clinic," the Temple of Health was redolent with orientalist imagery, its famous bedroom a fantasy space of libertine passion, carnal desire, and fleshy delights that, for a mere fifty pounds a night, catered to those seeking cures to infertility and impotence.[7] Add to this the misogynist and deviant perversions of the Marquis de Sade, the political skewering and caricaturing of Marie Antoinette as a sexually rapacious foreigner whose carnal appetites only served to further epitomize the inherently rotten and diseased core of the monarchy, the availability of classical erotic literature, the extensive international trade in licentious literature (the so-called *livres maux* and other "popular writings on sex"), as well as simple gossip, story, and conversation, and we quickly see that eighteenth-century culture was, quite literally, saturated with sex, a world in which seduction, through imagery, words, gestures, suggestions, comportment, and dress, was the order of the day, and in which discussions of sexuality took pride of place amongst the intelligentsia.[8]

But within this erotically charged social and cultural sphere was also a powerful culture of moral censure. The moralistic paintings of Jean-Baptiste Chardin present homely scenes of family, faith, nurturance, grace, and generosity. In stark contrast to the works produced by his compatriots, Watteau, Boucher, and Fragonard, Chardin explores the moral potential of childhood, innocence, and love. Jean-Baptiste

Greuze, too, chose to explore ideals of family and responsibility, producing such well-known visual morality tales as *The Wicked Son*, *The Father's Curse*, and *Filial Piety*. These visual signs formed the backdrop for extensive political, philosophical, and medical debates about the nature, function, and place of bodily pleasures in an ideal society.

Central to these debates was the relationship between sensuality, pleasure, class, and citizenship. Moral, medical, and legal discourses situated "proper" sexual conduct within the realm of heterosexual marriage.[9] Marriage, as *médecins-philosophes* such as Tissot argued, was integral to the bodily health of both men and women, to the extent that marriage was sometimes offered as a cure for the myriad ailments thought to plague widows and unmarried women.[10] Protestant theologians, meanwhile, believed that "sexual relations played an important part in a happy, chaste marriage ... Marital sex was not just allowable, it was good in itself."[11] Within this matrix, sex was understood as "purposive."[12] The end goal of so-called "natural" sexuality – that which promoted and enhanced the reproductive potential of married men and women – was procreation. In this way, sexual intercourse, properly directed, could be seen as a corporeal contribution to the general good of society, in the process cementing the normative power of the heterosexual family.[13] This ideological stance shaped many of the bodily experiences related in the previous chapter. But, as the letters to Tissot – and eighteenth-century erotic culture – demonstrate, very few sexual encounters could be captured and contained under the rubric of "purposive" reproductive sex. Sexual pleasure occupied a vast terrain. Pleasures were explored not only in the marital bed but also in shadowy doorways, extra-marital affairs, relationships with prostitutes, and even in the bedrooms and dormitories of schoolboys.

Medical and moral discourse around sexual pleasure was influenced by two popular publications, the anonymous English text, *Onania* (1716), which sold in the neighbourhood of thirty thousand copies within the first fifteen years after publication,[14] and Tissot's 1760 publication, *L'Onanisme*.[15] Tissot's work, originally published in Latin, enjoyed considerable success upon publication, appearing in endless reprints and translations throughout the second half of the century. Many correspondents make mention of it and, more interestingly, appear to take the letters he includes in it as models for their own writing.

But what, precisely, *was* onanism? The author of *Onania* offers a simple and concise definition: "Self-Pollution is that unnatural Practice, by which Persons of either Sex may defile their own Bodies, without the Assistance of others, whilst yielding to filthy Imaginations, they endeavour to initiate and procure to themselves that Sensation, which God has ordered to attend the carnal Commerce of the two Sexes for the Continuance of our Species."[16] Clearly evident here is the author's commitment to self-pollution as a moral rather than medical crime, an act that defiles not only the body but also, and more importantly, God's will. Bodies, the author notes, are "Temples of the Holy Spirit, because the Holy Spirit dwells in us, and pours forth his Benefits upon us, sanctifies us, and consecrates us to the Service of God; wherefore our Bodies partaking of this Honour, we are bound to preserve them in Purity, and to employ them to holy Purposes."[17] Crucially, for this author, onanism is not the solitary sin that its adherents would have everyone believe. Rather, it has pernicious – indeed, disastrous – social effects: this selfish practice actively undermines creation itself. In a hierarchy of sinful pleasures, which include "fornication and adultery," onanism is the most heinous of them all. As the author argues, self-pollution is "a Sin, not only against Nature, but a Sin that perverts and extinguishes Nature, and he who is guilty of it, is labouring at the Distruction of his Kind, and in a manner that strikes at the Creation it self."[18]

The question of reproduction is central to this author's arguments. Self-pollution, he argues, not only induces infertility but also, and perhaps more ominously, should the onanist manage to procreate, produces weak children. As he writes,

> In some Men of very strong Constitutions, the Mischiefs may not be so visible, and themselves perhaps capable of marrying; and yet the Blood and Spirits impair'd and the Seed render'd infertile, so as to make them unfit for Procreation, by its changing the Crasis of the spermatick Parts, making them become barren, as Land becomes poor by being over-till'd; and few of those who have been accustom'd to this Vice in their Youth, have ever much Reason to boast of the Fruits of their Marriage-Bed; for if by Nature's extraordinary Helps, they should get any Children, which happens not often, they are most commonly weakly little ones, that either die soon, or become tender, sickly People, always ailing and complaining; a Misery to Themselves, a Dishonour to humane Race, and a Scandal to their Parents.[19]

Interesting here is the author's insistence on the power of onanism to affect issues of inheritance and legacy: self-pollution impacts not only the individual but also the corporeal strength of future generations (and, although this is not explicitly stated, of the populace as a whole). Thus, even if there is no visible sign of disorder, the reproductive capacities of onanists – their penile performativity, if we recall the words of Cathy McClive – is still fundamentally compromised.[20]

In *L'Onanisme*, published almost half a century later, Tissot takes a very different approach. For one thing, onanism, as a practice, is much more loosely defined. Unlike the author of *Onania*, Tissot offers no explicit definition of the term. Rather, through his examples and arguments it becomes clear that his understanding of onanism is much broader than that proposed in the *Onania*. Tissot situates onanism within the context of generalized sexual excess, offering examples not only of solitary masturbators but also of precocious young men engaged in dalliances with servants, and even immoderate married couples indulging too freely in the pleasures of the marital bed. This suggests that, as Séverine Pilloud has observed, *onanism* was an umbrella term that captured a veritable panoply of sexual behaviours that went on outside the marital bed.[21] Also, unlike the anonymous author of *Onania*, Tissot shifts the focus from the moral to the medical.[22]

Both authors, however, draw on the works of others in order to support their individual arguments. While the author of *Onania* draws on the insights of moral and religious scholars, Tissot turns to the writings of famous physicians and philosophers, among them Hippocrates, Aetius, Sanctorius, Galen, Pliny, Lommisus, Tulpius, Hoffman, Boerhaave, Senac, and Ludwig. Drawing on the expertise of others allows both authors to assert the authority of their claims, in the process cementing their arguments for their readers. So, too, do both concur on the corporeal effects of the practice, however narrowly or broadly that practice was defined. The list of the corporeal after effects of onanism is lengthy and includes the following: consumption, loss of seminal liquid, infertility, lascivious or obscene dreams, weakness of breath, fevers, paleness, effeminacy, madness, imbecility, weight loss, disordered digestion, nocturnal emissions, liver problems, bodily incapacity, paralysis, laziness, loss of intellectual capacities, palsy, nervous disorders, fainting, epilepsy, lethargy, blindness, tremors, spasms, gonorrhoea, dropsy, gangrene, memory loss, disturbing dreams, pain, blindness, hearing loss, hoarseness of voice, excessive weeping, weak pulse, red face, tumours, deformity, convulsions, headaches, difficulty walking, numbness, loss of hearing, feverishness, excessive sexual desires, excessive circulation, vertigo, nightmares, insomnia, drowsiness, hypochondria, melancholy, palpitations, coughing, chest pains, intestinal problems, pox, facial disfigurement, loss of erectile function, premature ejaculation, urinary tract problems, testicular and penile tumours, hysteria, constipation, haemorrhoids, ulcers, fainting, diarrhoea, and death. In short, in the words of Michael Stolberg, "The masturbator lost his masculine strength and vigour, his control over the body and its orifices. Far from being self-contained, he became literally incontinent, and disgusting excretions were constantly flowing from him, in extreme cases from all openings at once."[23]

Although both authors insisted that onanism affected both men and women, their main focus was men. At issue for Tissot is the loss of seminal fluid, a beneficent, life-giving fluid that he compares to breast milk: "the seminal liquor … has so great an influence upon the corporeal powers, and upon perfect digestion, which repairs them, that physicians of all ages have been unanimously of opinion, that the loss of an ounce of this humour would weaken more than that of forty ounces of blood."[24] Interesting in both accounts are the roles of the imagination and the body in relation to the pursuit of sexual pleasure. Both authors insist on the agency of both imagination and body, an agency that has the capacity to wholly undermine the impulses of the rational mind. Chastity, the anonymous author of *Onania* proclaims, requires constant attention and vigilance. The imagination, he suggests, is particularly to be feared, for not only does it overwhelm a soul whose attentions should be directed towards the divine, but it also actively encourages similar unruliness in the body:

> The unchast [sic] Person has his Mind rarely free from lascivious and shameful Imaginations and Fancies. His Heart is a continual Spring of evil Thoughts, bubbling up in it every Moment: so that there needs only the Presence of an Object to inflame his Desire. Let him but see or hear any thing related to his beloved Sin, and his Lust is presently kindled by it. And only so, but, at other times when none of these Objects present themselves, his Memory serves to furnish him with such former Passages as had gratify'd his Sensuality; these he recalls to his Mind, and pleases himself with the Thoughts of them, instead of reflecting upon them, as he ought, with Sorrow of Heart, and Confusion of Face.[25]

Unruly bodies and imaginations are here imagined as active agents in the destruction of the self: they "pursue," "master," and "possess" the self to such an extent that the self is overwhelmed and ultimately forsaken by this dizzying area of images, ideas, and senses. Furthermore, because they were located within the self, they are particularly difficult to repel. Indeed, as the author of *Onania* opines, "when we have to do with Lust, the Enemy is within us."[26]

While refusing the overt conservative morality that infuses the *Onania*, Tissot nevertheless also insists on the formative role of the imagination. Citing the sixteenth-century Italian physician, Sanctorius, he observes that, "It is imagination, habit, and not nature, that importune [masturbators]. They drain nature both of that which is necessary, and also of that which she herself would have taken care to dispose of."[27] The imagination can directly excite the body, with unfortunate results: "When a person has habituated himself to confine his thoughts to one idea, he becomes incapable of any others; it's [sic] empire is fixed, it's [sic] reign is despotic! Those organs, which are incessantly irritated, contract a morbific disposition, which becomes a continual stimulus always present, independent of any external cause."[28] Tissot offers numerous compelling examples of this process of psychic and somatic unruliness. Consider, for example, a case described by M. Rast, le jeune, a doctor in Lyon: "A young man of Montpellier, a student in medicine, died of the excess of this kind of debauchery. The idea of his crime had made such an impression on his mind that he died in a kind of despair, fancying he saw hell opening on every side of him ready to receive him. A child of this city, at the age of between six and seven, instructed, as I imagine, by a servant maid, polluted himself so often, that a slow fever, which succeeded, finished him. His rage for this act was so great, the he could not be restrained from it the very last days of his life. When he was informed that he thereby hastened his death, he consoled himself, in saying, that he should sooner meet with his father, who died some months before."[29] In tone and approach, this case is very similar to one brought to Tissot's attention by a young medical student a number of years later.[30] Could this student's letter, then, be simply a way of situating himself not only within Tissot's presence but also within the presence of all the renowned doctors whom Tissot cites in his book? Certainly this assessment merits some consideration.

After sharing numerous examples drawn from the works of other doctors, Tissot recalls his own personal initiation into the realm of onanism. In a lengthy passage, he introduces the case of a suffering watchmaker, a man who masturbated several times a day and was unable to stop himself, even as evidence revealed the dangerous workings of this practice on his body. Tissot describes this unfortunate onanist as an object of horror:

> I found a being that less resembled a living creature, than a corpse, lying upon straw, meagre, pale, and filthy, casting forth an infectious stench; almost incapable of motion, a watry palish blood issued from his nose; slaver constantly flowed from his mouth: having a diarrhaea, he voided his excrement in the bed without knowing it: he had a continual flux of semen; his sore watry eyes were deadened to that degree, that he could not move them: his pulse was very small, quick, and frequent: it was with great difficulty he breathed, reduced almost to a skeleton, in every part except his feet, which became oedematous. The disorder of his mind was equal to that of his body; devoid of ideas and memory, incapable of connecting two sentences, without reflection, without being afflicted at his fate, without any other sensation than pain, which returned with every fit, at least, every third day. Far below the brute creation, he was a spectacle, the horrible sight of which cannot be conceived, and it was difficult to discover, that he had formerly made part of the human species.[31]

Unclean and infectious, this body broadcasts its disorder through excessive fluidity. This body is continually expelling itself: uncontrolled evacuations of semen, diarrhoea, blood, and water are mirrored by the equally uncontrolled ramblings of a disordered mind. Tissot's words – "being," "creature," "corpse," "skeleton" – suggest that he was unable to find the language to describe the tableau arrayed before him. A living tableau of Kristevan abjection, this watchmaker had ceased even to be human. Instead he was, as Tissot himself suggests, "a spectacle."

In formulating onanism as spectacle, Tissot inverts popular assumptions that onanism was a private (and in the case of masturbation, solitary) act. The disordered imagination and pleasure-seeking body were not private, intimate things that could be successfully hidden from public view. Rather, psychic and somatic horror manifested themselves in an array of highly visible bodily markers, all of which could be read by outsiders. In the process, bodily derangement and degeneration offered public evidence of private crimes. Is it any wonder that fear permeates so many of the letters addressed to Tissot?

In this climate, doctors, philosophers, and moralists lined up to condemn the frivolous debauchery and violent excesses of a social class otherwise perfectly positioned to provide the moral foundation and grounding for a virtuous polis.[32] The elite, such thinkers declared, had the capacity to show leadership. Instead, their commitment to superficial foppery, gallantry, and the pleasures of the flesh undermined, in a very real way, the broader concerns of the nation as a whole. Indeed, if we were to believe everything the moralists said, Europe was in trouble. The excessive debauchery among the elite classes, epitomized notably by the many ill-advised sexual exploits of Louis XV, the fabled dalliances of Catherine the Great, and the activities of Teresia Constantia Phillips – reputed to be "the most scandalous woman in England"[33] – all pointed to an environment dedicated wholly to the pleasures of the flesh and the fulfillment of carnal desire. "Purposive" sex occupied almost no place at all in the erotic imagination.

Pleasure, these jostlings suggest, was never merely pleasure. Rather, pleasure – and particularly the sensual pleasures of the flesh – was deeply and intensely political. Libertinage was associated not only with excessive sexual behaviours but also with perceived philosophical transgressions. And, as the caricaturists of late eighteenth-century France demonstrated in their lampooning of Marie Antoinette, sex and pleasure were directly implicated in questions of foreign affairs and concerns of the state.[34] Navigating discourses of pleasure thus required careful and close attention not only to questions of identity and subjectivity but also to the boundaries between acceptable and excessive pleasures.



Competing notions of pleasure – *plaisir* and *jouissance* – are central to the conceptual concerns of this chapter. Marie Mulvey Roberts observes that pleasure – as *plaisir* – was integral to notions of community in the eighteenth century: "As an expression of communality, pleasure was predicated upon conviviality, and institutions such as the playhouse, the club and the coffee-house were formed in order to consolidate the joys of social intercourse. But to what extent was pleasure stage-managed in order to make it socially, morally and politically acceptable? Was it, in part, a performance, or was it a moral desideratum in being allied to notions of social good, civic virtue and rationality?"[35] Roberts's questions touch on a fundamental tension – namely, the relationship between pleasure as bodily and social performance, on the one hand, and as consciously articulated moral virtue, on the other. Taking this line of questioning further, Roy Porter, drawing on the work of Bernard Mandeville and others, argues that pleasure was mobilized as a form of social discipline. In other words, it existed in order to manage social relations: "society ... was an engine form converting naked anti-social egoism into more peaceful and profitable ways for people to get what they wanted, at the cost of a bit of effort, some deferral of gratification and much ostentatious conformity ... Morality was the passport people had to display to prove that they were abiding by the social code. Honour and shame provided the motivations. Those playing by the rules of the game would be crowned in honour; rule-breakers would be covered in obliquy."[36]

An understanding of pleasure as a social good relies on the idea of reciprocity. That is, it depends on a conceptualization of pleasure as a shared experience. In this form, pleasure enables social cohesion. Indeed, *l'art de plaire* – the art of pleasing – as it was understood among the French elite of the period, required conscious commitment to the needs of the social environment as a whole.[37] The adulatory introductions that preface a majority of the letters to Tissot can be understood within this frame as well. In this light, pleasure can be productively linked with citizenship. As an act of citizenship, pleasure contributes to notions of imagined community. Coffee houses, clubs, salons, and other social organizations performed essential roles in the cultivation of pleasure.[38] As a social experience, pleasure enhanced individuals' understandings of themselves as members of a broader community, as part of a larger whole. Read this way, pleasure facilitated social identification. Eighteenth-century subjects sought out groups that catered to their tastes, and developed their social identities in the company of like-minded others.

As the century progressed, however, pleasure came to be more intimately linked with questions of morality. In the words of Roy Porter, "There was pleasure to be derived from altruism, sympathy, benevolence and sociability. Virtue was, in short, integral to a psychological pleasure – indeed its own reward."[39] Such, for example, is the theme of Sophie de Grouchy's *Lettres sur la sympathie*, published late in the century in response to Adam Smith's *Theory of Moral Sentiments*.[40] Here, Grouchy suggests not only that the individual is physically moved by the sight of the suffering of others to the extent that this evokes a sympathetic physical response, but that this embodied response propels the individual towards the alleviation of the social injustices that caused the original suffering.[41]

Pleasure as *jouissance*, however, is a different animal altogether. Unlike *plaisir*, *jouissance* performs no broader social function. Linked with ideas of possession and use – and here we might recall the possessive unruliness of the pleasure-seeking body as invoked by the anonymous author of the *Onania* – *jouissance* asserts the right of the individual to claim pleasure.[42] The definition offered by Antoine-Gaspard Boucher d'Argis in the *Encyclopédie* is helpful here: "*Jouissance* is ordinarily a synonym of possession."[43] Diderot, in another article, elaborates further on this, linking *jouissance* not only with possession but also with knowledge, stating, "*Jouissance*: To enjoy is to know, to experience, to feel the advantages of possessing. We often possess without enjoyment."[44] Interestingly, with its explicit links between knowledge and possession, this definition appears also to gesture towards the biblical fall.

Instead of gesturing towards reciprocity, then, *jouissance* appears to demand allegiance to the self. *Jouissance* does not build community. Rather, in the words of Roberts, "it disrupts the laws of reciprocity."[45] In so doing, it undermines the cohesion of the social order. Within this framework, *jouissance* is antithetical to notions of citizenship in that it places the needs of the individual above and beyond those of the community as a whole. For example, these notions underpin Gauteron's previously cited concerns with regard to social utility. That is, Gauteron's correspondence emerges, at least partially, from a fear that his commitment to self-pleasure has undermined his social responsibility to his community.

However, within this same matrix that linked pleasure (*plaisir*) with virtue and happiness, sexual pleasure (*jouissance*) could also be imagined as natural. Consider, for example, the subversive approach taken by Diderot in his *Encyclopédie* entry on *jouissance*. Unwilling to reassert the binary between moral good and bodily excess, Diderot situates *jouissance* both firmly within the realm of the sensual *and* as an engine for social good. As he writes,

If any perverse Man may have taken offence at my praise of the most august and the most prevalent of passions, I would invoke Nature before him. I would have her speak and she would say to him: Why do you blush upon hearing the name of an exquisite pleasure [*volupté*] when you do not blush for having felt attracted by it in the shadow of the night? Do you not know its aim and what you owe it? Do you think that your mother would have

    TELLING THE FLESH

risked her life in order to give you yours, if she had not attached an inexpressible charm to the embraces of her spouse? Be quiet, miserable one, and bear in mind that it is pleasure that pulled you out of oblivion.

The propagation of beings is the greatest goal of Nature. She solicits the two sexes imperiously in this aim, as soon as they have received what she designed for them in strength and in beauty. A vague and melancholic anxiety informs them of the moment; their mood becomes a mixture of pain and pleasure. That is when they listen to their senses, and they turn their awareness inward.

When an individual presents himself to another of the same species and a different sex, the feeling for all other needs is suspended; the heart palpitates; the limbs quiver; voluptuous images roam the brain; the torrents of the spirit flow into the nerves, irritate them and then move to the core of a new sense, which manifests itself and torments in turn. Vision is blurred, delirium is born; reason, a slave to instinct, contents itself with serving it, and Nature is satisfied.[46]

Here, Diderot offers a reading that overtly associates the pleasures of sexual excess (*jouissance*) with moral and social good (*plaisir*). Indeed, this excerpt offers a concrete example of Ludmilla Jordanova's assertion that "thought is an erotic act."[47] While this might be seen by conservative thinkers and moralists as a radical approach, it is clear that it resonated among certain elements of the eighteenth-century populace. After all, as the Comte d'Adhémar observed of his own bodily engagements with pleasure, how could something apparently so wrong feel so good?[48] So too would the Marquis de Sade later claim his right to sexual agency and freedom. Roy Porter observes that there was a "new accent on the legitimacy of pleasure – not as occasional release, aristocratic paganism or heavenly bliss, but as the routine entitlement of people at large to seek fulfillment in this world rather than only in heavenly salvation, to achieve the gratification of the senses not just the purification of the soul."[49] This conceptualization of pleasure as both legitimate – that is, as an earthly entitlement – *and* as a moral virtue – that is, as part of an active commitment to social good – underpins numerous letters to Tissot. Pleasure, then, was complex. Linked with contradictory impulses – benevolence, empathy, and virtue, on the one hand, and selfishness, voluptuousness, desire, and greed, on the other –

the concept of pleasure was challenging to navigate, and even more difficult to articulate.



What, then, might this mean for letters and their authors? As we know, letters were, in some cases, a vital site of erotic potential. Voltaire, for example, used illness as a conduit for erotic passion in his letters to Madame Denis.[50] Julie de Lespinasse, meanwhile, parlayed physical suffering into impassioned love letters to the Comte de Guibert.[51] We see something similar at play in libertine literature of the period, which often relies on epistolarity as a narrative device. Letters were also common props in libertine literature. In the words of Paul Young, they provided "opportunities for intimacy," propelling the voyeuristic nature of the libertine genre itself.[52] We need only consider such works as Choderlos de Laclos's *Les liaisons dangereuses* to get a sense of the potential of letters as vehicles for erotic exchange.

The letter, as an autoerotic gesture, enables the gaze. As a liminal space, the letter is both a stage upon which the correspondent performs his bodily pleasures and desires and the space in which such desires and pleasures are received. In this space, pleasure is both a somatic memory, recalled and reworked in textual form, and an emotional or psychic experience brought about through the acts of writing and reading. In writing, the correspondent words himself. The imagined audience, in response, asks him to read himself. In the process, the gaze is complicated and surveillance and voyeurism bring one another into existence.

As thresholds, letters bridge the gap between public and private and offer glimpses into carnal intimacy. But these thresholds are never wholly transparent. As is evident in Choderlos de Laclos's *Les liaisons dangereuses*, missing, misplaced, and misdirected letters highlight and increase the erotic tensions in the narrative. In the process, such plot devices trouble the whole concept of the gaze, complicating the relationships between observer and observed. Indeed, the letter appears to have been an ideal vehicle for the staging of eros, desire, passion, seduction, and the pleasures of the flesh.

The letters that individuals sent to Tissot are, of course, very different from those that would have been shared between Voltaire and Madame Denis, or Lespinasse and Guibert. They are also very different from those that framed larger fictional narratives. Nevertheless, they do form part of the same immense epistolary network – that extended conversation in writing – that marked eighteenth-century erotic sociability. As such they can – and should – be seen as sites for the staging of corporeal identity, as autobiographical traces that reveal the different ways that individual narrated pleasure-seeking and experiencing selves for the good doctor.

It is clear that the correspondents who wrote to Tissot were conversant with his treatise and his ideas, and it is likely that many had also encountered other treatises on moral and bodily chastity. A number made direct mention of Tissot's *L'Onanisme*. More significantly, many appear to have drawn on it as they shaped their own narratives. In both tone and language, the letters to Tissot mirror those included in his treatise. Indeed, it is almost as if the book has served not only as a medical work on the dangers of onanism but also as a treatise on the conventions of onanytic epistolarity. Thus, just as Madame de Sévigné's letters served as models of elite epistolary practice, so too did these letters serve as templates. In the process they shaped how individuals framed their experiences for Tissot as well as how they came to understand their bodily selves.[53]

We might take this one step further by postulating the possibility of specularity: in the encounter between treatise and letters, both readers and writers – at different times both Tissot (as author and as healer) and his audience (as readers and correspondents) – come to understand themselves through the specularity of the text itself. Letters, as noted in an earlier chapter, are fundamentally shaped by the explicit notion of an audience. That is, the audience powerfully affects both tone and content of the letter. But such a performative self-positioning also invites considerable self-reflection as the writer internalizes the recipient's gaze. From this perspective, letter writing itself might be understood as an autoerotic gesture that enables writers first to experience, then to write and finally to reconceive themselves through a doubled gaze: their own and that of the intended recipient. Given this doubled gaze, letters are an ideal venue in which to explore how it was that individuals understood and experienced their sexuality in an era of contradictions, an era that at once venerated the voluptuous sensuality of the flesh and simultaneously, denigrated it. Letters provide evidence of sexual practices and engagements, but they also offer something more; they reveal to us how it was that individuals understood and experienced bodily pleasures and torments. They tell stories of sensual and sexual selves navigating the social, cultural, and political mores of their period. Finally, such letters also tell us much about the language of sexual behaviour. In the transition from body to text, letters reveal much about the meanings ascribed to bodily pleasures, pains, and torments.

## SURVEILLANCE AND VOYEURISM: THEORIZING EPISTOLARY PLEASURE

I read your *Onanism* a bit too late, and I am left with some regrets ...
Capitaine Chateauneuf to Tissot, 26 July 1774[54]

Here, then, we come to the conceptual nub of the argument. What do I mean by the politics of pleasure? How is it that pleasure became a matter for politics? The letters to Tissot must be read at the point of encounter between moderation and excess, *plaisir* and *jouissance*. What I mean to say is this: the letters emerge from the very point at which the desire to seek bodily pleasures comes face to face with the equally strong moral need to discipline the social body – that is, when the illicit intimate pleasures evoked by Diderot in his *Encyclopédie* definition encounter the force of social discipline inherent in the art of pleasing. At this point of contact, letters perform a dual function in that they are both instruments of surveillance – confessional documents detailing activities of a criminal nature – and acts of voyeurism – spaces that enable the telling and retelling, imagining and reimagining of illicit passions and pleasures. While letters may, as I have argued in an earlier chapter, been understood as thresholds between sender and receiver, text and act, *plaisir* and *jouissance*, they also, as autoerotic gestures, map out the boundaries between surveillance and voyeurism. As thresholds, such letters are liminal spaces in which observer and observed are intimately intertwined with one another. In the words of Thomas Laqueur, it is about the space between *plaisir* and *jouissance*: "that part of human sexual life where potentially unlimited pleasure meets social restraint; where habit and the promise of just-one-more-time struggle with the dictates of conscience and good sense; where fantasy silences, if only for a moment, the reality principle; and where the autonomous self escapes from the erotically barren here and now into a luxuriant world of its own creation. It hovers between abjection and fulfillment."[55]

The imagery of the Möbius strip, introduced by Elizabeth Grosz as a way of conceptualizing the relationship between body and mind, can be useful in this instance as well. A series of unending curves, body and mind weave in and through one another, their relationship so deeply intertwined that they cannot separate themselves out. As Grosz writes,

> Bodies and minds are not two distinct substances or two kinds of attributes of a single substance but somewhere in between these two alternatives. The Möbius strip has the advantage of showing the inflection of mind into body and body into mind, the ways in which, through a kind of twisting or inversion, one becomes another. This model also provides a way of problematizing and rethinking the relations between the inside and the outside of the subject, its psychical interior and its corporeal exterior, by showing not their fundamental identity or reducibility but the torsion of the one into the other, the passage, vector, or uncontrollable drift of the inside into the outside and the outside into the inside.[56]

This model is highly evocative as a way of conceptualizing the relationship between *plaisir* and *jouissance*, the encounter between the "psychical interior and its corporeal exterior." It can also, in this regard, help to illuminate the point of contact between surveillance and voyeurism, concepts that are central to a theorization of the politics of pleasure. Indeed, just as body and mind are interwoven with one another, so too, are surveillance and voyeurism bound up with one another. The relationship between the two is such that it becomes challenging to figure out precisely where one ends and the other begins. One could, provocatively, suggest that they are, as Karen Barad has evocatively argued, entangled; they are "not simply intertwined with one another … but lack an independent, self-contained existence."[57] Like the loops of the Möbius strip, surveillance and voyeurism wind in and through one another, such that what is important is not one or the other but rather "the torsion of one into the other."[58]

## WRITING PLEASURE

Writing about sexual pleasure was almost wholly a male activity. In fact, one could argue that the experience and articulation of sexual pleasure were as integral to conventions of masculinity as they were marginal to normative understandings of femininity. The materials in the Fonds Tissot appear to bear this out: while many men make mention of sexual encounters, either in passing or as the central tenet of their letters, only a handful of women make explicit mention of matters of sexual concern.

In one form or another, sex entered into many letters concerning men's health. Correspondents describe the corporeal fallout from a broad range of sexual practices, from masturbation to extensive heterosexual engagements as well as incidences of gonorrhoea.[59] While the most obvious references can be found in the (almost always) guilt-ridden letters about masturbation, issues of sexual relations also make their way into far more "innocuous" (if you will) letters about a multitude of other ailments, from respiratory difficulties to nervous disorders. In many of these letters, references to sexual pleasure are much more oblique as would-be patients strive to position themselves favourably vis-à-vis the good doctor. Thus, individuals suggest that they are suffering the ill after effects of illicit activity as a result of the morally suspect actions of their wet nurses (even if they were nursed forty years previously). Such individuals (male or female) were, therefore, victims of another's poor decisions. Some male correspondents, meanwhile, will mention their years of sexual debauchery in passing, noting that they have suffered no ill effects as a result and, more importantly, that their *wives* have not suffered, a fact that is offered as proof that their own ailments are not of a sexual nature. Others will merely brush off youthful indiscretions.

In each of these cases, the goal is simple: to demonstrate an awareness of Tissot's understandings of the problems of sexual excess and to claim the moral high ground in response. What seems clear from these letters is a conscious positioning of a moral self, a performance and staging of identity that emphasizes the individual's worthiness to receive treatment from Tissot. In this sense, their autobiographical self-positioning appears, at first glance at least, to reflect the ideals of corporeal citizenship proposed by Tissot and thus to conform to the guidelines he has put forward. These are virtuous citizens who have either acknowledged the error of their ways and changed their behaviour, or they never engaged in illicit sexual pleasure to begin with. As a result, their ailments must have another source. Their sufferings must be symptomatic of an entirely different condition, a point I explore in more detail later in this chapter.

However, a closer examination of the letters suggests the need for a much more complex reading, one that moves beyond a pleasure/shame binary and instead attests to the ambiguity and ambivalence inherent in the oscillation between *plaisir* and *jouissance*, and further to the unstable relationship between bodily management, on the one hand, and bodily desire, on the other. Central to this examination is the agency of the pleasure-seeking body. In some letters, sexual pleasure is on the table, front and centre. Consider, for example, the complex self-positioning of one Gounon, who writes to Tissot in June 1773. He writes, "I was, bit by bit, victim of all the Passions. I love women with a fury. I have played [games] my whole life. I consume much wine and drink coffee constantly. The natural temperament of my soul has been to seize everything with passion."[60] On the one hand, Gounon presents himself as a "victim" of his passions and as an unfortunate accomplice to a body that appears to be inclined to excess. These excesses have had bodily effects: not only have they exacerbated his already overly emotional state but they have been the cause of a bout of venereal disease. These sufferings appear to offer corporeal proof of his apparently excessive and indiscriminate engagement in sensual pleasures. In this view, Gounon is, as he points out in his letter, a victim of "cruel passions."[61] On the other hand, however, Gounon appears unwilling to acquiesce fully to the chastened victim position: his passions may be excessive but they are *natural* to him. His physical and emotional sufferings are not the result of a wilful challenge to Nature, as both the *Onania* and *L'Onanisme* suggest. Rather, they are the outcome of a temperament that "has been to seize everything with passion." His condition and temperament are intrinsic aspects of his personal identity. Further, and more critically, this self-positioning asserts that Gounon is, by nature, a sensually desiring being. His actions, then, are not deviant; they stem from natural inclinations. This is a complex self positioning that at once acknowledges Tissot's vision of corporeal citizenship while also simultaneously challenging it in favour of an alternative bodily reading. For Gounon, corporeal citizenship is not about bodily management. Rather, it is about acknowledging the complexity of individual situations and the natural tendencies of the body. In this sense, corporeal citizenship is also about the conversation between patient and doctor, the interplay between different interpretations of bodily experience. For such individuals, citizenship appears to reside in the mutual reciprocity of the epistolary exchange – that is, in the very nature of the social contract itself.

In the sections that follow, I move from the often futile attempts to discipline an unruly body towards an acceptance, indeed sometimes valorization, of bodily pleasure. Then, I move into a section that asserts the unruly and volatile agency of bodies themselves. I assert that bodies actively seek pleasure, regardless of the views of individuals. Finally, I examine the question of female sexual pleasure in detail and the case of Madame de Chastenay in particular.

> As I have said a thousand times, it is by the imagination alone that the senses are awakened.
>
> Jean-Jacques Rousseau, *Emile, or on Education*

> At the age of 16, seduced by a young man, I abandoned myself to a vice that has, unfortunately, infected the youth of all countries.
>
> Krizler to Tissot, 12 November 1791[62]

Jean-Jacques Rousseau, the influential arbiter of eighteenth-century political morality, came to carnal knowledge while walking the streets of his beloved Geneva: "I have a horror of street walkers that has never worn off; I could not see a debauched person without disdain, even without fright: for my aversion to debauchery went that far, ever since the day, while going into Little Sacconex by a sunken road, on both sides I saw the holes in the ground where I was told that these people copulated. Also what I had seen of the couplings of dogs always came back to mind when I thought of these debauched people, and this memory alone made me sick to my stomach."[63] In this passage we see that, for all his professed sexual escapades, the Enlightenment's self-professed moral conscience nevertheless retained a certain prudishness about sexual behaviour. As Shane Agin so astutely observes, this initiation story relies on the juxtaposition of human with animal, in the process equating the act of sexual intercourse with animalistic desires – that is, with the corporeal actions of entities deemed incapable of rational thought.[64] These are, indeed, crude couplings, whose after effects reveal only the dark underbelly of human nature, reminding us that we are, at heart, nothing more than mere animals, fundamentally amoral beasts subject to the whims of uncontrollable urges and passions.

Sexual initiation is a common feature of the letters to Tissot. While many individuals mention this in passing, others make a point of explaining these early forays into carnality in detail. Like Rousseau, these correspondents stress their inability to control their bodily urges. Overtaken by corporeal desire, they are victims not only of their bodily weakness but also, frequently, of lascivious and lustful servants who are always eager to please. The situation of one Ousrard de Linière is a case in point: "Around the age of thirteen or fourteen, led by my friends' example, I developed the fatal habit of masturbation. I recall that it took violent movements to discover just a few drops of liquid that was still as clear as water. This lasted for a while, [but] I did not content myself with this. This [behaviour] was but a foreshadowing of another passion that would soon develop in me. The facility that I found with my mother's chambermaid emboldened me. I carried on a relationship with her for more than six months. I bathed frequently during this period. I was only 14 years old. Her departure ended the liaison and I was relatively calm until the age of 16."[65] This letter appears to situate Ousrard de Linière as a victim of his own passions and of the unruly passions of others. Pleasure, here, does not contribute to social stability. Rather, as *jouissance*, it undermines it.

But a closer look at the letter suggests that this young man's sexual preoccupations, which continued into his late teens during an extended stay in Paris, are part of a longer narrative of excessive behaviours that goes back to his childhood. Ousrard de Linière positions himself as a young man given to excessive passions and behaviours. As a child, he filled his days with play, but never in moderation: "games, excessive running and violent exercise" were the order of the day.[66] Later, as a twelve-year-old, he was introduced to a new passion: swimming. Here, too, he found himself unable to act in moderation: "At the age of twelve, having learned how to swim, I developed the habit of going swimming. This soon degenerated into a passion, and I found myself spending up to five or six hours in a row in the water, and often at the most inconvenient times."[67] Given this history, his later engagement with onanism appears to be part of a longer tendency towards excessive behaviours. The letter, as a whole, is a desperate plea for assistance from a man whom the author sees as a beacon of hope in an otherwise bleak situation: "Sensitive as you are to the sufferings of humanity, and having become, by the extent of your enlightenment, one of the greatest in the art of ending or comforting human suffering, I dare to address myself to you, Sir, in the sweet hope that you would take pity on an unfortunate man who, in the flower of his youth (21 years), has found himself prey (for the past two years) to the progress of an illness that is as obstinate as it is destructive. Reading your treatise on Onanism taught me about it, and its fatal consequences caused me to tremble. My only hope rests in you."[68]

As a result of his bodily excesses, this young man is unable, at a bodily level, to perform citizenship. Now in his prime, he finds himself not only prey to his excessive passions but also confronting a future of misery and horror. Had he been more measured in his behaviours, this young man might have been able to look forward to a more positive future, a life in which his pleasures could have been directed to the good of society as a whole. However, he fears that even though he has since committed himself to moderation and balance, it may already be too late. His early actions, evidence of a commitment to selfish pleasures, have resulted in a far more tragic situation. In many ways this letter would appear to confirm Stolberg's Foucauldian thesis. Surveillance and discipline are key words that might mark this narrative. So, too, is shame.

Shame is a powerful motivator in many letters to Tissot. In the words of Krizler, writing from a village near Lausanne, "I beg you, Sir, never to mention the cruel confession that I made to you … in the fear that this letter will, after my death, fall into strange hands and that my whole character will be judged as vulgar as a result of a youthful indiscretion."[69] Just as pleasure is embodied, so, too, is shame. Consider, for example, the case of Thomas Cranfurd. Writing from Naples in 1774, Cranfurd tells the following story: "I am 28 years old and I had the misfortune, before the age of reason (aged 10 or 11) to learn this unfortunate habit, the fatal effects of which you have made visible, for the good of mankind, with such strength and energy. Notwithstanding my frequent excesses, both in this area and in the course of everyday life, I enjoyed tolerably good health until my 24th year, when I suffered an attack of nerves and general languishing. In this state, having recklessly engaged in immoderate pleasures with a young woman for a period of a month, I soon began to suffer from nocturnal emissions, which often returned twice a night and soon led me to feel a cold sensation in my back and shoulders accompanied by weakening eyesight."[70]

Like other letters on this subject, this narrative begins with a precocious sexual initiation. This initiation, for which Cranfurd cannot be held responsible as it occurred "before the age of reason," subsequently sets the stage for later excessive behaviours in other areas of his life. Indeed, by organizing his letter as he does, Cranfurd gestures towards this history as the *source* of his later reckless behaviour; it is this original fall (in a biblical sense) that appears to have undermined his bodily control. First a victim of pleasure, he then becomes a willing participant, only to find his body marked by classic signs of onanytic degeneration. Pleasure, in this letter, is fundamentally troubled by the disciplinary power of onanism discourse and, as a consequence, this young man's corporeal identity has been compromised.

The corporeal effects of illicit pleasure could also manifest themselves in *other* bodies – that is, in bodies beyond those of the onanists themselves. The Chevalier de Peyrelongue, for example, who suffered from four episodes of gonorrhoea at the age of twenty and at the time of writing still occasionally suffered abrasions on his penis, cited his wife's apparent barrenness as evidence of his own physical infirmity: "I suffered from four bouts with gonorrhoea, from which I recovered as well as possible. No flows remain, but sometimes, small abrasions appear on my penis; however, these heal by themselves within 3 or 4 days. I should also add that for the past while, I have become very irritable and very worried and when I become violently angry, I experience serious pains in my chest and stomach … I have been married for three years, without having had any children. Because my wife had a child from a first marriage, it is clear to me that I must assign fault to my infirmities."[71] Corporeal stigmata, in this instance, mark not only the sufferer's body but also that of his partner, a fertile woman who finds that she can no longer become pregnant. Youthful bodily indiscretions have left an indelible mark, impacting the chevalier and his wife. In the process, Peyrelongue's actions have undermined his ability to perform masculinity, his own infertility antithetical to the performative requirements of reproductive masculinity as well as the parallel performatives required of his wife. In this way, Peyrelongue has, through his indiscriminate actions, compromised the corporeal citizenship of his family as a whole.

The tone that permeates such letters is common to many other letters on the topic. Although many correspondents stress that they were eventually able to extricate themselves from such situations, it is clear that they feel that the damage had been done. On the surface, then, such scenarios would appear to confirm the repressive power of Foucauldian confessional culture. But I would argue that such an approach does not go far enough. As Stolberg and others have noted, it is abundantly clear that those who wrote to Tissot were negotiating the repressive frameworks outlined not only in Tissot's framework on onanism, but also in relation to other documents of the period. But such narratives are not only about surveillance, even as this element stands out most prominently in a first reading. These narratives are *also* about pleasure. They are, like Diderot's subversive approach to *jouissance*, about the navigation, claiming, and articulation of sexual pleasure within the restrictive tenets of eighteenth-century moral belief. From this perspective, voyeurism, rather than surveillance, might be a more appropriate way of imagining them.

We might, for example, consider the case of young man named Rossary, who wrote Tissot a four-page letter in 1774. Like Ousrard

de Linière, Rossary finds his innocence compromised at the hands of
schoolmates:

> At the age of 16 or 17, I was taught how to masturbate, which my
> immature temperament had allowed me to ignore until that point
> … a too premature engagement with a practice more pernicious to
> young people than true pleasure hastened my naturally immature
> temperament. My school friends taught me early about an action
> about which I previously had no idea. This instruction excited
> my desires without satisfying them; and it was only after several
> frequently repeated lessons that I experienced a voluptuous tick-
> ling (but without ejaculation). Nature, aggravated, finally asserted
> itself, but with care. Ever-perceptive servants were quick to notice
> these changes in me and sought to share them, but they must have
> been little satisfied with my vigour. For the rest, I was only rarely
> with women, and even then only through the ease with which they
> lent themselves to my desires, rather than through incidences that
> led me to them. A natural shyness and further, an insurmountable
> horror that they would publicize our liaisons, and undoubtedly,
> my weak temperament, led me to be reserved in their presence.
> However, I manually stimulated myself frequently.[72]

Following a now recognizable formula, Rossary reports a relatively
traumatic initiation into sexual pleasure at the hands of other young
men. For Rossary, who acknowledged his immaturity, this was clearly
experienced as a loss of innocence. His innocence thus compromised,
he found himself prey to sexual advances from household staff whose
apparent clairvoyance enabled them to recognize his new state of sexual
awareness. Ultimately unable to psychologically bear the responsibilities of sexual relationships, he resorted instead to frequent masturbation. Habit became need and over a period of several years, he often
masturbated two or three times per day. Every time, he tried to repent
and made resolutions to change his behaviour, but all of this was to no
avail: "I finally became aware of the weakening of my strengths and
abilities, of erections that were less frequent and less full. I was still able
to recall them, but the damage was too deeply rooted. So I persisted
with a kind of despair; I understood my situation but habit had become
so powerful that I did not have the strength to resist."[73]

Until this point, Rossary's physiological concerns appear to confirm
Tissot's admonitions, as outlined in *L'Onanisme*. As Rossary continued

his activities, he found himself growing progressively softer, the virility and firmity that marked him as a man giving way to a softness that undermines otherwise naturalized sexual difference. In the process, Rossary also actively compromised his commitment to civic virtue: through his actions, he was not contributing to the social good; rather, by a commitment to the solitary pleasures of masturbation, he was merely feeding his bad habit. Rossary, however, takes pains to insist on a reading of corporeal virtue. As he indicates in his letter, he is a gentleman possessed of honesty, benevolence, and sensibility. Indeed, he can even provide written references that can attest to this: "I can tell you that in spite of this vice (into which I hope never again to fall), I am not a dishonourable man but that I enjoy the generosity and affection … of everyone I know, that I have an honourable, sensitive and grateful heart; that I have the strongest and most flattering recommendations and written attestations."[74] Rossary is, in other words, at heart a man of virtue, a moral citizen unfortunately overcome by bodily weakness.

But there are ruptures along the way. This letter is not solely about psychic and somatic distress; it is also about navigating pleasure. Rossary is clearly overwhelmed by his experiences. Sexual initiation, at an age when he did not feel ready for it, disturbed his natural temperament. Furthermore, his continued engagement with what he terms "*manualisation*" has fundamentally altered his physical abilities. Nevertheless, it is clear that Rossary enjoys masturbating. Masturbation is a safe outlet, one that allows him to indulge his sexual desires in the absence of amorous encounters with women, while also, simultaneously, granting him privacy. For Rossary, then, onanism is not just a convenient habit. Rather, it has become a need. Pleasure, in this framework, is fraught.

We can also take this further. Even as the objective of bodily discipline – that is, Rossary's desire to control his bodily behaviours – permeates the letter, it is clear that his body resists and refuses these interdictions. Rossary's body *seeks* pleasure, even if that pleasure is fleeting, illusory. This pleasure is addictive. He cannot stop himself from accessing it, even as he repeatedly tries to change his behaviours. A clue to his experience of pleasure can be found early in the letter. As a young initiate into the delights of pleasures of the flesh, Rossary experiences what he terms "*un chatouillement voluptueux*," a voluptuous – delicious, even – inner tickling. This is, in many ways, a very rich way of describing orgasm, a description that gets to the heart of a visceral engagement with the pleasures of the flesh. The language here is remarkably vibrant and evocative. Drawing on Baudelaire's idea of *volupté* – corporeal and sensual pleasure – his words recall the sensual flirtations central to so many of Fragonard's works: illicit pleasures derived from subtle glimpses under dress skirts, stolen kisses on balconies, and sexual innuendo during games of blind man's bluff. It also evokes links with the visual palette of artists like Boucher – in particular, the fleshy curves of Mademoiselle O'Malley erotically displayed in the intimate disarray of her boudoir. How, indeed, could a young man have possibly resisted such delights?

As an experience, tickling is something that overwhelms the whole body, and it is a memory that, in its recollection, continually asserts itself. As a bodily experience, a tickle is like a shiver. An involuntary response to external stimuli, it starts in one part of the body before quickly overwhelming all senses. In its eighteenth-century incarnation, tickling was also associated with the body. Tickling, the action of lightly touching another person, elicits an involuntary bodily response that usually provokes laughter. But tickling is not only a physical act, even as it results in physical pleasures. It is also an emotional state that can be brought about by flattery. To tickle, according to the *Dictionnaire de l'Académie française*, is to flatter the body and to excite the passions: "It is said that *Wine tickles the palate, the throat;* that *music, harmony tickle the ear, the ears*, in order to say that wine and music pleasurably flatter the senses."[75] Thus, tickling, as an emotional response to sensory stimulation, provokes a physical response, in the process uniting psyche and soma. Intriguingly, another example offered in this definition takes the idea further into the realm of self-pleasure: "Figuratively, one can say this of a man who excites himself to laughter, or who works to bring himself joy, even if there is no point to it, such as 'He tickles himself in order to make himself laugh.'"[76] Common to each of these applications is an association of the experience of tickling with that of sensual pleasure: tickling flatters, it excites, it brings joy. Furthermore, in its eighteenth-century incarnation, tickling is intimately linked with bodily agency. Indeed, it is one way that the body not only experiences pleasure but that it *claims* pleasure. Thus, tickling is both a social act – in the sense that one experiences bodily pleasure through flattery – but also, and this is significant in relation to questions of sexual pleasure, a private, intimate experience that can be enacted in and through one's own body. It is the promise of orgasm – of this voluptuous tickling – that makes it so hard for Rossary to resist temptation; indeed, in these instances, he revels in it.

The intimacy and privacy of tickling merits a closer look: although the tickle might emerge in the social, it is experienced *within* the body. Furthermore, it is an involuntary response; that is, it is the body asserting itself beyond the control of the individual. In this sense, the *chatouillement voluptueux* thus exists outside of regimens of control and surveillance. While such bodily responses can be reported as part of confessional culture, the experiences themselves cannot be denied. Once flattered, the body is determined to pleasure itself, and no amount of discipline can possibly control this. A *chatouillement voluptueux*, then, would appear to reveal a bodily resistance to the disciplinary power of surveillance and confessional culture. The story can be told, but the pleasures remain. In its articulation and re-articulation in epistolary form – a process that makes public the bodily intimacy of orgasm – tickling has much in common with voyeurism. Indeed, the voluptuous tickling offers an intriguing foreshadowing of Baudelaire's evocative imagery.

### SEEKING PLEASURE

While the correspondents cited in the previous section articulate their bodily pleasures through epistolary narratives of shame, others resist the discourses of bodily control propagated by doctors such as Tissot. Instead, they are far more overt in their claims to pleasure and in their understandings of the bodily agency. At the beginning of a medical consultation written on behalf of the Comte d'Adhémar, a forty-year-old man, the doctor observes the following: "He was born of healthy, temperate and strong parents who did not suffer from arthritic inflammations. He has never shown any visible sign of venereal disease although he has often run the risk."[77] We can infer from this a propensity or penchant for sexually excessive or risky behaviours. Indeed, the lengthy series of questions the correspondent poses to Tissot later in the letter bear this out. Nevertheless, it is clear that, unlike Ousrard de Linière and Rossary, this particular individual is neither ashamed of his dalliances nor convinced that they are the source of his problems. Unwilling to accept a prescription for sexual moderation, he challenges accepted wisdom by drawing from his own experiences: "Is moderate sexual commerce with women so very pernicious that it must be absolutely prohibited, and how could one believe that an evacuation that is so natural could possibly be the cause of a malady attributed to excess?

… The patient would like to note that during his different attacks … he engaged in sexual encounters with women, and far from feeling poorly as a result of this, he believed himself to feel better."[78]

Following a scientific method of careful and quantifiable corporeal observation, the Comte d'Adhémar offers bodily evidence that runs counter to prevailing medical opinion. Instead of resisting his body's authority, as the unfortunate Gauteron whose words opened this chapter might have done, the count uses bodily intransigence as proof that there must be something *else* at play. While Tissot and the medical establishment promoted narratives of bodily management and control, d'Adhémar's experiences, and his analysis of them, suggest an alternative reading that *embraces* rather than rejects the pleasures of the flesh. In so doing, he asserts full authority not only over his experiences but also over the narrative that results. While the conversation that emerges in a formal medical consultation is ostensibly between two medical professionals – in this case, the Count d'Adhémar's local doctor and Tissot – this particular conversation is very different. As an observer of his body's stories, d'Adhémar situates himself equally in relation to both his local doctor and Tissot. Unwilling to accept the moral reproach implied in his doctor's comments ("He has never shown any signs of venereal diseases although he has often run the risk"), d'Adhémar insists on his rights not only to self-diagnosis but perhaps more importantly to challenge the medical establishment. In so doing, he asserts corporeal citizenship not as acquiescence to medical opinion but rather as a site of critical self-reflection born of sustained engagement with and observation of the lived body and its stories.

So, too, does the Chevalier de Valpergue offer a resistant reading. Valpergue opens his letter with a litany of corporeal complaints: "In winter, and particularly when it is freezing, and during other seasons when it is windy or when the air is cold and penetrating, and finally, whenever there is some change of weather, I feel like a foreign body squeezes my lower abdomen, rises to my stomach and then to my head, [and this] causes precisely all of the effects of a bad head cold; I breathe with such great difficulty that I feel as though I am almost suffocating, a bad headache and sometimes heart palpitations; very sensitive tingling sensations in both sides of the nose, which excite sneezing and which, in turn give me such violent tremors that the whole machine is disordered."[79] Furthermore, the chevalier is also prone to emotional disturbance: "I am gloomy, and profoundly melancholy, continually occupied with painful thoughts that cause me much trouble, and the slightest contradiction makes me angry, even though I am, by nature, cold and peaceful ... I do not sleep at all, or rather, I sleep fitfully, my sleep accompanied by the most frightful dreams that wake me with a start and cause me much trouble."[80]

These psychic and somatic experiences – bodily disorder, emotional excess, disturbed sleep, and nightmares – could very easily be read under the rubric of onanism and, in fact, he indicates later in his letter that he "was not very wise during [his] youth, but not overly debauched,"[81] and that he suffered from numerous episodes of venereal disease. Read through the lens of onanism, Valpergue appears to have compromised any claim to corporeal citizenship. However, Valpergue resists a reading of onanism. While he acknowledges his poor choices, he also insists that these decisions are not the cause of his current suffering. His argument rests on bodily evidence: "It is true that I had some episodes of gonorrhoea, but they were always treated with much care and prudence and I do not believe that my sickness could have resulted from these actions, because I have no bodily mark or any pain, or any other things that would make me suspect this."[82] In writing this, Valpergue gestures towards common understandings of the period. While sexual acts were intimate and private, the diseases thought to result from excessive or indiscriminate sexual behaviours and the treatments that existed to cure them were highly visible; that is to say, disease and cure physically imprinted themselves on the body, visibly marking the suffering body. Disease and treatment stigmatized the body, making the nature of the suffering clear to all. For example, syphilis was, as Robert Weston has observed, "not only ... shocking in its manifestations, [but] with treatments which were also obnoxious ... a disease with implication of moral degradation."[83] Valpergue's letter is thus crafted in such a way as to situate himself, like the Count d'Adhémar, as a careful observer of his bodily experiences and a conscientious consumer of current medical theory. In so doing, it asserts Valpergue as a knower, as actively engaged in the production of knowledge. It also positions him as a corporeal citizen concerned with his bodily projects. But, significantly, this letter *also* reimagines the conventional narratives of onanism, in the process providing support for Valpergue's claim that although he was not particularly wise, he was also "not overly debauched." For Valpergue, in other words, sexual immoderation was not the source of permanent disability; it was simply part of his youthful experiences.

The narratives of the Comte d'Adhémar and the Chevalier de Valpergue suggest a critical engagement with the ideas presented in works such as the *Onania* and *L'Onanisme*. D'Adhémar and Valpergue are not content to accept conventional understandings at face value. Rather, by considering their own body histories, experiences and encounters, they argue for more complex readings that acknowledge the role of pleasure not only to the intimate experience of bodily subjectivity but also to the practice of corporeal citizenship.

## BODILY EXCESSES

I am discouraged; distracted from my work; unresponsive to
my desires and my resolve (especially in relation to my inner
feelings regarding my situation); alternately experiencing anguish,
hopelessness, desperation, hope and sometimes, satisfaction. Fearing
and sometimes desiring death; often, when going to bed, I dare to
hope that it will be for the last time.

Rossary to Tissot, 13 June 1774[84]

In a lengthy letter introduced previously, Martin, a twenty-one-year-old medical student, outlined the case of Claude Joseph Demeunier, a stubborn thirty-year-old "victim of onanism" now apparently close to death.[85] Demeunier apparently began masturbating at fourteen or fifteen, suffered from the ravages of excessive masturbation but refused to see the light. Instead, he consulted numerous "doctors, surgeons, charlatans and magicians"[86] about his sufferings, without actually revealing their cause. He knew the source of his infirmities but did not stop. On the contrary, he continued: "He refused to open his eyes to the danger in which he placed himself. Nor did the continual pain he experienced in the pubic area intimidate him."[87] Even as the situation worsened and Demeunier found himself unable to sleep, plagued with dreams and agitations, convulsions, involuntary rigidity, and spasms, he refused to stop. Indeed, he only started seeing the error of his ways in the two years prior to Martin's letter – in other words, fourteen years after his first experiences. With the unfortunate sufferer now close to death, Martin (the medical student) hopes that Tissot will "cast a compassionate eye on his pitiable state."[88]

Particularly intriguing here is the role that sight plays in this narrative.[89] Sight operates at numerous levels here. For Martin, Demeunier is an object of horror. The visual embodiment of the evils of onanism, Demeunier presents "a frightening portrait of a victim of onanism."[90] Martin, as the portrait artist, takes care to paint his portrait in detail:

     TELLING THE FLESH

"The sufferer, Claude Joseph Demeunier ... began the unfortunate practice of masturbation at the age of 14 or 15. The pollutions multiplied to three or four per day. Instead of sperm, they released pure blood, which soon made him melancholy and extremely thin. The instrument of his miseries became inflamed and was often in a state of very painful priapism after the subtle agitation; thoughts and dreams occasioned ejaculation. This considerable loss was such a blow to his nervous system that he was deprived of both movement and feeling for fifteen and sometimes twenty minutes after most of his pollutions. True but fruitless foreshadowings of his coming misfortunes!"[91] Martin also details further sufferings, including convulsions, troubled sleep, terrible dreams, loss of sensation, spasms, memory loss, pain, and impaired judgment.

But Demeunier, as an object of scrutiny, is not only exposed to Martin's horrified gaze. He is also, through Martin's intervention, exposed to a very different gaze: the beneficent gaze of Europe's most celebrated physician. From this perspective, Demeunier is not an object of horror but rather a pitiable creature worthy of compassion: "I hope ... that the sentiments of humanity that have led you to give a large number of excellent works to the public, will also led to you grant a compassionate eye on [this man's] pitiable state: without parents, without assets, without resources, he would like either to finish the miserable life that he has procured himself or to find ways to return to health, if not to a virile vigour, at the very least to be able to avoid indigence and starvation."[92] The eye, here, is not horrified; rather, it is generous, beneficent, compassionate. This eye does not turn away. Instead, it offers the possibility, however remote, of corporeal redemption.

Finally, Martin turns to Demeunier himself. Drawing on language that recalls the physical loss of sight understood to be one of the common effects of onanism, Martin evokes the metaphorical blindness of his patient, a man who "refused to open his eyes to the precipice he was causing himself."[93] Wilfully blind to both his sufferings and to the consequences of his actions, Demeunier appears to be an active participant in his own corporeal downfall.

Given Martin's age, twenty-one, it seems clear that much of this tale was recounted to him after the fact and that he, himself, was only ever witness to the end-stage ravages that appear to be consuming Demeunier's body. But there is something more intriguing at play. Unlike the letters penned by Gauteron, this letter is penned by an observer, not by the patient. Moral horror is here displaced from sufferer to witness. In bearing witness, Martin offers yet another "horrific tableau" that adds further weight to Tissot's perspective. But in positioning Demeunier's story as he has, Martin has also very effectively positioned himself, aligning his views and his approach directly with those of the good doctor. This is no insignificant matter when we consider that Martin himself is a medical student. In this case, the telling of sexual pleasure (and pain) becomes part of his autobiographical narrative of medicine – part of his identity as a doctor-in-waiting. Just as others were careful to position their behaviours favourably in relation to Tissot's beliefs and perspectives, so too does Martin take care to shape his story for his audience.

More important still is Martin's depiction of the lengths to which some individuals would go in order to secure bodily pleasure. Demeunier's narrative is one of both resistance and acquiescence. He completely refuses the conventional diagnosis of onanism, choosing instead to search high and low for alternative diagnoses. In so doing, he gives free rein to his body's agency, and this narrative offers an intriguing example of corporeal resistance through an insistence on pleasure. However, given his bodily disorders, this acquiescence is fundamentally troubled. Here pleasure is intermingled with pain, the combination of the two so seductive that Demeunier succumbs fully, apparently wholly unable to extricate himself from the morass in which he finds himself.

## BODILY AGENCY, BODILY IDENTITY, AND THE VIRTUOUS CITIZEN

Sexual commerce with women and even worse, masturbation, are very bad for my health; my sufferings are increasing.

Roussy to Tissot, 10 June 1774[94]

Bodily agency, as a troubled concept, is central to the Martin/Demeunier narrative. But it also emerges in other letters. I want to consider here the story of a young military man named Thomassin. This particular narrative is fascinating because of the extent to which one individual engages with the various meanings available to him, and from there, how he comes to his own bodily conclusions. According to his letter, Thomassin appears to be experiencing nocturnal emissions. But such bodily signs are not unambiguously read. Indeed, as his narrative progresses, three different meanings emerge. Throughout this narrative, it is clear that his body is exercising sexual agency. These various meanings, then, are mere interpretations of what is happening, almost insensibly, to him.

Thomassin began experiencing nocturnal emissions between the ages of thirteen and fourteen, while away at school. Upon his return home, his father, "more aware of the wickedness of schoolboys" than Thomassin, suspected masturbation.[95] As a result, "he tormented me cruelly to admit to a habit that I didn't have."[96] In spite of Thomassin's protestations, his father persisted: "He spied on my activities, and being unable to find any fault with them, he decided to check my sheets. He found evidence of an offense for which I played only a passive role ... and confronted me. Although I did not expect anything from this new form of proof, I was sternly lectured and threatened. I was given all the pious and religious books written on the matter."[97] In this part of his letter, Thomassin takes pains to position himself as a victim not only of his father's mistrust but also of his body's agency. Not only does he *experience* nocturnal emissions, but he is also *subject to* them. Furthermore, Thomassin offers alternative readings for the various sufferings that befall him – among them hearing loss. He notes that his loss of hearing cannot possibly be due to active engagement in masturbation on his part because it returns after he falls into a mountain crevice. Interestingly, his emissions also stop for a period after this. In presenting his case as he does, Thomassin moves the narrative, and his life story, away from onanism and its harmful after effects.

Thomassin's friends and classmates, meanwhile, apprised of the situation, locate the emissions within the framework of penile performativity – that is, as bodily evidence of masculinity: "'Proof of virility,' they told me. 'You need a woman.' I easily believed this false principle. I wanted to have affairs."[98] Still other friends, however, offered a third possibility. They saw his problems as signs of weakness and bodily relaxation. In his letters, Thomassin vacillated between these two differing poles of opinion. Again, as in the case of his earlier experiences with his father, Thomassin presents himself as a remarkably passive individual, subject not only to the whims of others but also to the whims of his body.

Ultimately, however, this narrative speaks to a clear sense of bodily agency. Like Rossary, cited earlier, Thomassin discovers that his body will act of its own accord, actively seeking pleasure even in the absence of conscious will on his part. Indeed, throughout this narrative, he positions himself as a passive innocent. But Thomassin's bodily agency is not clearly or easily definable. By the midway point in the letter, at least three different meanings have been put forward, and we have yet to get a full sense of Thomassin's personal reading of the situation. Given the uncertainty that surrounds nocturnal emission as a bodily sign, it is perhaps not surprising that Thomassin vacillates. Truth, as he understands it, comes to the fore in 1773. Worried about increasing emissions, he read Tissot's treatise: "finally, one beautiful day, opening your awful book on onanism, I stumbled upon the chapter that deals with this malady and I was not a little afraid of the sorry consequences of these emissions, and it was even worse when I came to recognize the fatal effects."[99]

The bodily logics at the heart of his nocturnal emissions are read very differently by Thomassin and his family. For his family, nocturnal emissions are signs of a bodily disorder wrought by masturbation. But Thomassin's narrative, informed by the varying opinions of his friends, is different. Tissot's definitive approach focuses yet another lens on the situation. In each of these cases, however, one thing remains clear: Thomassin details a body actively seeking pleasure, even in the face of mental resistance. For Thomassin, this bodily agency is unsettling, and, as his narrative progresses, it becomes threatening, horrifying in its unruliness and seeming uncontrollability. His body appears to be degenerating in front of his very eyes: "This strong body of robust appearance is weak and soft," he observes.[100] Ultimately frustrated by a deceiving body and a weak will, Thomassin expresses his deepest fears – that he, like Tissot's anonymous watchmaker, is losing grasp on humanity itself: "Finally, born of a healthy and strong mother and father, both very lively, I had reason to hope for a masculine character and a strong step. It is to you, Sir, that I address myself, that you might repair this disorder that has frustrated me. The operation will be difficult, but it is not beyond your abilities. Your enlightenment and your reputation are, for me, a certain guarantee. You know Nature, you can put my body back on the right track. You will return me to a health that will bring me liberty … you will return a citizen to a state of citizenship, and a man to humanity."[101] Thomassin's overt articulation of citizenship here indicates his own engagement with and commitment to ideals of bodily virtue. Interestingly, for Thomassin, bodily citizenship appears to be intimately linked with his ability to perform normative masculinity – a "masculine character and a strong step" – as well as to his ability to claim membership in humanity. Unfortunately, the agency of Thomassin's body is disruptive and actively troubles his moral desires.

This array of letters demonstrates that sexual pleasure was an ambivalent and complex space. While some, like Gounon, the Comte

d'Adhémar, and the Chevalier de Valpergue, were able to claim ownership of their pleasures, in the process questioning the dictates of medical
and moral authority, others, like Ousrard de Linière, Thomas Cranfurd,
and Rossary, struggled both to understand and to articulate their sexual
desires and bodily agency. Indeed, for some, like Gauteron, the terrain
of sexual pleasure was deeply fraught.

## GENDERING PLEASURE

But what of women's sexuality? What of their desires, their pleasures,
their struggles? This chapter has, for the most part, like the texts on
which it is based, tacitly linked the articulation and experience of sexual
pleasure with the male body and with the performance of masculine
identity. Indeed, in textual form, pleasures of the flesh are almost wholly
within the masculine domain. There are, in the Tissot collection, only
a few woman-authored letters that make direct reference to questions
of female sexual pleasure.[102] This is, no doubt, due to social and cultural restrictions of the period. The conscious articulation of a sexual
or pleasure-seeking self was, as we have seen, already a dangerous
prospect for men to explore. As a voluntarily anonymous correspondent commented, "Please excuse me, Sir, if I didn't sign my letter, but
you will agree with me that when one is guilty of a crime like the one
which I have just confessed, it is forgivable to be so ashamed as to
remain anonymous."[103] For women, it was likely too morally fraught
even to contemplate. While virility among men was accepted as long
as it was practiced in moderation, the articulation of a sexual desiring
self, for women, immediately undermined their social status and position, effectively denying them any possibility of civic agency. Instead,
such thoughts conjured direct associations with women of disreputable
character, among them actresses, prostitutes, and even, wet nurses.[104]
As Hanafi observes, norms of feminine modesty affected even medical
concerns unrelated to sexuality.[105]

Nevertheless, even as men asserted themselves as sexual subjects,
women peopled the landscape of sexual pleasure. Wives, lovers, par-
amours, prostitutes, slaves, and corrupters – all of these women are visible in the vast majority of male-authored narratives of pleasure: I loved
women, I enjoyed women, I used women, I sought out women. Women
are ever the objects of heterosexual male desire. Most often depicted as
anonymous bodies penetrated in the service of male sexual satisfaction,

they were also presented vicariously as sexual agents in their own right. From the letters, it is abundantly clear that women *were* sexually active and pleasure-seeking individuals.

Perhaps unsurprisingly, men's letters about sexual pleasure often present women as Eve-like characters: in offering a taste of the forbidden fruit, such women conspire to male moral downfall and, in some cases, to the corruption of otherwise morally upstanding innocents. Thus, correspondents introduce readers to the salacious actions of lascivious servants and domestics seeking actively to corrupt young bodies and minds. As we have seen, male-authored letters to Tissot, particularly those detailing precocious sexual initiations, rely on the presence of sexually aware and available women who are apparently more than happy to exercise their carnal powers over unsuspecting male innocents.

Interesting in this depiction are the obvious correlations that can be drawn between sexual agency, bodily assertiveness, and class. That sexual agency is imputed onto a servant body is, in this sense, to be expected. Servant bodies were, as numerous scholars have pointed out, disruptive bodies.[106] While they assured the proper functioning of elite homes and families, their bodily presence in these rarefied spaces highlighted the troubling and problematic porosity of the class system itself. Madame de Pompadour's social ascendancy might be read as the ultimate manifestation of this concern: hers was, and would always remain, a body out of place. The result of illicit dalliances, this body was later part of what was seen by many as a misbegotten alliance that threatened not only the cohesion of the family but the security of the state as a whole.[107] At a more mundane level, the porosity of class boundaries was most evocatively embodied in the form of the wet nurse, whose milk, as Melisa Klimazewski and others have argued, transmitted working class values into elite children.[108] Other correspondents, meanwhile, introduce the reader to apparently sexually rapacious young women whose previous encounters with other men might have undermined the health of the correspondent in question.[109] Even those who report no troubling health concerns recount active sexual histories that include numerous heterosexual liaisons with myriad partners.

Beyond the correspondence, libertine fictions, too, grant considerable power to female sexual agency. We might consider in this regard, the nefarious agency of Madame de Merteuil in *Les liaisons dangereuses*. Merteuil, fully versed in the arts of gallantry and seduction, attempts to orchestrate the moral corruption of a virginal young woman on the brink of marriage. In the process, Merteuil asserts her own vicarious pleasures, while also, ironically, assuring her social exile. Nor can any discussion of women's sexual agency ignore the political power and prowess of a woman like the Marquise de Pompadour, who not only deployed her bodily wiles in the service of social ascendance, but who was later reputed to have presided over her paramour's sexual appetites in the form of the infamous Parc-aux-cerfs. So, too, should we consider Olympe de Gouges, whose active resistance to narrow conventions of feminine propriety included the careful crafting of a pseudo-aristocratic identity and life story, the literary revelation of a troubled and unsavoury lineage, and later, the public assertion of women's rights to reproductive bodily authority and equal marriage.[110] Indeed, Pompadour and Gouges offer highly public examples of feminine sexual assertiveness and agency. All of these women, both fictional and historical, stands as a testament to women's sexual agency. Their actions demonstrate their keen abilities either to resist dominant narratives, or, at the very least, to navigate them in such a way as to assure their own needs. In each of these cases, they were able to use the sexed and gendered body to their own advantage, drawing creatively and subversively on dominant discourses of female sexuality in order to secure their own social positions. However, questions of desire and pleasure are rarely discussed in these cases; rather, these women wield their sexual bodies in the service of political gain. As such, while promising, these women's stories ultimately have little to contribute to a discussion of female bodily pleasure.

In the letters to Tissot, questions of female pleasure can only be vicariously gleaned. We are, for the most part, privy only to the narratives constructed by male sufferers of various forms of sexual dysfunction, all of whom were writing not only within a culture of moral disapproval but also under the gaze of a doctor who overtly linked excessive sexual practice with psychic and somatic disarray. Given this, it is risky indeed to draw uncritically on the obviously subjective portrayals of female sexual pleasure and sexual practice as found in male-authored letters. Assertions of female sexual agency and excess must be read in the context of an epistolary relationship that demanded the assertion of a morally-blameless corporeal self, even in the face of extensive evidence to the contrary. In addition to this, such assertions must also be carefully situated dominant discourses of femininity, which understood female sexual pleasure as perverse, deviant, and morally suspect – in short, well outside the realm of respectability. While the male-authored letters to Tissot might offer some insight into the question of female bodily pleasure, they, too, are ultimately an unsatisfactory source.

How, then, do we examine the thorny questions of female sexual pleasure and sexual agency? More relevant, for our purposes, are the insights shared by Madame Roland in her posthumously published *Memoirs*. As numerous scholars have noted, Roland is surprisingly frank in her depiction of sexual matters,[111] so much so that certain passages were expunged from early editions of the memoirs. Not only does Roland, in her memoirs, reference marital sexual relations, but she also reveals an early assault at the hands of an apprentice and more intriguingly in relation to the present study, references her adolescent engagement with sexual pleasure. In an extended passage that closely resembles the confessional tone and tenor of Gauteron's impassioned missives, Roland writes the following:

On May Day, when I was fourteen, my puberty burst upon me, effortlessly, like a rosebud opening under the rays of the spring sun … Before that time I had once or twice been woken in a rather surprising manner from a deep sleep. It had not been due to any imaginings on my part; I kept my imagination too firmly concentrated on serious matters, and my conscience was too strict a guardian over my curiosity for any unruly images to intrude. But in the warmth of sleep I experience an extraordinary surge of physical sensations, which through the agency of a healthy constitution and without any conscious participation by me, was like a sort of purification all of its own. My first reaction was a kind of fear. I had read in my *Philotée* that we are not permitted to derive any sort of pleasure from our bodies except in legitimate marriage. Recalling this precept I felt that I must be gravely at fault since the sensations I had experienced must certainly be described as pleasurable. Furthermore, the pleasure in question was undoubtedly one which would be most displeasing to the Spotless Lamb. So I fell into an agony of heart-searching, prayer and mortification. How was I to avoid such things happening again? For although I had not foreseen it, when it happened I had not done anything to check it. I began to watch myself very closely. If I noticed that any particular situation exposed me to temptation more than another, I avoided it. My anxiety was such that I sometimes woke up before the catastrophe; but if this did not happen I would leap to the foot of the bed, my cold, bare feet on the tiled floor, my arms stretched out to Heaven, and would pray to Our Lord and Saviour to protect me against the wiles of

     TELLING THE FLESH

the devil. I also imposed penances upon myself and occasionally put into practice the advice handed down to us by the Prophet King, probably merely as an oriental figure of speech, to mix ashes with our bread and to water it with our tears. Several times I poured cinders instead of salt on to my roast beef in penitence. This did me more harm than the nocturnal accidents for which it was intended to atone.[112]

As Dorinda Outram has observed, "Mme Roland's relationship with her own body was a focus on contradiction, and irreconcilable demands."[113] Her own experiences undermined any ability to assert an unambiguously moral virtuous feminine self, a factor that, according to Outram, fundamentally shaped her own understanding of her political importance vis-à-vis her husband's political roles.[114] Indeed, Roland's claiming of orgasm as "a sort of purification all of its own" is a particularly subversive reading that powerfully challenges even the most basic tenets of normative femininity.

Madame Roland's memoirs, penned over a five-month period prior to her execution in 1793, recall events that happened over two decades earlier. It is clear from her writing that she has come to terms with her early experiences. No longer a point of horror, her bodily agency is instead presented as "the agency of a healthy constitution," as a process just as natural to human development as menstruation. Madame Roland's adolescent horror stemmed, in large part, from the moral teachings she received as a child. As is evident from her narrative, the Catholic Church and her faith played a strong role in this. So, too, did literature. Roland references *Philothée*, a seventeenth-century book by the moral philosopher François de Sales. Subtitled *Introduction à la vie dévote*, the book encourages a practice of inner solitude, a practice of moral reflection and self control that, in the words of John D. Lyons, relied on the "deliberate use of the imagination to promote, on one hand, interiority and on the other hand, exterior conformity."[115] The individual seeking a devout life could actively cultivate inner peace, even in the midst of the various day-to-day activities that marked her life.

But as we have seen in Chapter 4, other literature, too, promoted the ideal of feminine moral virtue. In the work of Rousseau, for example, moral virtue is not just a practice of inner solitude but actively performative in nature. For Julie and Sophie, the heroines of two of his most influential works, embodied feminine virtue emerges through the active practice of femininity – that is, through a close engagement with the domestic virtues of home and family. Sophie and Julie were, first and foremost, to be wives and mothers, women whose virtue could be expressed through their bodily commitment to the needs of those in their care: for Rousseau, love and desire flowed from the maternal breast.[116] In this vision of gendered corporeal virtue, reproduction, which includes conception, pregnancy, delivery, and lactation, is not enough. As demonstrated earlier in this book, these bodily functions are infused with moral duties that envision the biological family as the cornerstone of a renewed polity founded on virtue. It is clear that those who wrote to Tissot responded to this vision. In the process, they often framed bodily selves as virtuous selves, asserting reproductive fecundity as a basis for corporeal belonging and citizenship.

A reading of female sexual agency, as it emerges in a series of four letters to Tissot from a single woman – Madame de Chastenay – is thus important to consider. After all, the writings of Madame Roland suggest that women were sexual agents in their own right and that their bodies, like those of their male counterparts, actively sought sexual pleasure. What, then, might the experiences of this particular woman add to this discussion? Catherine-Louise d'Herbouville, later Madame de Chastenay, was born in 1748 to an aristocratic family. The mother of the nineteenth-century memorialist and author Louise-Marie-Victoire de Chastenay, better known as Victorine de Chastenay, Madame de Chastenay emerges almost solely through the flattering tableaux penned by her daughter. According to Victorine de Chastenay, her mother was, as a young woman, a vision of delicate, porcelain beauty who resembled the Venus de Medici. A gentle blush stained her cheeks and she was possessed of an "enchanting smile and a fully French grace."[117] Furthermore, she embodied the principles of virtuous femininity: "She was going to be seventeen years old. Every day, she was more charming. She perfected herself in the arts of singing and harpsichord, she has an instinct for teaching, she bought the best books, and only opened them with pleasure."[118] So, too, was Madame de Chastenay an ideal mother: "From the moment I opened my eyes, Maman appeared to me a marvel of love and grace ... I found her charming and I loved her beauty. She undoubtedly inspired passions; I doubt, however, that any person shared the extent of my passion for her."[119] In her daughter's portraits, Madame de Chastenay emerges as a loving and beloved mother, a woman of beauty, grace, charm, generosity, and love who, together with her husband, presided over an idyllic family life in which young Victorine was given full rein to explore and develop her intellectual faculties.

   TELLING THE FLESH

Victorine de Chastenay also describes her mother as a woman given to nervous disorder. In a series of short passages, we read that Maman was apparently strongly subject to nervous malady.[120] As a result of this, she was surrounded by some of the leading lights in medicine: "Maman always believed herself to be sick and I could mention numerous celebrated physicians that we saw at home."[121] These doctors included Malouat, Bourdois, Portal, Corvisart, Fourcroy, and "the celebrated Tissot."[122] It is this nervous disorder that directs Madame de Chastenay to consult with Tissot. Madame de Chastenay sent Tissot a total of four documents, penned over a four-month period between November 1784 and February 1785.[123] Her first encounters – a letter and a medical consultation – are followed by two further letters in which she updates Tissot on her medical progress. The series as a whole offers remarkable detail and insight into the way that a single woman experienced and understood sexual pleasure, and how she relates these experiences to her social roles as wife and mother.

In a particularly revelatory passage, Madame de Chastenay writes, "I have a cold temperament when it comes to what might be termed intimate relations with my husband, but I have a vivid imagination, and, from the age of twelve, I abused myself often and excessively without knowing what I was doing. For the last several years, this practice has become increasingly rare because I fear the danger and also, because I have lost the habit. You see, Sir, I am offering you a confession."[124] What is interesting in this letter is Madame de Chastenay's assertion of her imagination as a site of pleasure. While her husband's advances leave her body cold, her vivid imagination ignites and enflames her bodily passions. For Madame de Chastenay, the pleasures of the flesh must first be imagined before they can be enacted through solitary engagements with the self.

Ironically, this description confirms the fears of moralists, who saw in novels and other imaginative works the source of social disorder. After all, we cannot know what went on in Madame de Chastenay's mind. We do not have access to her passions, her dreams, her erotic fantasies, or her desires. All that we know is that she did not desire her husband, a point that her daughter referenced, if rather obliquely, in her *Mémoires*. According to Victorine de Chastenay, "Maman's little taste for marriage" did not prevent her full involvement in the social and marital establishment of her children.[125]

Pleasure, for Madame de Chastenay, was therefore wholly autoerotic. Through her imagination, she was able to access carnal delight. But, as will become evident in the next chapter, such pleasure is never un-ambiguously experienced. For Madame de Chastenay, the pleasures of the imagination are fraught: "Please tell me sir, and prove to me that one cannot perish as a result of fear; that the imagination has never killed a single soul."[126] This statement, and, indeed the tormented nature of the letter as a whole, speaks to the contradictions inherent in the very idea of "imagination." As Mary McAlpin explains, "The term 'imagina-tion'… seems to be the closest equivalent in that period's lexicon to the Freudian unconscious, or it represented the mind's tendency to shoot off in undesirable directions in spite of the individual's best efforts to con-trol it. As such, it was the mental faculty that was the least connected to 'natural' sexuality, understood as desire instigated by the presence of a suitable partner."[127]

Madame de Chastenay's sexual agency rests on her insistence – not only over a period of several years but also with great frequency – on claiming sexual pleasure on her own terms and through her own body. One might even provocatively argue that her actions embody the poly-morphous sexuality articulated by Luce Irigaray in her foundational *This Sex Which Is Not One*. In a passage that evokes the sensuous-ness of both the imagination and the female body, Irigaray writes, "As for woman, she touches herself in and of herself without any need for mediation, and before there is any way to distinguish activity from pas-sivity. Woman 'touches herself' all the time, and moreover no one can forbid her to do so, for her genitals are formed of two lips in continu-ous contact. Thus, within herself, she is already two – but not divisible into one(s) – that caress each other."[128] But for women like Madame de Chastenay, such agency has been thwarted by the strictures placed on the practice by doctors like Tissot. As she indicates, she did not know what she was doing. In other words, her pleasure-seeking actions were, like those of numerous male onanists, blameless, the result of ignorance rather than of will.

However, having now acquired the knowledge gleaned from eating the forbidden fruit, Madame de Chastenay finds herself morally adrift. As a result, her imagination, previously a source of intimate pleasure, instead becomes a threatening entity, whose unruliness threatens to overwhelm her: "The idea comes to me that I will die immediately [and] if I am at the dinner table, I dare not eat anything further. Otherwise, I am ill at ease, and although I tell myself that I have had these thoughts 100,000 times, and nothing has come about, I am no less tormented … I have yet another concern which is perhaps better founded; and that is that I will go mad; because, ultimately, my thoughts are so very poorly reasoned and so unreasonable that my mind must be poorly organized."[129] Throughout her letter, Madame de Chastenay gives ample proof of her vivid imagination. But while this imagination fortified her early engagements with sexual pleasure, opening spaces of carnal delight in the otherwise barren terrain of her marital sexual relations, it is no longer a source of pleasure. Rather, it has become the foundation of her torment, even as she acknowledges that her fears have no basis in the reality that she is living.

Madame de Chastenay's troubles began after a conversation with her then four-year-old daughter: "She told me that she had dreamed that I was being placed into a hole."[130] The conversation appears to have shocked madame to such an extent that her thoughts took a turn towards the macabre. "I am almost always in a state of dying [*agonie*]," she writes. "And [although] persuaded that my health is good, I can still never be assured of my life for even fifteen minutes, because I constantly fear that my ideas, my thoughts [or] a conversation will cause me to experience a change that will kill me."[131] Thoughts of madness and death overwhelm her, interrupting even the most mundane daily activities.

Madame de Chastenay appears to be torn by the physical evidence of bodily health, on the one hand, and by a mind overcome with fears and useless rationalizations, on the other. This almost schizophrenic existence pits exterior against interior: "I offer myself beautiful rationalizations and I even tell myself that I am possessed of two different wills: one mad and the other rational."[132] Unlike Madame Roland, who constructed herself as "mistress of her imagination,"[133] Madame de Chastenay finds herself *subject to* her imagination. No longer in control of the pleasurable thoughts that occupied her younger years, she is instead prey to irrational thoughts that crowd her imagination, undermining her psychic being. Indeed, it is almost as if her youthful indiscretions have paved the way for imagination's ascendance.

Given this fraught self-positioning, is it at all possible for Madame de Chastenay to claim corporeal virtue? The structure and organization of Madame de Chastenay's letters might offer some insight into this. In the months following her original consultation with Tissot, Madame de Chastenay sent him two further letters updating him on her condition. Significantly, throughout the series of letters, Madame de Chastenay situates herself not primarily as an onanist but rather as a wife and mother. It is this domestic identity, in the form of her affectionate reference to her husband and children, that opens her first letter. Interestingly, it is also this identity that closes her second letter, where she cites her family's gratitude for Tissot's interventions: "My husband and my children offer you their sincere compliments."[134] So, too, do domestic concerns shape her interest in her health. As such, even as she details bodily occupations that should have wholly denied her access to the realms of corporeal citizenship, she couches these activities within a desire for health, a desire framed by an expressed interested in domestic virtue.

And yet, even this domestic identity is not unproblematic: Madame de Chastenay confesses that she should be "infinitely happy" as wife and mother, but she is desperately unhappy: "I lead an unhappy existence, when I should be infinitely happy. M. de Chastenay and my children lend sweetness to my inner life."[135] Can Madame de Chastenay realize her vision of domestic virtue? Can she move beyond her "unhappy existence"? Her vivid imagination – the source of her most intimate carnal pleasures – has also fundamentally destabilized the cohesion of her family. Nervous disorder, fuelled by a lengthy and inconsiderate engagement with the sensual pleasures of the imagination and the autoerotic pleasures of onanism, has corrupted her mental health, and in the process, the proper functioning of her family, all of whom are held hostage by her continued nervous sufferings.

Madame de Chastenay's letters demonstrate just how complex were the negotiations around questions of sexual pleasure and bodily agency. The individuals who contacted Tissot had to navigate social prescriptions and medical frameworks. They also had to live up to gendered expectations and family responsibilities. Furthermore, they needed to find productive ways to engage with the language and ideals of corporeal citizenship not only to elicit a positive reception with Tissot but also to resolve their own moral quandaries and to assert for themselves a positive, and virtuous, autobiographical subjectivity.

### RETURNING TO GAUTERON

> Conscience is the voice of the soul, the passions are the voice of the body. Is it strange that these voices often contradict each other? And then to which should we give heed?
>
> Rousseau, *Emile, or on Education*

But what, in the end, became of our afflicted hero, Gauteron? This was a question that nagged at me from the moment I first encountered his letters on my second trip to Lausanne. It is rare to find traces of these individuals beyond their encounters with Tissot. While aristocratic correspondents, like Madame de Chastenay may live forever in portraits or family trees, many others fall by the wayside, essentially lost to history, their voices only present in the letters to Tissot. But what might have become of individuals like Gauteron, our young man of learning?

Intriguingly, we find evidence of Gauteron's intellectual engagements in a number of publications dating from the late eighteenth and early nineteenth centuries. In 1787, five years before his first letter to Tissot, he was listed as a student at the Academy of Lausanne.[136] In 1795, he appears as one of three authors of a book of sentimental essays and commentaries on a variety of topics, from Swiss patriotism to the pleasures of the countryside, solitude, memory, consolation, and death.[137] Six years later, he is mentioned in Jean-Baptiste Pollin's evocative ode to *la vie champêtre, Le hameau de l'Agnelas*.[138] Here, Pollin paints a portrait of a man of extreme sensibility, a man who, perhaps unsurprisingly, takes pleasure in solitude, melancholy, the pleasures of the imagination, and the English spleen. Later, in 1808, Gauteron published a review of an agricultural fair at Hofwyl, near Berne.[139] More interesting still, however, was my discovery of a pair of letters Gauteron wrote to Philippe-Sirice Bridel in 1795 and 1807.[140] Bridel, a leading Calvinist luminary of the period, was a French pastor living in Basel at the time of Gauteron's first letter. By 1807, he had taken a more important position as pastor to the reformed souls of those living in the Montreux region of Switzerland. Posthumously, he is known less for his ministry than he is for his commitment to Swiss national identity. The author of a number of publications, Bridel advocated Swiss indigenous culture, championing what might be understood as bourgeois values: propriety, order, hard work, and frugality. The Swiss, Bridel argued, were a rural people, and this should be reflected in their national identity. Interestingly, these same ideals also shape Gauteron's publications.

Gauteron's 1795 letter is gathered together in a file that contains other letters addressed to Bridel that same year. His distinctive handwriting is easily recognizable. Also familiar in these letters is his style. Steeped in sensibility, this first letter to Bridel is very similar to that found in the letters to Tissot. While he makes no overt reference to the word itself, onanism lurks just below the surface, showing its morally reprehensible face in such words as "misfortune," "horror," "destruction," "fear," and "death." Indeed, this first letter is a letter of extreme moral disarray, revealing a young man experiencing suicidal thoughts and brought back only through the grace of a God who wants him to live: "I've seen it, this inexorable death, I've seen it from as close as one can get without becoming its victim, and like a tease, it didn't want anything from me except to keep its claws in those who would ask it to wait. For a long time I languished in an abyss of misfortune, and they … they told me that I was just trying to find reasons to speak of myself, to bring attention to myself, that I wanted to act as the hero of the novel, and they directed a thousand stupidities against me."[141] This maudlin engagement with his own misery, together with the annoyances of those who were subject to his complaints, also gives us other clues as to Gauteron's self-presentation. They suggest a committed engagement with the autoerotic specularity of life writing – that is, with the pleasures that one might access through telling, retelling, reworking, and re-thinking one's stories in and through different lenses and for different audiences. That Gauteron received some sort of narcissistic pleasure from his suffering, that he revelled in his shame, appears to have been a logical conclusion drawn by those around him.

By 1807, Gauteron was no longer a philosophy student. Instead, he was a pastor at a church in Tavanne, near Bienne, in Switzerland. Unlike the tortured missive he sent a dozen years previously, this letter is very different. This is not a letter of supplication; rather, it is a letter of profound appreciation. Gauteron writes that Bridel's words have had a profound impact on his life and that he has regularly drawn inspiration from Bridel's reply. So, too, does Gauteron blush when he thinks of what he dared to write and, further, when he is reminded of his other "reckless acts."[142] It turns out that Bridel has, in no small way, transformed Gauteron's life: "Together with Tissot, to whom I also found the strength to write during the same period and for the same reason (and in a tone that was likely very similar), you have been, through God's grace, the instrument that stopped me from following a career in the sciences, where I would have immediately damaged the tiny amount of debris which had escaped the drowning of my intellectual faculties, and put me on this path on which I should find my happiness by attaching myself to HE who reveals his glory and beneficence even through the smallest glass vessels created by his hands."[143] Looking back on his early years of excess, Gauteron now muses philosophically that it was good that he had suffered so much, for his sufferings taught him the lessons of unhappiness. From his current perspective, he is able to accept both his past and the uncertainty of the future by placing his trust entirely in God: "As long as my soul is united to this imperfect body I will no longer torment myself with the sins of the past or the uncertainties of the future ... Religion is the sole foundation of my happiness."[144] Gone is the torment. Gone are the struggles. Gone is the almost suicidal rhetoric. In its place is the peace of a true believer who puts his trust entirely in the hands of a supreme being. Health, in this sense, was not a physical state. Rather, Gauteron found healing in the grace of God, something that neither the intellectual climate nor the warm waters of Yverdon-les-Bains were able to offer.

Interesting, however, is Gauteron's reasoning: it is not his faith that has led him to this point; it is, rather, his suffering. Shame, in this sense, paved the way for redemption. The beneficent pleasures of divine grace were only possible through his sin: "It was good for me to have been thus afflicted; otherwise I would not have learned the lessons of evil, even as I imagined I could."[145] Ultimately, it is Gauteron's betraying, pleasure-seeking body that taught him the lessons he needed in order to follow his path to righteousness. Bodily shame, in this sense, powerfully experienced, worded, reworded, and reimagined through the specularity of all of his epistolary encounters, functions as the basis for spiritual pleasure and redemption.

What can we make of such letters? It is clear that the majority of Tissot's patients were fully aware that masturbation and various other crimes of the flesh were understood to be socially and morally unacceptable. And yet, at the same time, these letters reveal the extent to which illicit sexual activity was not only commonly practiced throughout this period but also enjoyed, regardless of Tissot's published views on the matter. Furthermore, such letters indicated that bodily pleasure was central to the correspondents' understandings of themselves as men and as citizens – that is, until a closer reading of Tissot's treatise disciplined them otherwise. These bodies had numerous stories to tell, stories that were variously experienced and variously understood. Finally, such letters suggest the extent to which the body itself actively sought out pleasure, even in the face of strong psychic resistance.

## CHAPTER SIX

# Neurographia: Writing Nervous Disorder

Please excuse the shape of my writing. When I am tormented by my sickness, I can find no expression nor anything enjoyable, and the character of my writing becomes completely unrecognizable.

Vauvilliers to Tissot, 15 May [1774][1]

For him, the moral affects the physical.

Unsigned to Tissot, [1776][2]

In May 1774, a man named Vauvilliers, secretary to Monsieur de Lamoignon, wrote a letter to Tissot.[3] In it, he touched on numerous topics, among them the challenges and annoyances of his current employment. However, he focused most intently on his nervous condition. Vauvilliers introduced himself as follows: "I am not quite thirty-five years old. I have a serious, melancholy and even somewhat savage temperament. I recall being quick to anger, although I am presently, either by reason or by study, at the point of appearing tranquil and moderate."[4] According to Vauvilliers, he enjoyed good health during childhood and into his adolescence. Things changed at the age of seventeen, when he witnessed a friend's sudden epileptic seizure. His horror at this sight was such that he experienced involuntary shivers throughout his body every time he encountered the "unfortunate victim of this cruel malady."[5] Even though Vauvilliers's friend later recovered, Vauvilliers found that he continued to experience the same corporeal reactions: "When I see only his hands; when one speaks his name to me, my whole body is affected by sharp involuntary trembling."[6] Since that time, things appear to have spiralled completely out of control. Vauvilliers suffers from vapours, vertigo, migraines, digestive problems, respiratory problems, and more. "I have," he concludes, "been reduced to a most sorry state."[7] Vauvilliers's extreme nervous sensibility and lively imagination have put him in a position of almost continual emotional and psychological terror. In the process, his body has become an instrument of this terror, his continued convulsions evidence of his mental anguish.

Vauvilliers's letter is one of many that treat a range of psychic and somatic experiences relevant to the broad category of nervous illness. From relatively vague experiences such as the vapours, to more specific concerns such as the trembling, migraines, digestive, and respiratory disorders that Vauvilliers recounts, nervous illness was a broad category that incorporated both psychic and somatic elements. In the case of nervous suffering, body and mind nurtured one another in what was, for some sufferers, a frenzy of uncontrollable bodily movements and psychic impulses.

Nervous disorder was ubiquitous among the European elite during this period. A "frothily fashionable"[8] disease, it tied doctor and patient into a complex, contradictory, intimate, and symbiotic relationship with one another. More importantly in relation to the conceptual interests that structure my study, nervous disorder also pushed at the limits of medical knowledge and, further, at the limits of understandings of corporeal citizenship and subjectivity. What role did nervous disorder play in the eighteenth-century social and cultural imaginary? How did the individuals who wrote to Tissot imagine the relationships between the vapours or nervous hypochondria with their tiresome but also seductive symptomatology, and the various convulsive disorders, potentially life-threatening and certainly life-altering states that appeared to undermine any notion of the human? At what point did sensibility, imagined by the Chevalier de Jaucourt in the *Encyclopédie* as a force for social good,[9] become a pathology? Furthermore, what happened at the point of no return – that is, at that tipping point when the vaporous individual actively in control of her or her bodily performance gave way to the convulsive individual, a monstrous entity seemingly controlled only by the irrational workings of a disordered body? These are the questions that have guided my work here.

The title for this chapter comes, most directly, from the work of Raymond Vieussens, a Montpellier-based anatomist active throughout the seventeenth century. Known for his work in cardiology, he also produced anatomical studies of the ear, the uterus, and the placenta. In 1675, he published *Neurographia universalis*, the first volume to express, in such a detailed way, the anatomy of the brain. In content and focus, it seems a fitting foil for the concerns I raise here. But I also titled this chapter "Neurographia" because the term points me in productive conceptual directions: neural writing and brain drawing. In this, I am indebted to the work of Sara Ahmed and Jackie Stacey, who, in their edited collection, *Thinking through the Skin*, point to the possibilities of "dermography" – that is, of not only writing *about* the skin, but of "think[ing] *with* or *through* the skin."[10] As they observe, "The word 'dermographia' is a medical term that means writing on, or marking, the skin. But here we use it to suggest that skin is itself also an effect of such marking … The skin is a writerly effect … Writing can [also] be thought of as skin, in the sense that what we write causes ripples and flows that 'skin us' into being; we write, we skin."[11] So, too, in this chapter, do I consider the possibility of neurographies, stories that take the brain as the basis for analysis, but also stories where the brain itself is the site of writing and imagining. In these letters, writing is intimately bound up with the imagination, the emotions, the nerves, the body – indeed, with all aspects of the brain and its workings. If, as Ahmed and Stacey argue, writing and the skin produce one another, so, too, in this chapter, do writing and the brain produce one another. Body and mind are deeply intertwined here, with the imagination, a central component of all writing, playing a key role linking them together.

This approach aligns itself with the broader conceptual concerns of this book as a whole, which, as I have also argued elsewhere, consider the body simultaneously as a surface to be written on and as a surface that writes itself.[12] As Michael Stolberg observes, the body is not only a text to be read but is "also a discrete entity which is ruled by laws of its own."[13] The Western philosophical imaginary has placed enormous value on the workings of the intellect; it is a capacity for reason and self-determination that defines the very category of human itself. These same capacities – reason, self-determination, individualism – also underpin notions of citizenship, as I have argued in Chapter 3. Notions of mapping, writing, and drawing the brain, therefore, appear to offer a productive entry point into understanding the human, and from there, the citizen.

Vieussens's work is part of a long trajectory of thinking and writing on the brain, a process that began with the intellectual musings of the Ancients and continues today. The brain remains one of the least understood of human organs but also, simultaneously, one of the most fascinating. The work of Norman Doidge, Oliver Sacks, and others has revealed to contemporary popular audiences the mysterious workings of the brain; the writings of Siri Hustvedt and Lauren Slater, meanwhile, point us to the limitations of language.[14] In its return to materialism, contemporary feminist theory, too, has turned toward the brain and brain science as productive sites of inquiry.[15] We are, then, it would seem, in the grips of a general neurography. Seeking to map neural stories, we are, ourselves, engaged in a sort of *neurographia universalis*: we map, we graph, we write the brain, in each iteration struggling to articulate its complexities and contradictions.

So, too, did those who wrote to Tissot struggle. For some, neurological disturbance was a prime site for self-fashioning, an ideal locus for the presentation of a sensitive, feeling, emotional, creative, and, above all, elite, self. For such individuals, nervous disorder was productive and generative, a site of agency and authority. In this form, it was a vehicle of sensibility, a social obligation, a social entrée, and a point of honour. It enhanced the presentation of a creative, sensitive, and imaginative self, and, as Tissot observes, it also provided sufferers with ways to manage the sometimes debilitating frenzy of elite social encounters: chronic melancholia was a justifiable reason to pull back from social obligations. But for others, nervous disorder was profoundly debilitating, not only to themselves but also to their families and to their communities. In these instances, nervous disorders, particularly when they manifested themselves in convulsions, were points of horror, states in which the unruly body took full control over the self.

I have argued elsewhere that corporeal understandings during this period might be viewed through a specular lens. I have suggested that the suffering body can be seen as a mirror that reflects and refracts images of the self.[16] Elite individuals were acutely aware of the performative power of their bodies and they harnessed this power in their correspondence with Tissot.[17] However, such corporeal mirrors are not always flattering. As the letter from Vauvilliers suggests, regarding the self through the lens of the other can be a discomfiting and uncomfortable experience. In this iteration, the convulsive, suffering body must be seen not only as spectacle – a reading manifest perhaps most evocatively in the case of the *Convulsionnaires de Saint-Médard* in Paris and the patients at Bethlem in London[18] – but also as *specular*, a spectacle, that is, that reflected the potential weaknesses of the self, and from there, the weaknesses of society as a whole.[19] As Roy Porter has observed of the patients at Bethlem hospital, "patients were meant to serve as object lessons, living exemplars to the penalties consequent upon vice and disorder."[20] This is abundantly evident in the letters addressed to Tissot, in which the witnessing of nervous illness, and particularly those sufferings that manifested themselves in convulsions, was as corporeally relevant as experiencing nervous disorder. In the words of Leigh Wetherall-Dickson, the act of witnessing was an integral part of the experience of melancholy, one form of nervous disorder: "Depressed states … can be looked at as a relationship between the individual and society, but also how society affects individuals and how they perceive themselves."[21] Nervous disorder, more than any other sufferings recounted in the letters to Tissot, must therefore be read through a social lens.[22] It can never be solely an individual experience. Furthermore, I would argue that nervous disorder is unique because it pushes at the limits of the cognitive self to such an extent that in numerous instances, its stories can only be told by those who are witness to, rather than suffering from, it. This uneasy and troubled relationship between performer and spectator – specifically, between the convulsive individual and the witness who records the events in letters to Tissot – is central to this chapter.

I use the term *neurographia* to capture the diversity of experiences within the broad category of neurological disorder, from what doctors imagined simply as hypochondria to those they recognized as dangerous pathological conditions, and from what individuals experienced as vapours to what they witnessed as convulsions. More specifically, I look at how correspondents mapped the workings of the brain, and I consider what these mappings might suggest about how they understood selves and subjectivities. I am particularly interested in the ways that the individuals who wrote to Tissot navigated questions of bodily citizenship in relation to nervous disorder. To what extent was nervous disorder productive, a site of creative agency in the articulation of the self? By contrast, to what extent was nervous disorder experienced and understood as a point of horror, the point at which meaning itself collapsed? Thus, while in previous chapters, we encountered instances where individuals wrestled with the unruliness of their bodies, here I introduce cases where the body itself takes over – that is, where it moves completely beyond the control of the mind. In these instances, autobiographical subjectivity emerges – as it does for Vauvilliers, whose experiences introduce this chapter – through the vicarious experiences of witnesses, whose own bodies and psyches take on the sufferings of others. Furthermore, as the letter from Vauvilliers indicates, nervous disorders tapped into deeply held social anxieties. Such anxieties, which included material and philosophical engagements with questions of lineage and inheritance, such as those found in Chapter 4, as well as individual concerns about madness, reflected larger scale demographic concerns linked with population health, broadly speaking, as well as economic concerns and the perceived political needs of the nation.[23]

Wetherall-Dickson has argued that autobiography is never solely about the articulation of an ideal self. As she writes, "If one aspect of autobiography is about definitions of the self, another is about elucidating the dangers to, and disturbance of, that self."[24] During the eighteenth century, nervous disorder came to be understood as an essential marker of identity; it was integral to the performance and presentation of the elite self throughout this period. On the one hand, nervous disorder was, at least among the elite, an accepted space for the performance of excess, an embodied manifestation of sensibility. On the other, however, nervous disorder tested the limits of discourses of sensibility, in the process highlighting the limitations of self-fashioning. There is, therefore, a continual vacillation between a productive and a pathological disorder and it is on this axis that this chapter turns. I begin this chapter by considering nervous disorder as an umbrella pathology and link the emergence of nervous disorder with sensibility and with notions of imagination. I then move into a discussion of its role and function as a fashionable disease and as a productive site for the staging of the self. From here, I turn from experience to witnessing, and move into an examination of convulsive disorders, including epilepsy. I consider in particular the specular function of the convulsive body, and the ways that this body tells corporeal autobiographies.

### IMAGINING NERVOUS ILLNESS

Nervous disorder, as an umbrella category, covered a vast terrain during the eighteenth century. A term that shifted in meaning in the course of this period, it came to include, at various points, not only such conventional diagnoses as the vapours, hypochondria, and hysteria, but also such conditions as spleen and melancholia as well as menstrual disorders, convulsive disorders, and epilepsy.[25] According to Elizabeth A. Williams, nervous disorder "included disruptions of virtually every bodily function, as well as a harrowing array of emotional and mental states."[26] Stolberg points out that "Almost any symptom in any body could now be attributed to the nerves, since, as Tissot noted 'the nerves are everywhere.'"[27] In other words, the whole body was up for grabs. This totalizing impulse had important psychic and somatic ramifications. On the one hand, nervous disorder offered numerous possibilities for self-fashioning, and in the guise of sensibility, also produced numerous social obligations. But, on the other hand, it also offered material opportunities for physicians, who were able not only to extend their professional reach and client base but also their social status through a conscious and concentrated focus on nervous disorder. Furthermore, imagining nervous disorder through the lens of medical pathology framed it as a social disease that had the capacity to undermine the population's health – and with it, political and ideological aspirations – at a grand level. Nervous disorder was thus inextricably linked with questions of corporeal citizenship.

Nervous sufferings manifested themselves in a broad range of symptoms. In the letters, sufferers and witness reference a wide array of ailments. At a corporeal level, these included headaches, digestive problems, respiratory problems, and convulsions. But correspondents also reference emotional suffering, citing such states as obstinacy, sorrow, disinterest, and, most prominently, fear.[28] Thus, the Chevalier de Valpergue, writing in July 1776, describes in detail his emotional character, physical sufferings, and his body history. He also recounts his dream states: "I do not sleep at all, or rather; my sleep is fitful, accompanied by terrifying dreams that wake me with a start and cause me considerable trouble."[29] Medical publications, too, referenced a wide range of possible symptoms, with individual authors promoting individual understandings and approaches. This broad lexicon suggests that while doctors themselves might have been, at least at an individual level, very precise about their understandings, it is entirely likely that readers would have come away with a much less coherent understanding of the medical implications and meanings of their sufferings. This broad symptomatology, what Wetherall-Dickson refers to as a "shared lexicon of symptoms," was common currency that could be drawn upon and then individually interpreted and deployed in performances of self.[30] However, an over consumption of medical treatises could not only lead to confusion, but it could also, as one correspondent notes, lead directly to hypochondria: "I take pleasure in reading medical texts [but] I have learned that this inclination, for those who do not do it systematically … was proof of hypochondriac condition."[31]

According to doctors and moralists alike, nervous disorder could be attributed to numerous causes. Michael Stolberg offers a concise overview of the presumptive causes of nervous disorders: "Lack of exercise,

overly spiced food, fashionable stimulants such as coffee, tea, chocolate, and tobacco, a reversal of the natural succession of sleeping and
waking through night-time festivities, constant erotic stimulation due
to intensive social contact between the sexes, the excitement of gam-
bling, the artificial stimulation of the imagination through music, novels
and drama, and innumerable other unnatural influences put the nervous
system in a state of continual tension and excitement and harmed the
entire organism."[32] Interesting in this overview is the role of the imagination in fostering nervous illness. Such an approach builds on Tissot's
arguments, which linked overindulgence in intellectual study and imaginative engagements with the inability to properly fulfill one's social
roles, but also, as noted in Chapters 4 and 5, on ideologies propagated
by Tissot's compatriot, Jean-Jacques Rousseau.

Equally interesting, however, is the direct causal link that many
doctors, including Tissot, drew between excessive living and nervous
disorder.[33] According to eighteenth-century doctors, moralists, and
commentators, Europe was "in the grip of a nervous epidemic."[34] The
extent of this epidemic – George Cheyne estimated that one-third of
the British population was suffering from it[35] – had potentially profound political implications. Nervous disorder could, if left unchecked,
undermine not only the health of the populace but also the strength and
power of the state.

Nervous suffering was framed as a particularly classed disorder that
ran rampant through the cities while sparing the "cruder nervous system[s]" of labourers and peasants in the countryside.[36] The definition
of "vapours," as found in the *Encyclopédie*, is bitingly apropos: "It is
worth noting that the vapours generally attack persons who are lazy
in body, who tire easily in the course of manual labour, but who think
and dream a lot: ambitious people who are enterprising, with a lively
mind, and strong lovers of the good things in life, men of letters, people
of quality, religious men, devout people, individuals weakened by debauchery or by too much concentration, lazy women who eat too much,
are some of the people subject to the vapours."[37]

Similar understandings lie at the heart of Tissot's medical-philoso-
phical vision as well. According to Antoinette Emch-Dériaz, Tissot
imagined his work on nervous disorders, which would later come to
include the *Traité de l'épilepsie* as well as four other published volumes
and numerous planned but unfinished chapters that remained unpublished, as an extension of ideas he first presented in *L'Onanisme*.[38] In

these works, Tissot outlined the anatomy of nervous disorder as well as its characteristics, its causes (both moral and physical), the range of possible treatments, and prognosis.[39]

At heart, Tissot understood nervous disorders as "lifestyle diseases," sufferings that arose from social malaise and from individual inabilities to moderate actions and behaviours in all aspects of their lives. Nervous disorder was a manifestation of excess – in diet, in sexual activity, in social engagements. Tissot felt that nervous disorder was occasioned by wilful neglect of healthful practices – namely, by the lifestyle of excessive indulgence practiced by the urban elite. In this, he was not alone. Tissot's admonishments echoed those of the medical generation that immediately preceded his own, including George Cheyne and Robert Whytt, both of whom pinpointed luxury and excess as foundational causes of nervous disorder.[40] Particularly intriguing in the critiques levelled by these doctors is the language they used. In his publications, Tissot draws on such words as "luxury" and "excess." Whytt, meanwhile, focuses on "strong desire" and Cheyne targets "those who fare daintily and live voluptuously."[41] Nervous suffering, then, is directly linked to sensual excesses. It is about pleasure, desire, voluptuousness and about an excessive engagement in the broader pleasures of the flesh – dietary, social, intellectual, and sexual. These ideas are already familiar to us in relation to the debates around onanism. Numerous scholars have also explored links with the pleasures of consumption.[42] In this way, the medical profession as a whole contributed actively to what Anne C. Vila has referred to as a "larger debate over the decadence of civilization."[43] Tissot's published oeuvre as a whole situates itself firmly within these debates: his quartet of writings on public health takes decadence as a central organizing factor and, in addition to this, reveals his interest in challenging and reimagining what constituted "civilization" during this period.

Tissot believed that nervous disorder could transcend generations: a psychically weak parent could later give birth to a psychically weak child. But this was not the only concern. Nervous disorder fundamentally compromised marriage prospects, and, from there, the continuation of the family name and line. A childhood diagnosis of nervous disorder, of any variety, was often understood as a death knell for the family line as a whole. Within this context, it is entirely unsurprising that a doctor writing on behalf of a twenty-two-year-old man with epilepsy refers to it as a "scourge of humanity."[44]

   TELLING THE FLESH

Nervous disorder manifested itself in both psychic and somatic ways. At a corporeal level, nervous disorder was often associated with digestive disorders and problems. Vila notes that philosophers such as Voltaire, Diderot, and others "seemed … to regard the Republic of Letters as an institution plagued with indigestion – both the metaphorical indigestions induced by the flood of books issuing forth from writers great and small, and the literal indigestion that torment those who indulged in high living, the pursuit of learning or both at once."[45] Indeed, Fredrik Albritton Jonsson points to the threat of what he terms "gastric rebellion" during this period: "During the eighteenth century, the stomachs of the British upper ranks threatened to turn on their owners and devour them from the inside."[46] This gastric excess is perhaps most clearly embodied in the person of Voltaire, a man whose imaginative capacity was seemingly fuelled by his extensive corporeal frailties.[47] As Vila observes, Voltaire "live[d] out the experience of his own, digestively troubled carnality."[48]

This notion of what Elizabeth A. Williams terms "psycho-gastric illness" later came to dominate medical understandings and underpins the medical philosophy of Philippe Pinel (1745–1826), the so-called father of modern psychiatry.[49] Although the work of Pinel is not directly relevant to this study, one aspect of his medical philosophy is worth considering. Pinel believed that hunger "was a fundamental cause of mania."[50] For Pinel, this hunger was literal; that is, it was a corporeal experience associated with inadequate material sustenance. But this formulation also suggests an alternative reading that might accord more directly with Tissot's corporeal vision. In this alternative reading, nervous disorder emerges as a form of mental hunger, a bodily manifestation of emotional distress in the face of a culture of indulgence and excess. Certainly, this reading appears to tie into the work of Roy Porter, who links mental distress with anxieties surrounding consumption, and to the observations of Fredrik Albritton Jonsson, who contends that "the elite stomach [was understood as] the symbolic stage for wider anxieties about the bodily causes of disorder … The vision of a corrupt and enfeebled elite threatened by mindless convulsions was performed by organs and vital fluids in a gastric drama which illuminated the precarious foundation of genteel authority in the uncertain mastery of the private body."[51] Hunger, in these instances, is not about nutritive sustenance. Rather, it is conceptual – the social hunger for a renewed, morally sound society. In the words of Michael Stolberg, "there is much evidence to suggest that the vapours and nervous complaints can similarly be understood in retrospect as an 'idiom of distress,' as a reaction to individual or collective trauma, fears, disappointments, or constraints. In fact, the patients themselves frequently attributed their diseases to what we would call emotional trauma or psychological distress."[52] In these iterations, psychic hunger fuelled bodily disorder.

Furthermore, while nervous disorders were occasioned by improper or immoderate lifestyles, they could also emerge, as Antoinette Emch-Dériaz notes, when there was a misalignment between social expectations and individual temperament.[53] Such a reading would accord with Elspeth Probyn's critical analysis of the concept of shame. Shame, Probyn observes, can manifest itself as bodily dis-ease; it is, she observes, "the body's sense of being out of place."[54] Thus shame is an embodied articulation of one's inability to reconcile the private self with the requirements of a social reality. Given the medical stigma that surrounded nervous disorder during this period, shame – in its iteration as "being out of place" – is worth considering.

The relationship between body and mind is thus integral to an understanding of nervous disorder during this period. Doctors and philosophers imagined the body as an interconnected web, with the veins and nerves serving as channels that connected all the disparate parts into a whole. Consider, for example, George Cheyne's evocative description, early in his influential 1733 publication, *The English Malady*. Cheyne writes that the human body is "a Machine of infinite Number and Variety of different Channels and Pipes, filled with various and different Liquors and Fluids, perpetually running, glideing or creeping forward, or returning backward, in a constant circle."[55] This description suggests an entity that is continually in motion, an efficient system of highways and feeder routes that move fluids and other products through the body. It is an image that resonates also with La Mettrie's *L'homme machine*, in which he describes the human body as a clock, an image later taken up by one of Tissot's correspondents as well.[56] Further, this imagery offers an intriguing counterpoint to Tissot's onanytic watchmaker, introduced in Chapter 5.

This conceptualization is also fundamental to the work of Denis Diderot, particularly as represented in *Le rêve de d'Alembert*. In an approach that rivals contemporary dynamic systems and entanglement theories,[57] Diderot posits the nervous system as an interconnected spider's web of threads, which "vibrate [and] transmit to the common centre a multitude of sensations often discordant, disconnected and muddled."[58] For Diderot, this interconnectivity was volatile: while sensibility animated the web, it could also undermine the social order. In the process, sensibility was transformed from a morally beneficent force that facilitated social cohesion into an out-of-control solipsistic behaviour that threatened the very social cohesion it was meant to support.[59] To follow Diderot's metaphor, if the web was not directed by the workings of a rational mind – that is, by the conscious engagements of the corporeal citizen – chaos could ensue. No longer was the spider in control of his web. Rather, it was "alerted, excited and darts here or there."[60]

In the words of Clark Lawlor, psyche and soma were "mutually interactive … disorders in one lead to disorders in the other."[61] Thus, just as a disordered body could lead to a disordered mind – as, for example, in the case of onanists, whose sufferings progressed from physical into mental sufferings – so, too, could a disordered mind, through an excessive engagement with the passions, lead to a disordered body. Fundamental to medical thought was the notion of symbiosis: body and mind were not disparate entities; rather, each informed the other.

Interestingly, this complex symbiotic relationship between mind and body might also be mapped onto the doctor–patient relationship during this period. In this relationship, one might imagine the physician as mind – as the entity that, through careful forethought and consideration, guided corporeal proceedings – and the patient as the body, the potentially unruly entity that, through decadent living, resisted containment. Such a reading would also accord with what Vila observes as the "veiled autobiographical quality" of Tissot's *De la santé des gens de lettres*.[62] Prior to this publication, Tissot was himself also subject to the symptoms of nervous disorder. Located at the juncture between bodily experience and professional practice, he bridged the mind/body divide.

This symbiotic relationship linked doctor and patient intimately with one another not only in relation to medical diagnosis and cure but also to the material practice of medicine itself. While Tissot and other doctors moralized extensively on the subjects of decadence, excess, and the dangers of high living, and while they often held suffering individuals personally responsible for their own nervous ailments, they also relied on those same suffering individuals for their own material wealth and well-being. Hypochondria, melancholia, the vapours, and convulsive disorders were lucrative, and numerous physicians profited handsomely from the epidemic. In addition to building international practices that drew clientele from around Europe and beyond, doctors like Tissot extended their medical reach through the publication of numerous works on the topic of nervous disorder. As Allan Ingram observes, they drew their social and political authority – their citizenship – from their overtly public commitment to the health and well-being of the populace as a whole. Not only were they the medical gatekeepers of sanity, they were also "pilot[s], steering the ship of state, or at least the ark of sanity, through the choppy waters of mental disorder to the safe harbor, soundness of mind, the sane haven of a clear brain."[63] In this way, physicians situated themselves firmly as Diderotian spiders in full control of ever-expanding webs.

But the elite, too, found themselves in a curious position. Their social status required an engagement with emotional sensibility and sensitivity. Sensual refinement, as numerous scholars have indicated, was a hallmark of elite identity. In the words of Fredrik Albritton Jonsson,

> For the established elite as well as the upwardly mobile sort, sensibility emerged as a new form of cultural capital ... Such sensibility justified moral and aesthetic judgment in the name of nervous superiority. Exquisite nerves not only magnified the power of the senses, but also increased the strength of the imagination and the moral sentiments. This superiority was properly demonstrated in bodily performances like embraces, tears, swooning, and olfactory sensitivity. The conceit of sensibility broadened the corporeal basis of the elite, offering the authority of nervous refinement as an alternative to aristocratic birth and blood. Indeed, it formed a cultural and literary code, elaborated in numerous genres ... These models of sensibility could be assimilated and performed by anyone with sufficient attention to its gestures and language as well as education, income, and leisure to sustain such social theatrics.[64]

From this perspective, even as Tissot took the elite to task for their inability to fulfill their social functions as role models for society, the elite themselves came to understand heightened psychic and somatic sensibility as intrinsic to the performance of elite identity. Put differently, nervous disorder was central to notions of elite corporeal citizenship. The elite individual manifested his or her social belonging through the performance of heightened sensibility.

Such a framing meant that elite identity – as performance – was fundamentally at odds with medical narratives. In other words, the performance of elite corporeal citizenship appeared to rest necessarily on a rejection of Tissot's vision of corporeal citizenship. These contradictions presented members of the elite with a curious paradox. On the one hand, the elite correspondent needed to understand nervous disorder as a productive site of self-fashioning. On the other hand, however, they had to engage with the pathologizing language of medical narratives. If they wanted to assert their right to be heard by Europe's most famous doctor, they had to understand their nervous sensibilities as fundamentally detrimental to their health. Thus, within the contours of this symbiotic relationship, Tissot's correspondents had to toe a fine line that required them to simultaneously perform and reject nervous disorder. Could they navigate this thorny, contradiction-filled space in such a way as to honour the foundational elements of their classed social identity while also acquiescing to established medical and philosophical opinions? Was it possible for them to play both sides of the equation?

It is obvious that numerous correspondents were aware of the need to tread carefully. Some found their allegiances divided as they sought to reconcile the oppositional requirements of social and medical corporeal citizenship. Thus, for example, young women, as members of the social elite, were expected to fully conform to the corporeal norms of their station; indeed, their membership in their social community demanded it. And yet these norms, which included quiet, docile, domestic lives with little exercise – consider a husband's belief that his wife's vaginal discharge increased after their marriage, possibly because she lived a sedentary life and stayed in bed too long[65] – simultaneously exiled young women from Tissot's corporeal vision, situating them instead as obstacles to social renewal.[66] As Antoinette Emch-Dériaz explains, "In the way young girls were raised, Tissot discerned the reasons for their subsequent nervous disorders. Their inactivity, be it physical, intellectual or sexual, led to hysteria or vapors, which for Tissot was hardly surprising as inactivity was not the norm of a healthy life."[67] In such letters, psychic disorder is often framed as being the result of social disorder.[68] Furthermore, as noted in Chapter 4, political machinations within elite families could provoke nervous disorder in family members slighted in the process. In this way, elite nervous identity was both innate to the elite condition *and* a product of elite moral disarray. In these iterations, psychic disorder was a manifestation of social disorder, an embodied response to moral and legal injustice.[69]

The body/mind symbiosis offers an attractive way of imagining doctor–patient relations and, further, of imagining the amorphous nature of relations of power within this relationship. But a return to Diderot's spider metaphor also allows something further: a consideration of the web as a whole. As noted previously, the Diderotian spider web can be a beneficent and balanced structure. However, it is also, as Diderot himself observed, prone to instability and corruption. Such webs were always threatened by the excesses of the individual threads that linked them together. If we take the physician-as-spider metaphor forward, then individual correspondents might be positioned as threads that both supported the power and authority of the spider, while simultaneously, through their moral and corporeal weaknesses, undermining the strength and cohesions of the web. Convulsions, tremblings, faintings, migraines, madness – each of these potentially undermined the structural integrity of the whole.

### FASHIONING THE NERVOUS SELF

I would readily agree with you, Sir, that there is something strange
about my situation, but of what are hypochondriacs not capable?

M. Gochuat to Tissot, 1 November 1785[70]

Nervous disorder as a social experience performed distinct functions. Among the elite, who were particularly predisposed to nervous suffering, these disorders could be alternately – and in the case of some sufferers, simultaneously – productive and disabling. Particularly interesting in relation to this chapter is the notion of the tipping point: at what point did beneficent moral sensibility – a corporeal stance that fostered social cohesion and articulated group membership – tip into something much more sinister, a possible fatal bodily disorder that was the result of what Foucault terms "falling ill from feeling too much"?[71] Stated differently, at what point did the corporeally beneficent citizen, who drew her inspiration and meaning from a productive engagement with sensibility, transform into a corporeal monster, a failed citizen whose excessive sensibilities not only undermined her health but also threatened the health and prosperity of society as a whole?

As a fashionable disease, nervous disorder marked the boundaries of elite identity. It could also be strategically deployed to manage the requirements of elite social life and was productive at the level of the imagination. Finally, nervous disorder could function as an effective site

     TELLING THE FLESH

of resistance. Many of the health concerns cited in previous chapters in relation to kinship and sexuality could also be read wholly under the rubric of nervous disorder as resistance; in other words, they represented corporeal responses to psychic distress.

As an iteration of elite identity, nervous disorder offered a somatic way of identifying the sensibilities of the truly elite. In the process, bodily weakness was reimagined as a site of aristocratic possibility and agency – as the articulation of a properly and appropriately sentimental self. Within this framework, nervous disorder, at least of the vaporous variety, was linked directly to notions of imagined community: it offered an ideal way to perform bodily citizenship and to enact one's membership within the community of the elite. As noted previously, the performance of nervous disorder also offered a unique opportunity to claim membership in the community of patients associated with Tissot, which was a vital social cachet. As a performative gesture, then, nervous disorder thus served to situate individuals within a specific social milieu and from there granted them an entrée into the benefits of this community.

As something understood to be integral to the elite condition, nervous disorder enabled individuals to manage the obligations of elite social life. Sabine Arnaud, Michael Stolberg, and others observe that nervous disorder could be strategically deployed. In other words, it can be productively understood as a social instrument that enabled individuals to both enact membership and to subtly disrupt the contours of normative social behaviours while still operating within them.[72] As Arnaud observes, "The vapours are a vehicle by which to pursue one's interests while observing society's conventions. They permit periodic departures from propriety while an appearance of conformity is maintained. The body therefore becomes a material that the vaporous sculpt to their benefit. They develop the vapours as a bodily discipline that can be used to please others, solicit attention, indicate preference, or command respect."[73] In this sense, the vapours could be an enabling rather than disabling experience that allowed individuals to manage the demands of elite social responsibility and obligation.

In the Tissot correspondence, this appears to be particularly true of women's complaints. Thus, while some women appear to have deployed nervous illness as a way of escaping the requirements of their class, gender, and social condition, others appeared to be suffering as a result of being deprived of necessary social engagements. Consider, for example, the case of a woman living in Turin. The correspondent, in this case her husband, situates his wife's suffering in relation to her social situation: "She is sweet, very sensitive, committed to her husband and strongly wedded to her domestic occupations, taking part – with pleasure – in upstanding diversions, enjoying the company of sensitive individuals and suffering from being located in an isolated place (and as a result, deprived of the company of refined and upstanding individuals)."[74] From this account, the correspondent's wife emerges as a model of exemplary elite femininity, a woman who was clearly committed to her gendered social positioning and thrived on the social obligations relevant to her position. Through this lens, social deprivation can be read as an underlying cause for her current emotional distress, which he defines as *chagrin* – grief, sorrow, or heartache.

Ironically, while Tissot's narrative engagement with nervous disorder, founded on notions of excess and indulgence, would suggest a body and mind that were out of control, an approach that takes into consideration the performative function of nervous disorder enables a very different reading. The successful performance of a vaporous subjectivity relies not on excess but rather on what Arnaud refers to as "an insistence on complete and continuous control over expressions."[75] Here, nervous disorder – as tool – required full mastery of the signs and symptoms, such that they could be effectively deployed in all social occasions, from the theatre to the boudoir. Indeed, nervous suffering was an ideal vehicle for the presentation of self.[76] This reading of the performative nature of nervous suffering fits within the broader spectrum of elite tools of social navigation, from the art of pleasing so central to etiquette treatises of the era, to treatises on epistolarity. Such tools were of particular relevance for elite women, who generally had much less social room to manoeuvre than their male counterparts. Careful and strategic social negotiations enabled women to more effectively and deftly navigate the power structures that limited their social spheres. Nervous disorder, in its manifestation as the vapours or hysteria, appeared to extend the discourse of normative femininity, allowing women to operate more strategically in their own best interests, even as they appeared to conform fully to gendered expectations of their social positioning.[77]

Nervous disorder was also productive at the level of the imagination. As Lawlor has observed, "Melancholy detached one from society just enough to liberate the imagination, and indeed body, from social constraints that might be inconvenient to the creative process."[78] The vapours could remove one from the potentially stultifying confines of social obligation, opening up a space for different iterations and articulations of the self. Nervous disorder was, as the letters to Tissot make clear, a chronic condition from which it was difficult to extricate oneself. But this chronicity did not necessarily limit the possibilities of self expression; in some cases, nervous suffering functioned as an ideal platform for the presentation of the creative, imaginative self: "Chronic diseases favour the development of thought and writing: dying of consumption or suffering from melancholy … might inspire a poet to compose a sonnet sequence … Melancholy's chronicity and the tendency to introspection and imaginative inspiration were a happy combination for the creative person. The 'story' of melancholy's progress as a disease process has its own characters or symptoms, if one can put it like that, but the time taken for melancholy to develop is a core element in the connection between literary-artistic people and this condition."[79] Monsieur Puihabilié, who wrote to Tissot in 1770, for example, appears to revel in his nervous disorder, actively claiming a hypochondriac condition as part of his identity.[80] Puihabilié, who is in full command of his senses – "understanding, judgement, imagination, memory" – for about two-thirds of every month, nevertheless finds himself overcome with nervous suffering at regular intervals:

Sometimes, and always when I am thinking about it the least, I find myself stopped suddenly in my tracks. I cannot understand, I cannot hear, so to speak. That which was easy in my eyes becomes a difficulty without equal; there's a darkness and an embarrassment in my ideas, a dryness of imagination, an aridity, nonsense … I cannot, strictly speaking, put four lines together. I search for the word, the thought, I erase, I return, and I finish by dropping everything with a sense of despair that, you can imagine, would strike someone who did not experience it continually. These episodes occur every eight, ten or twelve days: thus, there are four, five, or six days where I do not wish to be in the world. I sequester myself as much as possible. I bury myself and seek distraction in amusing or instructive books … but it is impossible to find. In vain, I also go to shows or on walks … everything displeases, worries, saddens and hurts me. Every time [this happens] it appears to me that this condition will last forever and that I will never recover.[81]

Finally, nervous disorder could manifest itself as a creative site of resistance. Thus, it offered a unique way to escape what some experienced as rigid social requirements. Consider, for example, the case of an anonymous woman. In her corporeal habits, this woman modeled the requirements of her station. At least at the outset, she offers the image of reproductive fecundity: she is the ideal mother and wife. The anonymous letter begins as follows: "Madame the patient is 40 years old, of a decent constitution, possessed of a sanguine temperament and a lively and sensitive character. Married at the age of 18, and mother to 14 children, which she had over a 17- or 18-year period."[82] In bodily history and background, this woman is an ideal corporeal citizen. Her body and mind appear healthy and her reproductive virtuosity – fourteen children in a seventeen- to eighteen-year period – is virtually without parallel in all the correspondence to Tissot. However, we soon learn this woman has suffered from a form of delirium for the past seven or eight years. The correspondent writes, "The delirium from which she has suffered since last November was preceded by … considerable worrying, agitations, sadness, moralizing, ennui, disobedience, and indifference to her environment, with the exception of those persons who should be most dear to her."[83] During this period this woman also became, in the words of the anonymous correspondent, intractable and furious.

Interesting here is the fact that this woman's sufferings appear to actively undermine her otherwise virtuoso performance of normative femininity through reproductive fecundity. In her delirium, she behaved in decidedly unfeminine ways: she was difficult, argumentative, intractable. There is, therefore, a slippage between the gendered corporeal virtue suggested by her fecundity and apparent good health, and the gender failures inherent her current mental state. Another reading would suggest that her emotional excesses appear to mirror, at a psychic level, her reproductive excess; that is, her fecundity is no longer a virtuoso performance of motherhood but rather it must be read as a first symptom of corporeal excess. In this framing corporeal citizenship has gone too far, a condition then mirrored in her delirium. After all, the delirium precludes her ability to perform her maternal virtuosity and, as a result, offers a form of resistance to otherwise accepted social and maternal obligations. In this way, psychic distress could, as Heather Meek has observed, highlight "the depressed social condition of eighteenth-century women – what Mary Wollstonecraft would term, in 1798, the 'wrongs of woman.'"[84] Given the prevalence of nervous disorder among elite women during this period, the condition might be understood under the rubric of what Lauren Berlant has articulated as "slow death" – "the physical wearing out of a population and the deterioration of a people that is nearly a defining condition of their experience and historical existence."[85]

In either reading, nervous illness appears to offer an escape from the continued obligations expected of this mother's social positioning. Indeed, this woman's reproductive virtuosity must be read not only through the number of children to which she gave birth but also through the time it took to sustain fourteen pregnancies and births. Until the onset of her delirium, Madame was almost continually pregnant. Might this delirium then be understood as an escape from these continued reproductive obligations? Does her agitation come from a desire to withdraw from the expectations of her social environment, a desire that manifests itself in the form of excessive nervous malady? In this reading, nervous illness can be seen as an act of resistance, a way of actively thwarting both corporeal and social expectations.

So, too, might we read another anonymous case through the mode of escape or resistance. An undated letter begins as follows: "On 16 February 1772 at 10 o'clock at night, my sister had, for the first time, one of those convulsive attacks that have so strongly alarmed us: her mouth was all askew, her arms akimbo, she expelled much saliva, and experienced a sort of suffocation, and completely lost consciousness. The 10th of April at 6 o'clock in the morning, the domestic servants imprudently all left at once to go to church. My sister, who perceived that she was alone, was overcome by fear; she threw herself from her bed and went to search for help at the other end of the apartment where she hoped to find someone. Having arrived at the salon, she was attacked by a second incident. A servant returned and found her unconscious on the floor."[86]

To those who were witness to her convulsions, this young woman's sufferings appeared to transform her into an almost unrecognizable creature: "She told me that she was clearly able to hear the prayers that were recited on her behalf, but that she was forced to cry out without any rational thought, just as a watch is forced to run so long as the spring is wound. She wanted to speak, but because her tongue was overcome, we heard only inarticulate sounds that resembled howls that continued until her convulsions became so violent that she lost consciousness."[87]

This description details common aspects of convulsions: howling, saliva, respiratory difficulties, bodily rigidity, and loss of consciousness. More intriguing are the observations regarding this young woman's moral character. At time of writing, this sufferer was unmarried and twenty years old, but she had a rigidity in her body that, to her sister's mind, was "uncommon to a woman who has been delicately raised … It seems to be that she would be less strong if she felt better. One cannot perceive, either in her arms or in any other part of her body ... that flexibility so natural to her sex and her age."[88] In other words, her bodily bearing – rigid, stiff, strong – undermined the expected requirements of normative femininity. At a fundamental level, she appeared incapable of performing the proper young woman.

Nervous disorder could also, as Clark Lawlor has observed, legitimate otherwise forbidden desires. Female sexual desire, for example, could be authorized in the venue of spiritual or religious melancholy. So too might the vapours announce a corporeally virtuous response to otherwise improper or aberrant desires. Thus, for example, Madame de Chastenay's previously cited mental distress occasioned by her onanytic habits, originally introduced in Chapter 5, might be read not only as a form of corporeal punishment for bodily sin but also as a form of repentance, an acknowledgement at a psychic level that the behaviour was not acceptable. In this reading, nervous disorder might be understood as a form of atonement and a gesture towards corporeal redemption. Furthermore, such an approach might also legitimate female textual agency. Melancholy, in other words, can authorize text and, further, authorize a desiring self.

The notion of illness as escape appears to function along specifically gendered lines; while nervous suffering was common to both men and women of the elite, it rarely appears to have functioned as a mode of escape for men; rather, it appears to be intimately linked with women. While the letters to Tissot offer an entry point into a particularly select group of correspondents and cannot, therefore, be read as the experiences of all individuals during this period, it is worth noting that the performance of illness appears to have been one of the more socially acceptable ways for women to retreat from the gendered requirements of their social station.

### HORROR

The most terrifying illnesses are those perceived not just as lethal but as dehumanizing, literally so.

Susan Sontag, *AIDS and Its Metaphors*

While nervous disorder was productively deployed in the performance of mental and bodily sensibility, it could also, as numerous scholars have observed, transform itself into a dangerous pathology that not only undermined the health and well-being of the individual but also of the family and, from there, society as a whole. In this reading, nervous disorder must be understood as a form of social horror, a monstrous disease that threatened the very nature of the human itself. In 1769, Madame Chevallier de Bouchet contacted Tissot on behalf of her son, a twenty-eight-year-old man "suspected" of having epilepsy. This individual appears to have experienced a relatively disease-free childhood. Apart from a bout of smallpox at the age of ten, from which he recovered fully (and which left no physical marks on his body), he was healthy. His mother acknowledged that he was born with a delicate constitution but also notes that he was nursed by a "strong and healthy woman."[89] The problems began when he was a teenager. He began experiencing convulsions, which were diagnosed as nervous disorder, at the age of fourteen or fifteen. Interestingly, this young man did not lose consciousness during his seizures. Rather, his mother states that "he appeared, on the contrary, stronger than usual during his episodes of convulsion. He spoke and was fully conscious."[90] However, as the years progressed, the seizures became both more frequent and more violent, such that the young man was now experiencing "trembling, convulsions, flushing, and finally paleness [all of which] followed one after another in succession. His eyes were fixed and open, he lost consciousness entirely."[91]

To what might we attribute this acceleration of symptoms? Madame Chevallier de Bouchet hints at some possible causes. It seems that her son had not lived a completely blameless life. As a mathematics student in Paris, he studied hard, thus, perhaps, falling victim to the various problems that Tissot outlines in his *De la santé des gens de lettres*. It was during this time that he was first diagnosed as epileptic. But the worst was yet to come. Following his studies he entered into military service where, "left to his own devices (and those of his peers) and although born with a sweet and moderate temperament, he abandoned himself to every excess of youth: wine, liqueurs, coffee, late nights and, above all, women."[92] Although he returned to a more regulated life, his convulsive episodes continued, and with greater frequency and violence than before. No longer did they appear to make him stronger; rather, they transformed him into an insensible being devoid of both reason and consciousness. The convulsions also transformed his emotional state. Madame Chevallier de Bouchet indicates that her son "is strongly affected, either by pain or by pleasure, a sentiment to which he has become particularly susceptible since his illness."[93]

As this consultation suggests, epilepsy, or presumed epilepsy, was fearsome in its presentation. This convulsive disorder undermined all accepted notions of what it meant to be human, what it meant to be a citizen. This young man was not the ideal citizen envisaged by Aristotle. Rather, during his seizures, he was grotesque, monstrous – a being that displayed the inner torment of the suffering body. In her letter, Madame Chevallier de Bouchet articulates the Dr Jekyll and Mr Hyde character of epilepsy. While her son was, at heart, a gentle, happy, tranquil man of moderation, his seizures transformed him into another creature entirely: no longer fully human, his eyes were fixed, his body rigid. His whole being was taken over with trembling and convulsions, and during these periods, he was pale and thin.

This letter tells us a considerable amount about morality, horror, and fear. At issue is not only the convulsive suffering itself but the larger context in which that suffering takes place: the health of the individual is deeply intertwined with the health of the family and the community as a whole. So, too, is it a reflection of the individual's perceived moral agency and authority. What happens when nervous disorder goes too far – that is, when the fashionable sufferings of the vaporous elite turn into the violent, irrational thrashings of a convulsive creature? At what point does sensibility become pathology? How is autobiographical sub-jectivity understood in the apparent absence of rational thought? What might this mean for notions of corporeal citizenship?

The turn towards convulsions and seizures, episodes in which suffering individuals appear to have lost full control of their psychic and somatic functions, appears to have been understood by many correspondents as a point of no return. Convulsive disorders, which included, but were not exclusive to, epilepsy, provoked fearful responses from concerned family members and friends. But what might it have been that provoked this level of horror?

Fashionable performances of nervous suffering relied on the narrative agency of the sufferer; that is, suffering individuals were understood to be in complete control of their bodily performances. But for convul-sive individuals, narrative agency shifted. No longer was the individ-ual in control of the body; rather, the body had come to control the performance. This process consequently transformed the conventional relationship between sufferer and society, performer and audience. Where fashionable disorder accorded performative agency and author-ity to sufferers, convulsive horror required the narrative intervention of observers. Indeed, the traditional relationship between observer and observed is, in this iteration, completely inverted. While the hypochondriacs or vaporous individuals could still observe and comment on their own bodies, witnesses to convulsive episodes were put in the position of narrating the meanings of a body beset by actions that were, unlike their own performances of sensibility and hypochondriacal excess, unintentional. Put more simply, the elite hypochondriac was suffering but still in control of his psychic and somatic narrative. The convulsive individual, however, no longer had the capacity to tell her own story. Narrative control shifted from sufferer to observer. Important here is the transition from corporeal citizenship as performed and embodied as an act of individual agency to corporeal witness, the observation of corporeal distress and the effect of this distress on the subjectivity of the witness.

This conceptual shift in focus from performer to audience cannot be underestimated. Indeed, it powerfully undermines conventional understandings of citizenship, which rely on the notion of the individual human agent, a rational, autonomous individual capable of acting on his or her own behalf. Such narratives also push up against Tissot's understandings of corporeal citizenship: while Tissot insisted on the role of the body in the performance of citizenship, he also insisted strongly on the careful moderation of that body – that is, on the active role of a sound, healthy, rational, and reasoned mind in the management of bodily behaviours. Central to the act of corporeal witnessing is the witness's encounter with an uncomfortable truth: the convulsing body undermined the authority of the mind in the construction of the self. Instead, the unruliness of the convulsive body asserted the body as an agent in its own right. In the process, convulsive individuals, through the apparently involuntary thrashings of their bodies, challenged the accepted social order at a fundamental level. In these episodes, agency appears to be enacted through the body alone. The rational self appears to have had no say in the proceedings at all.

The case of the Comtesse de Non, first introduced in the previous chapter, offers an exemplary instance of this process.[94] According to her husband, the countess lived a sedentary life, like most women of her social station and condition. Mother to five children, but nurse to none, she had been experiencing the vapours for the past three years. These sufferings, which appear to have emerged after a miscarriage that preceded the birth of her fifth child, were considerable. At the time of writing, the countess suffered from weakened health and had fallen into a deep melancholy. The Comtesse de Non's melancholy manifested itself in profoundly somatic ways. In addition to experiencing a loss of appetite and suffering from an inability to support her body weight, she also suffered from vertigo, yawning, a bad taste in her mouth, a dry tongue, teeth grinding, dry skin, a continual chill, swelling in her legs, numbness in her arms and fingers, constipation, and impaired vision. Indeed, her whole body appears to have become a site of nervous sensibility, to the extent that "the smallest disagreeable sound, the friction of certain bodies, like that of a body against silk fabric, [or] a fork that slides awkwardly on a plate, excited in her an unbearable feeling."[95] In this particular instance, the nervous disorder appears to have manifested itself as a response to emotional grief: the stillbirth of a child. For the Comtesse de Non, sensibility moved beyond the purely fashionable and into a form of dangerous pathology. What might have begun as a corporeal experience of grief following a stillbirth instead progressed into a state of nervous agony. Nervous suffering affected almost all parts of this suffering woman's body: her limbs, her skin, her tongue, her vision, her mind. Her body, both inside and out, was overwhelmed by its senses.[96]

A convulsive body also challenged the performative underpinnings of nervous disorder. If, as Arnaud has suggested, nervous suffering could be understood as a form of extreme body mastery, a conscious marshalling of the signs, then the fully convulsive body would appear to be a grotesque inversion of this process, a monstrous parody or mockery that undermined the very nature of elite self-fashioning.

We should not underestimate the mirroring imperative so central to elite social relations during this period. If the elite self was understood, as conduct books of the time asserted, as a mirror that reflected the beauty of the social order, then the convulsive self – a body in turmoil – reflected not the beauty and moral rightness of the social order but rather a fundamentally disordered social space. In other words, elite convulsive bodies were specular entities that embodied, in their monstrous performances, the rotten and diseased core of elite society, and, in the process, also confirmed Tissot's suspicions about the elite. These acts of corporeal witnessing were, therefore, fraught. While observers wanted to accurately recount the details of the episodes they witnessed, this witnessing was also, by its very nature, profoundly autobiographical. That is, in witnessing the sufferings of others, they also, as Vauvilliers's letter suggests, bore witness to their own mental and corporeal weaknesses. Convulsive bodies were spectacles whose thrashing limbs, rolling eyes, and subhuman vocalizations displayed their corporeal instability. Such spectacles were simultaneously fascinating and repellent, provoking curiosity and fear in equal parts. The *Convulsion-naires de St Médard*, for example, were so popular that one could rent chairs to watch them convulsing in public. But they also simultaneously sparked fear and concern about the possibility of an epidemic.[97] So, too, might we consider the case of four siblings who succumbed, one after the other, to a trembling disorder in a process that seems to suggest the possibility of convulsive contagion.[98]

Unruly, convulsing bodies, as both specular and spectacular, challenged notions of citizenship. Not only were they suggestive of a lack of control and a social undoing, but they also gestured towards the notion of a compromised self, a self not only beholden to but *captive* to the will of a recalcitrant and otherwise resistant body. Furthermore, they challenged the very notion of Enlightenment itself. In the words of Roy Porter, "Why had the progress of civilization apparently led to the increase of mental instability and suicide?"[99] Consider, for example, the following two descriptions of convulsions, as penned by witnesses:

> Finally, a few weeks later, while sleeping with a younger sister in her mother's room, one morning before daybreak, the mother heard an extreme commotion in her daughters' bed. She got up and found her eldest with her eyes closed, in some sort of a trance, so heavy that she could never have placed her daughter's head on the pillow; [the mother] called out with loud cries, believing that this was some form of apoplexy, when the young person was returned to herself. She could not speak, having cut her tongue against her teeth.[100]

> I saw him during one of his episodes. [The episode] came as quickly as it left. The convulsions pass through and across the face. The right side was trembling with rapid movements … he did not lose consciousness because he could tell me what happened during the episode. [But] when he wanted to start speaking, he was completely unable to shape the words. After the episode, his right side remained paralysed for a few minutes, and then the warmth, strength and movement returned and he spoke as if he had had no episode at all.[101]

Each of these examples details bodily behaviours that challenge notions of the human: stiff limbs and facial features, a sleep-like trance from which it is difficult to wake; excessive, almost animal-like saliva production; and teeth gnashing to the point of serious tongue injury. Such descriptions are common in letters dealing with nervous, convulsive, or epileptic disorders. The witness observes a body that completely defies rational principles: it trembles and it stiffens; individuals are unable to speak, their own voices strangled in a body that resists rational impulses. These were not genteel members of the elite; rather, they were monstrous creatures whose behaviours fully exceeded the human.

Convulsions could, in some instances, completely undermine any possible notion of corporeal citizenship. The following example, detailing the sufferings of a seventeen-and-a-half-year-old girl, is particularly evocative: "On the 17th of June ... while seated next to a table where she was working with a young *demoiselle*, she suddenly lost consciousness, her eyes rolled and she fell to the ground, her limbs clenched stiffly ... Her face became purplish red in colour, her lips swelled, [and] she was in this state for several minutes ... She spewed globules of thick saliva. At the end of the convulsion, she had heart palpitations and vomited worms."[102] This description is vivid and horrifying. Throughout the convulsive episode, this young woman – otherwise a vision of appropriate femininity working quietly at a table with another young woman – loses all connections with the feminine; indeed, she loses all connections with the human. Instead, with her purple face, her swollen, saliva-spewing lips and her rolling eyes, she is presented as a monster. The *coup de grâce* is the expulsion of worms from the inside of the body. No longer associated with the virtuous propriety of normative femininity, this woman's violent, convulsing, worm-filled body instead evokes comparisons to the mythical Medusa.

For many of those who wrote to Tissot, moral agency appears to derive from an engagement with the will, a notion central to the idea of the rational, self-actualizing citizen. So, too, was the notion of the will central to public health discourses during this period. Health, according to physicians like Tissot, was the result of the active engagements of a rational, self-actualizing subject in bodily practices of moderation and balance undertaken in order to ensure good health. Corporeal failure, then, could be imputed to a lack of will, a reading that places moral blame directly on the shoulders of sufferers, a notion I have discussed earlier in this book.

But convulsive disorders like epilepsy could challenge the very notion of the will. Seizures were not the actions of men of reason or will; rather, they operated wholly outside accepted norms of bodily behaviour. Thus, in seeking to favourably present the sufferings of family or community members, correspondents engaged in sometimes complex manoeuvres to assure the moral agency of the sufferers. Convulsive disorders were, therefore, particularly challenging to navigate within discourses of corporeal citizenship. For many individuals, convulsions had no apparent moral or physical cause. Correspondents needed to assert the credibility of the suffering they witnessed while also assuring the corporeal virtue of the suffering individuals. In this regard, we might consider the following narrative, penned on behalf of a suffering grocer: "There is a man in my district who has been attacked by some sort of illness. This man is 41 years old, [has been] married 15 years, [and is the] father of 4 children. [He] has not been ill since childhood. It's been about 12 years since he was [first] attacked by the *mal*. He is a grocer by profession. The first time he perceived this malady he was working all night at his job. The next morning he had a small dispute with his neighbour, who made him angry, and he fell unconscious to the ground."[103] Interesting here is the tension between the perceived moral virtue of the grocer and his bodily disarray. According to the narrator, this grocer was a committed father and husband (as evidenced by his long marriage and reproductive fecundity) who worked hard at his profession. He had been "working all night at his job." He was, then, in all respects, a virtuous corporeal citizen whose sufferings emerged only after a small disagreement with a neighbour. This representation serves simultaneously to situate the grocer as a moral agent and to externalize the convulsive sufferings. If the suffering did not inhere in the grocer's being, then his moral virtue – the basis of his corporeal citizenship – remained intact, even in the face of bodily disorder. While the body appears to have lost control of itself, the person as moral agent was unblemished.[104]

So, too, does an anonymous correspondent reflect on the convulsive behaviours of an eleven-year-old boy: "the word *convulsive* is possibly incorrect to explain movements that are not directed by the will, because they sometimes occur at night while sleeping … and too often to be nature. But they are not enough nor violent enough nor of the necessary activity to qualify as convulsions: they are not accompanied by a loss of consciousness or *alienation d'esprit*."[105] Interesting here are the apparent connections this correspondent makes between the will and notions of sleep and wakefulness. Thus, the will is associated with a state of alertness. Lack of will, meanwhile, is associated with sleep, a state in which the rational mind is not necessarily in control of bodily behaviours. While these erratic movements, which the correspondent hesitates to categorize as true convulsions, could suggest a compromised corporeal citizen, the fact that they occur during sleep and are not easily defined, offers a different conclusion: as with the previous example, the suffering individual is an unfortunate victim of a disordered body. His moral core – his corporeal citizenship – remains intact.

However, the convulsing body, like the pox-filled face of the syphilitic individual, could also function as irrefutable proof of moral disarray. The case of a thirty-six-year-old man whose seizures appear to be linked to his sexual behaviour offers some insight into this.[106] The correspondent, Dr Sidenier, writes that this man contracted venereal gonorrhoea at the age of eighteen. Two further episodes, both the result of "*un commerce impur*," followed. According to the correspondent, these immoderate and poorly considered actions had consequences: "the patient was surprised, immediately after intercourse, by his first epileptic seizure."[107] While this attack was short, lasting just fifteen minutes, the next one – at twelve hours in length – was much more extensive. The descriptions travel well-traversed territory: "a loss of consciousness and of memory, an inflamed face almost purple in colour, rigidity in all limbs, foaming at the mouth and clenching the jaw so tightly that the tongue was wounded."[108] This particular case offers some insight into the nature and meanings accorded to moral weakness. For some sufferers, convulsions appear to be the result of immoderate behaviours. In such instances, it is possible that convulsions were read as corporeal manifestations – and public corporeal manifestations, at that – of corporeal excess. In this way, convulsions exiled such individuals from the possibilities of corporeal citizenship.

These diverse examples suggest that convulsive disorders challenged conventional understandings. If, as doctors and moralists suggested, health was the result of individual responsibilization – that is, if it was the result of the individual's active engagement with moderation – then those who lived lives of moderation, controlled their animal and visceral tendencies, and committed themselves to living responsibly, could expect to live healthy, fulfilled lives, their psychic and somatic health a testament to their civic virtue. However, bodies did not always comply with such directives. One girl was raised with great care, and with great ease, and grew into a strong young woman who "enjoyed the most perfect health."[109] She and her parents were equally engaged with her development, with the written consultation making reference both to a mutually agreed upon educational plan and a convent education. This family background suggests thoughtful and considered parenting,

　TELLING THE FLESH

a performance of maternal and paternal corporeal citizenship embodied in the health of a strong young woman. However, at the age of thirteen, her body began to display traits that did not reflect this careful upbringing. Her first episode – a short episode of fainting – had no discernible cause whatsoever, and her sufferings only continued. While one doctor suggested menstrual irregularity as a cause, the other, less hopeful, diagnosed her sufferings, which also included a flushed face followed by extreme paleness, a body that appeared to swell up, and a dilated oesophagus, as epilepsy.

What were eighteenth-century individuals to make of such experiences? Letters such as these make it clear that illnesses could not all be blamed on individual excesses or mistakes. How, then, was one to understand or work with illness? What could one do? How could they reconcile the promise of health with the reality of suffering? And on whom could they lay the blame for apparent corporeal failures? Not only did this girl's convulsive body undermine any parental claims to corporeal virtue, but it also undermined the pronouncements of medical authorities such as Tissot, whose works proclaimed the health benefits of moderation, who all but promised that good health would naturally follow from a commitment to the principles laid out in his books. Claire Colebrook has observed that "the living of one's self requires that one be a subject."[110] Neurographia, the writing of nervous disorder, fundamentally challenges the boundaries of the human and the boundaries of the citizen subject. In the Epilogue, I interrogate these limits and consider critically the limitations of storytelling, citizenship, and the self.

# The Limits of Storytelling

As long as we are able to label others as post-persons, however, we can whisper to each other and to ourselves that, at least for now, we remain human.

James Overboe, "Ableist Limits on Self-narration: The Concept of Post-Personhood"

How does one know what is normal? Is normality … simply a matter of what the majority thinks it is? And is to depart from that normality therefore inevitably to attract a definition of madness?

Allan Ingram, "Deciphering Difference: A Study in Medical Literacy"

In *The Still Point of the Turning World*, Emily Rapp's 2013 memoir of loving and losing her young son, Ronan, who suffered from Tay-Sachs Disease, Rapp writes,

An elaborate taxonomy of transformation exists in our culture. Change your body, change your life, take charge of your financial future, stop wrinkles. Americans are driven by future-directed resolutions. We thrive on the idea of change, the business of ambition … But Ronan would never speak, or write, or do much with his hands besides spin the little lizard inside the plastic egg on his bouncer, turn the pages of a soft book and bat the chimes of his dragon toy. He had, literally, no future. How did we understand the meaning and purpose of Ronan's life in a society – like most societies – that was dedicated to progress and achievement, where going back was synonymous with failure? Where the longer life was seen as the more successful one, the one worth fighting for? If you were unable to tell your own story, did it mean you didn't have one to tell?[1]

What does it mean to have no future? What does it mean to have no story? Where does the citizen – the human – reside, if not in the stories that she tells? And in a storytelling world, what does it mean for those of us who have stories to tell to be confronted by the horror of silence? How do we make meaning when the stories we encounter don't fit the narrative structures we have put in place for them? When they are opaque? Resistant? When they are not really stories at all? What do we do in the face of absence?

It seems to me that many of the correspondents who wrote to Tissot did so out of a desire for an audience – out of a desire to tell their story and to have that story heard. Telling their stories made their sufferings real, moving them from the realm of personal experience into a shared communal space. Telling their stories allowed them membership in an imagined community of sufferers, all seeking succour, empathy, understanding, healing. But bodily storytelling also did something more: it allowed them access to a privileged space of bodily citizenship; it moved them into the realm occupied by Europe's most famous physician.

But among the archival materials in the Fonds Tissot are also, as we have seen, many letters from those incapable of telling their own stories, letters from family members, doctors, and other observers detailing the irrational and unruly bodily behaviours of those under their care. These are stories of profound psychic distress, madness, and cognitive impairment, what Tissot and other doctors term variously as *folie*, *imbécilité*, *hystérie*, *fureur*. These are stories that do not – and cannot – follow conventional patterns. They resist easy telling. They confound. They disturb. They challenge. In many cases, these are stories with no futures. In their telling, we, as readers are forced to confront the limitations of narrative as a vehicle for the telling of selves. In these stories, it is only the body that remains, only the body that tells stories at all. But in this uncharted space, we come to terms with our inability to grasp bodily meanings, and from there, the meanings of the lives shaped by such bodily workings. How, indeed, do we understand the meaning and purpose of lives like these? What stories do they tell? And how might they trouble the very notion of citizenship – and the human – itself?

In the vast majority of documents addressed to Tissot, the voices of the sick and suffering are readily available. Even in letters penned by family members, community members, or doctors, the suffering individual's perspective is usually quite clearly discernible. These are patients who speak, letter writers who listen, and body stories that can, then, enter relatively easily into language. As distinctive forms of life writing, such letters can, as I have argued throughout this book, be seen as conscious iterations of the self during an era increasingly interested and intrigued by the possibilities of self-revelation and confession. Furthermore, as articulations of the self, these letters offer insight not only into the experience of illness and suffering but into broader philosophical questions about what it means to write, what it means to claim a voice, what it means to be a citizen, what it means to be human. In other words, such letters support my arguments about the relationships between letters, bodies, lives, and claims to citizenship.

But the letters about cognitive impairment and mental derangement stop me in my tracks. My usual conceptual and methodological tools fail and I am forced to rethink my arguments. In a world that values stories, what happens to those who cannot, for whatever reason, tell them? And further, what happens to questions of citizenship, justice, and politics when these terms exclude the very terms they were designed to include? In Chapter 6, I explored the realm of nervous suffering, considering the relationships between the vapours – a form of suffering predicated on the sufferer's complete control of his or her bodily performance – and convulsive disorders – sufferings in which the body itself took centre stage. In this Epilogue, I take this further to consider the limitations of corporeal storytelling. In it, I take seriously the concerns raised by Susanna Egan regarding the limitations of storytelling: "If creating and rehearsing and developing one's own story is so crucial to self or identity, then must we assume that [those who cannot tell their own stories] have no selves?"[2] If our world is made up of stories, then what happens to those who have no stories to tell, or to those who are incapable of telling their stories? Does this mean, as Egan queries, "that such people have no selves"? Or is it, rather, that we may need to learn to listen differently, to imagine different stories, with different outcomes?

The conceptual quandary that lurks just beneath the surface of this study as a whole has been productively articulated by Peter Cryle: "What is a knowledge of the body other than an aggregation of perceptions mediated by language? How can we refer to the flesh without doing it in words?"[3] There is, indeed, an almost insurmountable divide between body and text, a chasm that may be impossible to traverse. Does the body exist at all without language? And if it doesn't, what might that mean for the whole concept of bodily subjectivity? Is it even possible to consider the body as an agentive entity busy with its own projects? I am somewhat comforted by Egan's words: "I note that the

   TELLING THE FLESH

word 'corpus' refers both to the human body and to a body of work."[4] For Egan, there is a symbiotic relationship between the two: body and text are inextricably intertwined; what is of interest is not the separation that divides lived identity from textual identity but rather the relationship that unifies the two. And yet, I find such an argument ultimately unfulfilling. While it neatly extracts me from my initial quandary, I am left with another: If bodies and selves and lives and texts are linked, then what happens when that linkage is broken? That is, what happens to the stories of those who cannot write? What happens to those whose bodies overwhelm their narrative capacities, those for whom the body and its workings are the only stories that remain? This is a question that has been central to those working on the ethics of life writing, and it is one that also runs through this book: If lives are stories, and stories are the basis for selfhood, does that mean that those who have no stories have no claim to selfhood? Where is political agency – citizenship – located if not in the stories we tell about ourselves? Such questions gesture towards the very limits of storytelling, suggesting the possibility that some stories can never be told and, as a result, that some selves must remain eternally compromised.

In this Epilogue, I consider the limits of storytelling and, with them, the limits of the human. If, as Aristotle observed, the citizen and the human are fundamentally interwoven, then what does this mean for the question of bodily citizenship? Ultimately, I argue that it is not citizenship that is the problem but rather that it is our dependence on language, which I understand here as words, phrases, and sentences organized into normative patterns, that makes this project impossible. Returning to Carol Bacchi and Chris Beasley's notion of "social flesh," I gesture towards the possibility of imagining language otherwise – that is, of moving towards a framework that acknowledges that the fracturing of the self, usually approached with horror, might be productively reimagined using a geographical lens: fractures break, but in their breaking, they reveal new knowledge.

## ARCHIVAL LIMITS: TEARS, INVOLUNTARY LAUGHTER, AGITATION, AND SONG

There are numerous stories of mental derangement and cognitive impairment in the correspondence. Desperate letters from parents whose children appeared to develop normally only to regress into a form of imbecility.[5] Letters from spouses.[6] Letters from doctors and others cataloguing, in detail, the bodily symptoms of madness.[7] Each of these letters reveals the limits of the human. In so doing they highlight the vulnerability of the very category of the human, the point at which the concept itself disintegrates. What remains for those who are witness to the seemingly insensible babbling, jerking bodily movements, sighs, tears, and disturbing laughter of their family members and friends? How do we make any sense at all of their stories? Put more simply, what do we do with cases such as these?

I am, in this epilogue, interested in questions of speech, language, and discourse – that is, in examining how it is that the body comes into language, and what this might mean for research into selves and identities that exist *beyond* language. In other words, I want to understand the performance of the autobiographical self in the cases where the body's narrative is *all* that we have available to us. This is, therefore, not just to follow ideas put forward by Philippe Lejeune, "the autobiography of those who do not write,"[8] but, rather, "the autobiography of those who do not – for the most part – even speak." How might we analyze these narratives? How do we read autobiographies in the virtual absence of "text"? And what might this mean for questions of citizenship, for notions of the human?

The Fonds Tissot includes a series of letters concerning the health of Mademoiselle Disque. The correspondence in question consists of a series of twelve letters written by three different doctors between 1768 and 1769, with a single outlying letter from 1772.[9] From their arrangement, it would appear that the first nine letters, directed to an unknown correspondent, likely the Marquis du Manoir, Mademoiselle Disque's uncle,[10] were later forwarded to Tissot along with the final letter, which summarizes the situation and the patient's medical history. The patient, Mademoiselle Disque, aged approximately twenty-three in the first letter, appears to suffer from some form of nervous malady, an illness which is referred to variously as *fureur*, *imbécilité*, *affections mélancoliques*, and *manie*. The story of her illness is narrated by three doctors: Cosnier, Pomme, and Souquet. Cosnier was a doctor in the Faculty of Medicine, Paris. Pomme, meanwhile, author of a foundational treatise on nervous disorders, the *Affections vapoureuses des deux sexes* (1763), is best known as a specialist in the area of nervous disorder. Souquet, finally, appears to have been Disque's local doctor in Boulogne. In this series of letters, Cosnier and Pomme appear to be jointly responsible for Disque's care in Paris.

In contrast to the vast majority of letters addressed to Tissot, Mademoiselle Disque speaks coherently only once in the letters; that is to say that we hear her actual words and ideas at only one point in the course of the whole correspondence. In the second letter of the series, dated 22 December 1768, Cosnier notes that she speaks only to express her desire to return to Boulogne, and that this desire is so great that it has caused her profound agitation. As a result of this, she has lost much sleep.[11] Apart from this, Mademoiselle Disque is said to communicate; she is said to have an active mind; she is said to speak at times, but as readers, we have no idea what she says, how she says it, where she says it, or why she says it. In addition to this, her doctors note that she sings, laughs, trembles, convulses, faints, strikes herself, and stays mute, all bodily responses commonly associated with the broad category of hysteria. For the most part, then, we, as readers, do not have access to her "voice," to a speaking subject. Mademoiselle Disque does not speak in ways that make it possible for those around her to understand. The only comments that her doctors can share are those of her body's workings. In other words, her voice, in the absence of what we might term "rational discourse," exists only in her madness, in the extra-textual elements that are so present that they are no longer extra, but rather, the text itself. As autobiographical fragments, these letters are difficult to read, and even more difficult to analyze. As a researcher, I must, then, proceed with caution.

It is fair to begin by stating that the autobiography that emerges from this series of ten letters is not that of the patient, but rather, that of the doctors who were witness to her condition. In telling the story of Mademoiselle Disque, Cosnier, Pomme, and Souquet reveal their own stories and their own histories. These letters are ways of seeing that tell us much more about the producer than about what they purport to see. This means that we are left only with what they, as elite, eighteenth-century, male doctors, found relevant or important. Thus, we are told that Mademoiselle Disque spoke more than once but we are not privy to what she said.[12] Perhaps she just kept on reiterating her desire to travel to another region. Perhaps she said something else entirely. We know that, according to her doctors, "her mind was active,"[13] but we do not know how this was assessed or measured. Perhaps they observed her responses to external stimuli. Perhaps she wrote. Perhaps she read books. We are told that she sang.[14] But we do not know what or how she sang. Perhaps she sang with words; perhaps she only hummed tuneless melodies. The doctors inform us that she laughed, shivered, and descended into a form of mania or fury.[15] Perhaps her laughter was not inconsequential, perhaps her shivers were not irrational, or perhaps they were. We are also told that there is no rhyme or reason to her speech, song, and tears, but we are also told that she raves in an almost methodical manner and that she writes scraps of letters that appear remarkably rational.[16] There are, therefore, some things that we know, but so many more, particularly in relation to issues of language, speech, and discourse, that we will never know. The stories that remain are those of the people who observed her actions, their observations shaped by their own personal and professional histories.

While I do not want to, as I have indicated previously, paint a picture of the oppressive power of the medical gaze over the disciplined body of the docile patient, I do want to recognize and be attentive to Robert McRuer's assertion that able-bodiedness, "still largely masquerades as a nonidentity, as the natural order of things."[17] That is to say, just as compulsory heterosexuality produces marginalized sexual practices and identities (as we have seen in Chapter 5), so, too, does compulsory able-bodiedness produce disability. In the process, able-bodiedness is not only the taken-for-granted norm against which aberrations are measured. Susan Wendell has observed that "the public world is the world of strength, the positive (valued) body, performance and production, the able-bodied and youth."[18] As numerous scholars in disability studies have pointed out, this able-bodied norm – and the foundational frameworks that continue to sustain bodily injustice – remains completely uninterrogated.

The narrative of Mademoiselle Disque also requires me to be attentive to Judith Butler's argument, articulated in her essay, "Violence, Mourning, Politics."[19] Here, she considers the inherent vulnerability of the body: "The body implies mortality, vulnerability, agency: the skin and the flesh expose us to the gaze of others, but also to touch, and to violence. Although we struggle for rights over our own bodies, the very bodies for which we struggle are not quite ever only our own. The body has its invariably public dimension. Constituted as a social phenomenon in the public sphere, my body is and is not mine. Given over from the start to the world of others, it bears their imprint, is formed within the crucible of social life; only later, and with some uncertainty, do I lay claim to my body as my own, if, in fact, I ever do."[20] To me, this suggests a need to consider carefully the stories that I read, and in particular, to consider carefully those stories that have been narrated by others. These are stories informed by social relations; stories shaped by intersecting webs of class, sex, gender, sexuality, and ability, webs that shape not only the experiences of patients and doctors (or family or other observers), but also the shape of the text. Finally, these webs also, and inevitably, inform my own reading and analysis of the text.

All of this leads me to an impossible situation. I began this book by arguing that stories matter. Implicit in this statement is the notion of language – words, strung together to make meaning. As a general rule, we assume that language happens in words and that we are all capable of communicating in a common language that will somehow be accessible. But what does this mean for those who lack access to this common language? Does this common language even exist? The definition of language is, itself, not neutral. After all, as Jasbir Puar observes, "The ability to understand language is also where human/nonhuman animal distinctions, as well as human/technology distinctions have long been drawn."[21] James Overboe also stresses the political nature of conventional understandings of language: "Language is political because the forming of grammatically correct sentences is, for the normal individual, the prerequisite for any submission to social laws. If one cannot do so, or is ignorant of grammaticality, one belongs in a special institution."[22] So, too, are the stories of Mademoiselle Disque and others silenced. Defined in and through the medical gaze, their humanity is fundamentally compromised. In the words of G. Thomas Couser, "Individuals with disabilities that preclude or interfere with self-representation are ... doubly vulnerable subjects."[23] How then, will I ever recover the story, the voice, of Mademoiselle Disque and others like her? Where will I locate them within the category of the human? Can I make a case for corporeal citizenship at all?

## STORYTELLING, SUBJECTIVITY, AND CITIZENSHIP

> Why are we so afraid of the body? Is it because it's a mess,
> unpredictable, mortal, unreliable? ... A paradox: we pretend we don't
> need it, that it's our minds that matter, and yet the body is the thing we
> can't ignore and that knocks our thinking minds flat to the floor.
>
> Emily Rapp, *The Still Point of the Turning World*

As I have intimated throughout this book, I want to argue for the possibility of bodily storytelling and from there, bodily subjectivity. Thus, if, as Sidonie Smith and Julia Watson argue, "experience is discursive, embedded in the languages of everyday life and the knowledge produced at everyday sites,"[24] then we can and should see the body as productive of discourse. Through its workings it produces and circulates knowledge about itself. But at the same time, I must acknowledge that within our systems of understanding, it is only through the body's engagement with language – and here I use language as we conventionally understand it – that the body's workings take on meaning. But what happens if we take the idea of the discursive body seriously? To what extent might we be able to assert that it is through bodily function, or dysfunction, that the subject comes into being, that meaning is created in her life? The question is, are we equipped to handle such forms of subjectivity?

It is abundantly clear that the conventional tools of the autobiography scholar – words and writing – are inadequate. Even an engagement with epistolarity lets me down in the case of Mademoiselle Disque. The biggest problem, indeed, is that I have no recourse to conventional language in these letters, and both autobiography and epistolarity are premised primarily on textual representation. In these letters, I am left only with the workings of the body – the body's stories, the body's language, the body's speech, the body's narrative, the body's discourse. And from these words alone – narrative, story, speech, discourse – it is quite obvious that even language itself fails me. How can I talk about the body having language, the body having speech? Because how will I ever know what it is saying? And while this query gives me an opening, in that it enables me to say that I can learn a new language, I am still confounded by Butler's assertion that the body takes on meaning only in social relationships, that it can come to life only through its entry into language. Just as Mademoiselle Disque's bodily workings are available to us only through the interventions of her doctors, so too are my experiences of my body are shaped by my social world. They do not *precede* the social; they are part of the social.

In Chapter 3, I postulated that writing could be understood as an act of citizenship. As Margaret Rose Torrell observes, echoing ideas put forward by G. Thomas Couser, this is particularly true of communities that have been traditionally disenfranchised within conventional models of citizenship. Autobiography, these scholars argue, has "emancipatory potential"; it "gives a disabled writer a forum in which she can construct her disabled identity on her own terms."[25] But these letters demonstrate that my insistence on language, on the coherence of the written word, is insufficient. Furthermore, it can further perpetuate the very frameworks it seeks to disrupt. That is, writing excludes from citizenship the very individuals who would seemingly have most to gain. Do I, in my founding assumptions, play into the further production rather than dismantling of disability? Do I contribute to rather than disrupt the norms on which Western notions of the human are premised?

Here I must take seriously Overboe's critical response to *The Diving Bell and the Butterfly*, Jean-Dominique Bauby's hauntingly intimate account of a life lived within Locked-in Syndrome (LIS). For Bauby, communication is only possible through the intervention of others. It is entirely dependent on two factors: whether those around him recognize his blinking as communication and whether they choose to engage with this form of communication.[26] According to Overboe, the diving bell, often posited as a symbol of Bauby's bodily limitations, must be differently conceived: "The diving bell, for me, does not represent Bauby's imprisonment by LIS but rather the oppressive practices of those who usually privilege an able-bodied perspective. They see the problems of lack of communication, of lesser embodiment and absence of selfhood, as residing with Bauby as a result of LIS. In contrast, I see the problem as lying in such readers' inability to understand his attempts at communication, their failure to appreciate his embodiment, and finally their refusal to recognize his selfhood. His desire to open up the cocoon is reaffirmed in his continuing efforts to try to communicate with others."[27]

Perhaps, then, the answer might be found in listening otherwise, in speaking otherwise, in crafting a new language for the body, one that is attentive not only to social convention, but one that tries to dig deeply into the body and its workings. Perhaps, the answer is to take seriously the workings of the body on their own terms, to consider carefully and thoughtfully the relationship between body and story, body and speech, body and language. Perhaps we need to focus not so much on the words themselves but on the crafting of body narratives, on the minutiae of corporeal experience. And perhaps we need to take seriously the narratives offered by the body, to recognize that the body is an active entity capable of telling its own stories even as it functions simultaneously as a stage upon which the identities of both doctor and patient are performed. In this sense, I cannot take these letters at an individual level. I must consider them relation to other letters of the period, letters that may or may not have dealt with similar health concerns but that are situated within similar understandings of lived bodily experience, letters that reveal individuals grappling with how best to describe, in conventional language, what they are experiencing and what their bodies are telling them.

What is evident throughout the letters in the Fond Tissot is a struggle to define, in conventional language, what is happening to the body. "Sickness," as Roy Porter observes, "inevitably puts language under strain. We have a pain: we grope for the right word to convey the nature and intensity of the feeling, and to clarify just where under the skin it is located."[28] Einat Avraham would agree: "Illness autobiographies are illuminating precisely because they enact one of the major obstacles in the attempt to reconcile the current frameworks that contain the body, for they grapple – urgently and pragmatically – with the felt incongruity between the culturally tractable body and the experientially unruly yet constraining body."[29] It seems that it is not the body that is unable to tell its stories; it is the limitation of language to comprehend them. And yet, this storytelling body is essential if we want to capture the stories of young women like Mademoiselle Disque and, further, if we are to engage with broader understandings of citizenship. Indeed, the workings of Disque's body – the laughter, crying, shivering, convulsions – are *all* I have to work with. Throughout these letters, I get a sense of the body revealing itself. The difficulty lies in deciphering its messages. The limitations are not in the body but rather in how we perceive – and have perceived – the body and its stories.

In a 2007 book chapter, Overboe reflects on the relationships between bodies, citizenship, and selves. He suggests that people with disabilities move into a state of "post-personhood" that "comes about when circumstances of disease, disability, or trauma are perceived to rob an individual of his or her personhood."[30] Post-personhood is a state that exists outside of the human but that has been defined by and is thus irrevocably affected by the human. Post-personhood is thus fundamentally shaped by the unwillingness or inability of the able-bodied human subject to engage with its others. In Overboe's words, "it is not the person experiencing post-personhood that has the failure to communicate. It is the 'uncomfortableness' of the privileged persons, not the abject other, that causes communication to break down between persons and post-persons. Consequently, what is required is the political will for a paradigm shift that begins to see post-persons as persons who communicate differently."[31]

As I observed in the Introduction, what Tissot's correspondents did with their bodies – and what their bodies did for them – mattered. Improper bodily acts and experiences could, within a framework of corporeal virtue, relegate an individual to the category of the post-person or failed citizen, a negative and fundamentally transgressive identity that threatened the coherence of the polis as a whole. But while membership in the imagined community of corporeal virtue was desirable, it was, as we have seen, tenuous. Belonging was fragile, uncertain, and ambiguous. For some, it was wholly impossible.

The letters to Tissot can be productively understood as acts of citizenship, spaces in which suffering individuals could navigate the ideologies of corporeal citizenship and through which they could assert their individual claims to belonging. Here, the comments of feminist philosopher, Rosalyn Diprose, may be relevant: "to understand the word, writing, meaning, simply in terms of a metaphor that stands above, on or about, the work being addressed, or above the body that the work is about, is to miss what matters. The word, spoken or written (scientific or sociological) is not *on* or *about* its matter, as if separate from it. The word does come before a particular body, but not to shape it simply into a seamless socially recognised whole ... Rather, the word is also always *of* a body, written in blood, sweat and tears."[32] Diprose gestures towards the essential entanglement of word and flesh; each, it seems, produces the other. Such thinking returns me to Egan's previously cited reassurances: "'corpus' refers both to the human body and to a body of work."[33]

These epistolary spaces were fraught in that they required individuals to balance multiple allegiances: from their responsibilities to their gender, marital status, career and social station, to those they owed to Tissot as the arbiter of bodily health and citizenship. But these letters also suggest that corporeal citizenship is not a stable or static concept; rather, it is fluid, mobile, and dynamic. In the language they use, the details they include, the questions they ask, the stories they tell and those they leave untold, Tissot's correspondents understand citizenship as a process that emerges in the course of their conversations with Tissot. In their exchanges, letters as thresholds enable a continuing dialogue between the doctor and his suffering patients. As stages for the performance of self, letters also enable a dialogue between suffering individuals and their bodies, allowing individuals grappling with bodily dis-ease to both critically interrogate the meanings of their bodily sufferings and navigate the ideologies of corporeal virtue.

The letters to Tissot thus offer a material evocation of Bacchi and Beasley's notion of corporeal citizenship as "social flesh" – that is, a fleshy citizenship that emerges not within the constrained boundaries of the rational, autonomous, disembodied individual but rather in the intersubjective encounters *between* embodied selves. They offer the possibility of an imagined community that comes into being at the points at which bodies touch, meet, and acknowledge one another. Such an approach can be profoundly transformative. As Beasley and Bacchi observe, "Invoking social flesh, insisting on our embodied fleshly intersubjectivity … renders the normative 'strange'"[34] and thus paves the way for a reimagining of social relations. Beginning from the perspective of social flesh recuperates the bodily experiences, actions, and sufferings of the otherwise failed citizens who populate the epistolary landscape of the Tissot correspondence: onanists like François Louis Gauteron, Thomassin, Claude Joseph Demeunier, and Madame de Chastenay; reproductively troubled mothers like Madame Tollot and Madame Moreau de La Villegille; and convulsives like the Comtesse de Non. So, too, can it facilitate a rethinking of the seemingly incoherent ramblings of Mademoiselle de Disque, situating them not as exemplars of failed citizenship but rather as openings to new intersubjective conversations and thus as beginnings of new stories.

When the body is the only script available to us, we cannot just look away and pick up another, more easily decipherable story. Rather, we need to open our ears, our eyes, our minds, and, indeed, our bodies to a range of alternative possibilities. We need to consider autobiographical tracings that exist beyond of our experiences, beyond our language, and beyond our comfort zones. Social flesh does not ask us to renounce the connections between storytelling, citizenship, and the human. Rather, it asks us to listen otherwise and to take seriously the active role of the intersubjective, fleshy body in these conversations.

INTRODUCTION

1  This material is slowly becoming more easily accessible to researchers and the general public. Many of the letters of Hans Sloane, for example, are now available online, thanks to the work of Lisa W. Smith and her colleagues (see Sir Hans Sloane's Correspondence Online, https://drc.usask.ca/projects/sloaneletters/doku.php). Scholars at the University of Glasgow, meanwhile, are working to produce a digital database of all of William Cullen's letters (The Cullent Project, http://www.cullenproject.ac.uk/index.php). So, too, did scholars at the Institut universitaire d'histoire de la médecine et de la santé publique in Lausanne (among them Séverine Pilloud, Micheline Louis-Courvoisier, and Vincent Barras) publish a digital edition of Tissot's letters in 2013.

2  Rieder, "Patients and Words."

3  See, for example, Wild, *Medicine-by-Post*, as well as the myriad works by Séverine Pilloud and Micheline Louis-Courvoisier.

4  Ephron, *Heartburn*, 176–7.

5  P. Dumonceaux takes this further, asserting the power of the written word to "fix" truth ("Le XVIIe siècle," 296).

6  Marais, *Pièces de viole*, 101–2. For more on the programmatic elements of this work, see Vigroux, "Marin Marais et *Le tableau de l'opération de la taille*"; Franklin, "Surgery, note by note."

7  Burney, *Journals and Letters*, 6:597. Burney's letter has been the subject of much critical study. See, for example, Epstein, "Writing the Unspeakable"; Kaye, "'This Breast – It's Me'"; Pécastaings, "Frances Burney's Mastectomy."

8  Burney, *Journals and Letters*, 6:611.

9  Ibid.

10  King, *The Truth About Stories*, 9.

11  Qtd in Tissot, *De la médecine civile*, 82.

12  Tissot, *Advice to the people in general*, xix–xx.

13  Pilloud, "Tourisme médical."

14  Tissot, *De la médecine civile*.

15 For more on the popularization of medicine through the *Avis*, see Singy, "The Popularization of Medicine." For more on the changing face of medicine, see Murphy, "The French Medical Profession"; Coleman, "The People's Health"; Goubert, "1770–1830"; Porter, "Modernité et médecine." For more on the popularization of medicine in general in this period, see the various chapters in Roy Porter's edited collection, *The Popularization of Medicine*.

16 Tissot, *De la santé des gens de lettres*, 183–4; Tissot, *An essay on the disorders of people of fashion*, 144. For more on the relationships between physiology, morality and maternal breastfeeding, see Boon, "Mothers and Others."

17 Emch-Dériaz, *Tissot: Physician of the Enlightentment*, 130. Emch-Dériaz is the only contemporary biographer of Tissot and her book-length study has been essential to situating the correspondence within a broader context. For more on Tissot as a medical educator, see Emch-Dériaz, "L'enseignement clinique."

18 Tissot, *Advice to the People in General*, 579.

19 Mademoiselle de Zerbst, undated [1769], Bibliothèque cantonale et universitaire de Lausanne [hereafter BCU], Fonds Tissot, IS3784/II/149.01. 01.05. All translations from the Tissot letters are my own, unless the original letter is in English.

20 Madame de Bombelles, Marquise de Louvois, 29 October 1784, BCU, Fonds Tissot, IS3784/II/144.03.04.18.

21 Rouvière, 26 May 1783, BCU, IS3784/II/144.03.03.24.

22 Stolberg, "An Unmanly Vice."

23 Louis-Courvoisier and Mauron, "'He found me very well.'" See also, Louis-Courvoisier, "Qu'est-ce qu'un malade sans son corps?" Other sources indicate that the total is somewhere around 1,200 (Louis-Courvoisier and Pilloud, "Consulting by Letter in the Eighteenth Century," 72) or even under 1,000 (Teysseire, "Mort du roi," 51). My own calculations come to a number between 1,200 and 1,300.

24 Louis-Courvoisier and Mauron, "'He found me very well,'" 9. Again, numbers are in dispute. Louis-Courvoiser and Pilloud cite "more than 800 authors" in "Consulting by Letter in the Eighteenth Century" (73), while Nahema Hanafi, in "Le cancer à travers les consultations épistolaires envoyées au Docteur Tissot," offers a more precise "934" (97).

25 See C. Neider Doria Cassa, 30 September 1780, BCU, IS3784/II/144. 03.02.02, and Rouvière, 26 May 1783, BCU, IS3784/II/144.03.03.24. Nahema Hanafi notes that lay letters written by suffering individuals can be quantitatively organized as follows in relation to country of origin: 50 percent from France; 19 percent Switzerland; 6 percent Germany; 6 percent Italy; 5 percent Europe; and 14 percent no mention ("Des plumes singulières", 47n11). While this enumeration can be helpful, it nevertheless misses the often more complex geographic life trajectories that brought individuals into contact with Tissot.

26 Louis-Courvoisier and Pilloud observe that "the great majority of Tissot's patients were members of the social elite" and, as a result, would have had a relatively strong mastery of medical language of the period ("Le malade et son entourage," 942).

27 Louis-Courvoisier and Mauron, "'He found me very well,'" 9.

28 Ibid. See also Louis-Courvoisier, "Qu'est-ce qu'un malade sans son corps?" 302.

29 Pilloud, in her 2013 study, identifies four main types: consultation letters, consultation memoirs, letters of introduction, and medical consultations (*Les mots du corps*, 38). At the level of methodology, I situate all of these documents under the general rubric of epistolarity as they are, in my reading, all framed by the same objectives, goals, and purposes that structure epistolary culture more broadly speaking. Furthermore, my grouping is framed by the discernible differences between lay and professional documents. I discuss epistolarity in greater detail in Chapter 1.

30 J. Pierre Gay, 21 January 1773, BCU, IS3784/II/144.02.02.09.

31 Bastian, 1 March 1773, BCU, IS3784/II/144.02.02.11.

32 Louis-Courvoisier, "Le malade et son entourage"; Pilloud, "Mettre les maux en mots."

33 Pardo-Tomás and Martínez-Vidal, "Stories of Disease Written by Patients and Lay Mediators in the Spanish Republic of Letters," 474.

34 Drs Cosnier, Pomme, and Souquet, Letters to Samuel Auguste Tissot, 19 December 1768 to 29 June 1772, BCU, IS3784/II/144.04.08.22 to IS3784/II/144.04.08.33.

35 [d'Hervilly family], Letters to Samuel Auguste Tissot, BCU, IS3784/II/144.02.02.16 to IS3784/II/144.02.02.24.

36 Dupan de Saussure, 18 August 1784, BCU, IS3784/II/144.03.04.23.

37 Pilloud and Louis-Courvoisier, "The Intimate Experience of the Body," 454.

38 Ibid. Again, there are some discrepancies here, which may be related to the way letters are counted. In another article, Pilloud and Louis-Courvoisier state that "about 60% of patients" do not write letters on their own behalf ("Le malade et son entourage," 940), a figure that does not fully accord with the 450/1,300 who do write on their own behalf, cited in Pilloud and Louis-Courvoisier's "The Intimate Experience of the Body" (454). Hanafi offers "close to 500" ("Le cancer," 97).

39 Stolberg, "Medical Popularization," 90.

40 Withey, *Physick and the Family*, 99.

41 Weston, *Medical Consulting by Letter*; Withey, *Physick and the Family*, 36–42.

42 It is also important to consider that while literacy rates increased dramatically from the beginning to the end of the eighteenth century, less than 50 percent of the male population and just over 25 percent of the female populate was literate by the end of the century (Weston, *Medical Consulting by Letter*, 151).

43 Meek, "Medical Women and Hysterical Doctors," 2.

44 Young, *On Female Body Experience*, 17.

45 Hanafi, "Le cancer," 96.

46 Bossis, "Atelier no. 4," 457.

47 Plummer, *Documents of Life*, 55.

48 Hanafi, "Le cancer," 96.

49 Ousrard de Linière, 17 August 1772, BCU, Fonds Tissot, IS3784/II/144.01.07.26.

50 See, for example, a letter from Polier de Loÿs to Tissot, dated from Lausanne, 8 February 1792, in which he makes specific reference to "les malheurs du temps," particularly in relation to those individuals whose business is tied to France (8 February 1792, BCU, Fonds Tissot, IS3784/II/144.05.04.14).

51 Smith, "Reassessing the Role of the Family"; Smith, "'La raillerie' des femmes"; Smith, "The Body Embarrrassed?"; Smith, "The Relative Duties of a Man"; Smith, "'An Account of Unaccountable Distemper.'"

52 Rieder and Barras, "Écrire sa maladie." For more on the idea of medicine as a social experience, see, for example, Churchill, *Female Patients*; McClive and Pellegrin, eds., *Femmes en fleurs, femme en corps*; Withey, *Physick and the Family*.

53 Unsigned [Mother of Princess de Vaudemont], undated, BCU, Fonds Tissot, IS3784/II/144.03.02.28.

54 Mademoiselle de Charitte, 22 May 1773, BCU, Fonds Tissot, IS3784/II/144.02.01.26.

55 Roussy, undated, BCU, Fonds Tissot, IS3784/II/144.02.05.25.

56 Madame de La Millière, 1 March 1767, BCU, Fonds Tissot, IS3784/II/144.02, hors série.

57 Hanisch, "The Personal is Political."

58 Egan, *Burdens of Proof*, 15.

59 Beasley and Bacchi, "Envisioning a New Politics."

## CHAPTER ONE

1 Hartmann, 19 June 1792, BCU, Fonds Tissot, IS3784/II/144.05.05.32. See also, Monsieur Dauphin, who observes that his body is a "true barometer" susceptible to all changes in weather (Dauphin, [1772], BCU, Fonds Tissot, IS3784/II/144.01.07.06).

2 Bruckner, undated, BCU, Fonds Tissot, IS3784/II/144.04.01.15.

3 Slater, *Lying*, 221.

4 Weston, *Medical Consulting by Letter*, 10–11.

5 Hanafi, "Le cancer," 96.

6 Darnton, *The Great Cat Massacre*, 262.

7 Ibid., 4.

8 Porter, "The Patient's Point of View."

9 See, for example, Baker, "Hearing and Writing Women's Voices."

10 Withey, *Physick and the Family*, 122.

11 Duden, *The Woman Beneath the Skin*. See also Duden's *Disembodying Women* and Roper, "Slipping out of View."

12 Butler, *Gender Trouble*; Butler, *Bodies That Matter*.

13 Barras and Dinges, *Maladies en lettres*; Barras and Louis-Courvoisier, "Tissot et la médecine des Lumières"; Louis-Courvoisier and Pilloud, "Consulting by Letter in the 18th Century"; Pilloud and Louis-Courvoisier, "The Intimate Experience of the Body in the Eighteenth Century"; Louis-Courvoisier, "Le malade et son médecin"; Louis-Courvoisier, "'Il me trouva très bien'"; Louis-Courvoisier, "Quelques traces de liens familiaux"; Louis-Courvoisier, "Qu'est-ce qu'un malade sans son corps?"; Louis-Courvoisier and Mauron, "'He found me very well'"; Rieder and Barras, "Écrire sa maladie au siècle des lumières"; Rieder and Louis-Courvoisier, "Enlightened Physicians"; Barras and Rieder, "Corps et sujet"; Pilloud, Hächler, and Barras, "Consulter par lettre au XVIIIe siècle"; Rieder, "Patients and Words"; Rieder, "La rencontre thérapeutique"; Pilloud, *Les mots du corps*; Pilloud, *Documenter l'histoire de la santé*; Pilloud, "Tourisme médical"; Pilloud, "Marges interprétatives"; Stolberg, *Experiencing Illness and the Sick Body*; Stolberg, "Medical Popularization"; Stolberg, "An Unmanly Vice"; Stolberg, "Self-Pollution, Moral Reform, and the Venereal Trade"; Stolberg, "A Woman's Hell?"; Stolberg, "Les lettres de patients."

14 Lejeune, *On Autobiography*; Smith, *A Poetics of Women's Autobiograpy*; Smith and Watson, *Getting a Life*; Smith and Watson, *Interfaces*; Smith, *Subjectivity, Identity, and the Body*; Couser, *Recovering Bodies*; Couser, *Vulnerable Subjects*; Couser, *Signifying Bodies*; Eakin, *The Ethics of Life Writing*; Eakin, *How Our Lives Become Stories*; Kadar, Warley, Perrault and Egan, *Tracing the Autobiographical*; Kadar, *Essays on Life Writing*; Brant, *Eighteenth-Century Letters*; Goodman, *Becoming a Woman*; Grassi, *L'Art de la lettre*; Grassi, "Epistolières aux XVIIIe siècle"; Bland and Cross, *Gender and Politics*; Didier, "Ecrire pour se trouver"; Earle, *Epistolary Selves*; Gilroy and Verhoeven, *Epistolary Histories*; Altman, *Epistolarity*; Cook, *Epistolary Bodies*; Redford, *The Converse of the Pen*.

15 Ahmed and Stacey, *Thinking through the Skin*; Birke, *Feminism and the Biological Body*; Gatens, *Imaginary Bodies*; Grosz, *Time and Perversion*; Grosz, *Volatile Bodies*; Kirby, *Tellling Flesh*; Murray, "(Un/Be)Coming Out?"; Murray, "Normative Imperatives"; Prosser, *Second Skins*; Prosser, "Skin Memories"; Wendell, *The Rejected Body*.

16 Boon, *The Life of Madame Necker*.

17 See, for example, Ruberg, "The Letter as Medicine"; Rankin, "Duchess, Heal Thyself"; Wild, "Doctor–Patient Correspondence"; Pardó-Tomás and Martinez-Vidal, "Stories of Disease"; Churchill, "Bodily Differences?: Gender, Race, and Class"; Smith, "Reassessing the Role of the Family"; Smith, "The Relative Duties of a Man"; Smith, "'An Account of Unaccountable Distemper'"; Shuttleton, "'Not the meanest part of my

works'"; Steinke, "Maladie en context"; Redien-Collot, "Discours médical et pratique poétique"; Götz, "La maladie comme effet"; Grenon, "'J'ai appris à souffrir'"; Rieder, "Correspondances historiographiques."

18 Pilloud, "Tourisme médical."

19 Pilloud and Louis-Courvoisier, "The Intimate Experience of the Body"; Louis-Courvoisier and Mauron, "'He found me very well'"; Louis-Courvoisier, "Le malade et son médecin"; Louis-Courvoisier, "Quelques traces de liens familiaux"; Louis-Courvoisier and Pilloud, "Consulting by Letter in the Eighteenth Century"; Louis-Courvoisier, "Qu'est-ce qu'un malade sans son corps?"

20 Louis-Courvoisier, "Qu'est-ce qu'un malade sans son corps?"

21 Barras and Rieder, "Corps et sujet"; Barras and Louis-Courvoisier, "Tissot et la médecine des Lumières"; Barras, Hächler, and Pilloud, "Consulter par lettre au XVIIIe siècle"; Barras and Gaist, "Petit dossier Tissot."

22 Rieder, "La rencontre thérapeutique"; Rieder and Louis-Courvoisier, "Enlightened Physicians"; Rieder, "Patients and Words."

23 Singy, "Le pouvoir de la science"; Singy, "The Popularization of Medicine"; Singy, "Friction of the Genitals"; Teysseire, "Mort du roi et troubles féminins"; Hanafi, "Le cancer"; Hanafi, "Les mères et les médecins"; Hanafi, "Des plumes singulières"; Hanafi, "Pudeurs des souffrants"; Hanafi, "'Le fruit de nos entrailles'"; Stolberg, "An Unmanly Vice"; Stolberg, "Self-Pollution, Moral Reform, and the Venereal Trade"; Stolberg, "A Woman's Hell?"; Emch-Dériaz, *Tissot: Physician of the Enlightenment*.

24 Belsey, "Textual Analysis as a Research Method."

25 Ibid., 164.

26 Lejeune, *On Autobiography*, 5.

27 Thomas Cranfurd, 28 October 1774, BCU, Fonds Tissot, IS3784/II/144. 02.05.09.

28 Madame Morozzo, 23 March 1773, BCU, Fonds Tissot, IS3784/II/144. 02.03.11.

29 Comte d'Halgouet, 17 November 1776, BCU, Fonds Tissot, IS3784/II/ 144.02.07.07.

30 Pilloud, *Les mots du corps*.

31 Baecque, *The Body Politic*; Baecque, *Glory and Terror*; Outram, *The Body and the French Revolution*; Fermon, *Domesticating Passions*.

32 Stolberg, *Experiencing Illness*; Withey, *Physick and the Family*; Churchill, *Female Patients*; Weston, *Medical Consulting by Letter*.

33 Smith, "Reassessing the Role of the Family"; Smith, "'An Account of Unaccountable Distemper'"; Weston, *Medical Consulting by Letter*; Withey, *Physick and the Family*; Wild, "Doctor–Patient Correspondence."

34 Anselment, "'The Want of Health'"; Dawson, "Voltaire's Complaint"; Götz, "La maladie comme conme effet"; Grenon, "'J'ai appris à souffrir'"; Ingram, Sim, Lawlor, Terry, Baker, and Wetherall-Dickson, *Melancholy Experience*; Ingram, "Deciphering Difference"; Ingram, "Identifying the Insane"; Ingram, "Resisting Insanity"; Ingram, "Steering Toward Sanity";

Ingram, "Time and Tense"; Magrath, "'Rags of Mortality'"; Meek, "[W]hat Fatigues"; Meek, "Medical Women and Hysterical Men"; Meek, "Of Wandering Wombs"; Pardo-Tómas and Martínez-Vidal, "Stories of Disease"; Rankin, "Duchess, Heal Thyself"; Smith, "'An Account of Unaccountable Distemper'"; Smith, "The Body Embarrassed?"; Sturzer, "Love and Disease."

35 Stolberg, *Experiencing Illness and the Sick Body*.

36 See, for example, Boon, "Epistolary Labours"; Boon, "Gender, Class and Epistolary Suffering"; Boon, "Mothers and Others"; Churchill, *Female Patients in Early Modern Britain*; Churchill, "Bodily Differences"; Churchill, "The Medical Practice of the Sexed Body"; Louis-Courvoisier and Mauron, "'He found me very well'"; Louis-Courvoisier, "Que faut-il ne pas dire à qui?"; McClive, "Blood and Expertise"; McClive, "L'âge des fleurs"; McClive, "Masculinity on Trial"; McClive, "Menstrual Knowledge and Medical Practice"; McClive, "Quand les fleurs s'arrêtent"; Redien-Collot, "Discours médical et pratique poétique"; Ruberg, "The Letter as Medicine"; Smith, "La raillerie des femmes"; Smith, "Reassessing the Role of the Family"; Smith, "The Relative Duties of a Man"; Stolberg, "A Woman's Hell?"; Stolberg, "An Unmanly Vice"; Weston, *Medical Consulting by Letter*; Withey, *Physick and the Family*; Weston, "Epistolary Consultations"; Wild, "Doctor–Patient Correspondence"; Broomhall, *Women's Medical Work*.

37 Duden, *Woman Beneath the Skin*; Louis-Courvoisier and Pilloud, "Consulting by Letter"; Louis-Courvoisier, "Qu'est-ce qu'un malade sans son corps?"; Pilloud, "Mettre les maux en mots"; Pilloud and Louis-Courvoisier, "The Intimate Experience of the Body"; Wolff, "Perspectives on Patients' History."

38 Stolberg, "Self-Pollution, Moral Reform, and the Venereal Trade"; Stolberg, "An Unmanly Vice"; Stolberg, "The Monthly Malady"; Stolberg, "A Woman's Hell?"; Rankin, "Duchess, Heal Thyself."

39 Weston, *Medical Consulting by Letter*, 4; Pilloud, *Les mots du corps*, 30. Other scholars, however, have situated medical letters within the context of epistolarity more generally speaking. See, for example, Rieder, "Correspondances historiographiques."

40 Rieder, "Patients and Words," 215–16.

41 Louis-Courvoisier, "Qu'est-ce qu'un malade sans son corps?" 300, translation mine.

42 Louis-Courvoisier and Pilloud, "Le malade et son entourage," 942. See also Smith, "Reassessing the Role of the Family"; Broomhall, *Women's Medical Work*.

43 Monsieur Lasseire, 22 April 1778, BCU, Fonds Tissot, IS3784/II/149.01.01.25.

44 Ibid.

45 Madame de La Fosse Joly, 19 February 1779, BCU, Fonds Tissot, IS3784/II/149.01.01.21.

46 Unsigned [on behalf of M. de Germigny], undated, BCU, Fonds Tissot, IS3784/II/144.04.04.30.

47 Rublack, "Fluxes."

48 Monsieur Gringet, 4 January 1784, BCU, Fonds Tissot, IS3784/II/144.03.04.21.

49 Ibid.

50 Ibid.

51 Ibid.

52 Louis-Courvoisier, "Qu'est-ce qu'un malade sans son corps?" 299, translation mine.

53 Butler, *Bodies that Matter*.

54 Weston, *Medical Consulting by Letter*, 4.

55 Richardson, "Writing: A Method of Inquiry," 516.

56 Lejeune, *On Autobiography*, 4.

57 Rousseau, *The Confessions and Correspondence*, 5.

58 Schaffer and Smith, *Human Rights and Narrated Lives*; Smith, *A Poetics of Women's Autobiography*; Smith, *Subjectivity, Identity, and the Body*; Smith and Watson, *Getting a Life*; Smith, Watson, and Corbett, "De/Colonizing the Subject."

59 Woolf, *A Room of One's Own*.

60 Armstrong, "Racism: Racial Exclusivity and Cultural Supremacy."

61 Smith and Watson, *Getting a Life*; Smith, *Interfaces*.

62 Berger, *Ways of Seeing*.

63 Gilmore, *Autobiographics*; Kadar, Warley, Perreault, and Egan, *Tracing the Autobiographical*, 1.

64 Eakin, *How Our Lives Become Stories*; Eakin, *The Ethics of Life Writing*; Couser, *Vulnerable Subjects*.

65 Translation mine.

66 Bossis, "Atelier no. 4," 457.

67 Brant, *Eighteenth-Century Letters*, 13.

68 Stanley, "The Epistolarium," 203.

69 Earle, *Epistolary Selves*; Gilroy and Verhoeven, *Epistolary Histories*; How, *Epistolary Spaces*; Cook, *Epistolary Bodies*. Journal special issues include *Yale French Studies* 71 (1986); *Eighteenth-Century Life* 35, no. 1 (2011); *Life Writing* 8, no. 2 (2011).

70 Earle, *Epistolary Selves*, 1.

71 Cook cited in Berg, "Truly Yours," 41.

72 Schneider, *The Culture of Epistolarity*, 13.

73 Brant, *Eighteenth-Century Letters*, 2.

74 *OED Online*, s.v. "Threshold."

75 Redford, *The Converse of the Pen*, 2.

76 Françoise Valérien de Mérande, 4 October 1783, BCU, Fonds Tissot, IS3784/II/144.03.03.14.

77 Goodman, *Becoming a Woman*.

78 Ballaster, "Economics of Ethical Conversation," 121.

79  Ibid., 121. I explore this notion further in "Does a Dutiful Wife Write?"
80  Madame Carbounié de Castelgaillard, [1775], BCU, Fonds Tissot, 1S3784/
    11/146.01.04.19.
81  Mademoiselle Morozzo, Comtesse de Valfenere, 19 May 1773, BCU,
    Fonds Tissot, 1S3784/11/144.02.03.12.
82  Brant, *Eighteenth-Century Letters*, 3.
83  Grassi, "Epistolières aux XVIIIe siècle," 94.
84  Bland and Cross, *Gender and Politics in the Age of Letter Writing*, 5, ital-
    ics original.
85  Fraser qtd in ibid., 8.
86  Ibid., 7.
87  Dumonceaux, "Le XVIIe siècle," 289.
88  Gilroy and Verhoeven, *Epistolary Histories*, 14–15.
89  Bakhtin qtd in ibid., 14.
90  Ibid., 19.
91  Coligny and Kueffer, 17 September 1774, BCU, Fonds Tissot, 1S3784/11/
    144.02.05.08.
92  Haggarty, "'The Ceremonial Letter for Letter,'" 152.
93  Ibid., 161.
94  See, for example, the letters penned by François Louis Gauteron (BCU,
    Fonds Tissot, 1S3784/11/144.05.05.19–1S3784/11/144.05.05.23) and Chil-
    laud l'aîné (4 May 1790 and 15 May 1790. BCU, Fonds Tissot, 1S3784/
    11/144.05.02.29 and 1S3784/11/144.05.02.30).
95  Thomassin, 8 May 1776, BCU, Fonds Tissot, 1S3784/11/144.02.08.14.
96  Joan DeJean, in her article, "(Love) Letters: Madeleine de Scudéry and
    the Epistolary Impulse," considers the ways in which the newly founded
    postal system shaped identities within Scudéry's circle.
97  Berg, "Truly Yours," 41.
98  Altman, *Epistolarity: Approaches to a Form*, 89.
99  Stanley, Salter, and Dampier, "The Epistolary Pact," 264.
100 Barton and Hall, *Letter Writing as a Social Practice*.
101 Barton and Hall, Introduction to *Letter Writing as a Social Practice*, 6.
102 Foley, "'Your Letter Is Divine,'" 239.
103 Russell, "Life's Illusions," 153.
104 Stanley, Salter, and Dampier, "The Epistolary Pact," 278.
105 Barbazan, Letters to Samuel Auguste Tissot, 28 February 1772, undated, 5
    October 1772, undated, 20 August 1773, undated, and 12 December 1773,
    BCU, Fonds Tissot, 1S3784/11/149.01.04.16 to 1S3784/11/149.01.04.22.
106 Avrahami, *The Invading Body*, 3.
107 Woolf, "On Being Ill," 3–4.
108 Stanley, Salter, and Dampier, "The Epistolary Pact," 265.
109 Ibid.
110 Russell, "Life's Illusions," 154, italics original.
111 Burton, "An Assemblage/Before Me."
112 Stanley, "The Epistolary Gift," 136.

113  McGrath, "The Other Body," 29.

114  Magrath, "'Rags of Mortality,'" 255.

115  Kadar, Warley, Perreault, and Egan, *Tracing the Autobiographical*.

116  Beauvoir, *The Second Sex*, 65.

117  Tyler, "Skin-Tight," 77. See also Prosser, *Second Skins*.

118  Magrath, "'Rags of Mortality,'" 255.

119  Qtd in Poustie, "Re-theorising Letters and 'Letterness,'" 23. See also MacKenzie, *Sent as a Gift*, 5.

120  Prosser, "Skin Memories," 52.

121  Unsigned, undated, BCU, Fonds Tissot, IS3784/II/149.01.07.14.

122  Gounon (in the hands of his wife, Madame Gounon Laborde), 11 June 1773, BCU, Fonds Tissot, IS3784/II/144.02.02.08.

123  Prosser, "Skin Memories," 65.

124  Tyler, "Skin-Tight," 76.

125  Steedman, *Dust: The Archive and Cultural History*, 74.

126  Douglas, *Uneasy Sensations*, xxii.

127  Pilloud and Louis-Courvoisier, "The Intimate Experience of the Body," 452.

128  Ibid., 452.

129  Smith, "An Account of Unaccountable Distemper," 466.

130  Schaffer and Smith, *Human Rights and Narrated Lives*, 7–8.

131  Portelli, *The Death of Luigi Trastulli*.

132  Ibid., 1.

133  Schaffer and Smith, *Human Rights and Narrated Lives*, 7–8.

134  Qtd in Ibid., 66.

**CHAPTER TWO**

1  BCU, Fonds Tissot, IS3784/II/149.01.05.11.

2  Chevalier de Soran, 17–23 October 1771, BCU, Fonds Tissot, IS3784/II/144.04.08.11.

3  Ibid.

4  Gounon (in the hand of his wife, Madame Gounon Laborde), [1773], BCU, Fonds Tissot, IS3784/II/144.02.02.08.

5  Vauvilliers, 15 May [1774], BCU, Fonds Tissot, IS3784/II/144.02.04.27; Madame Jequier, 15 August 1774, BCU, Fonds Tissot, IS3784/II/144.02.05.14.

6  Madame la Comtesse de Wedel, 12 November 1784, BCU, Fonds Tissot, IS3784/II/144.03.05.01.

7  Egan, *Burdens of Proof*, 31.

8  Canning, "The Body as Method?"

9  Grosz, *Space, Time, and Perversion*, 103.

10  Kirby, "Natural Convers(at)ions," 221.

11  Sontag, *Illness as Metaphor*; Woolf, "On Being Ill."

12  BCU, Fonds Tissot, IS3784/II/149.01.02.10.

13  Weston, *Medical Consulting by Letter*, 147–8.

14  Vess, *Medical Revolution in France*, 11.

15  Porter, *Disease, Medicine and Society*, 17.

16  See, for example, diarrhoea experienced by an anonymous correspondent (undated, BCU, Fonds Tissot, IS3784/II/144.03.05.23) and the interminable vaginal bleeding experienced by Madame la Comtesse de Wedel (Letters to Samuel Auguste Tissot, 12 November 1784 and 28 January 1785, BCU, Fonds Tissot, IS3784/II/144.03.05.01 and IS3784/II/144.03.05.02).

17  See, for example, Mme de Corselles, who is exhausted as a resulted of inexplicable, continually interrupted sleep (17 January 1790, BCU, Fonds Tissot, IS3784/II/144.05.02.26); and an anonymous sixteen-year-old girl, who has been experiencing convulsions, which began after having been knocked to the ground by a soldier fleeing a superior who had challenged him to a duel (Monsieur Bon, Consultation to Samuel Auguste Tissot, [1790], BCU, Fonds Tissot, IS3784/II/144.05.02.36).

18  Desbordes, 10 August [year unclear], BCU, Fonds Tissot, IS3784/II/149.01.03.05.

19  Weston, *Medical Consulting by Letter*, 4.

20  Suzanne Fleischman, "I Am …, I Have …, I Suffer from…," 5.

21  *Dictionnaire de l'Académie française*, 1st ed. s.v. "Maladie."

22  *Dictionnaire de l'Académie française*, 4th ed., s.v. "Maladie," translation mine.

23  Diderot and d'Alembert, *Encyclopédie*, s.v. "Maladie s.f. Médc," translation mine.

24  Ibid.

25  *Dictionnaire de l'Académie française*. 4th ed., s.v. "Sain."

26  *Encyclopedia of Diderot & d'Alembert, Collaborative Translation Project*, s.v. "Health," trans. Victoria Meyer, http://creativecommons.org/licenses/by-nc-nd/3.0/.

27  Comte d'Adhémar and Dr de Vergennez, Consultation to Samuel Auguste Tissot, [1777], BCU, Fonds Tissot, IS3784/II/144.03.01.11.

28  Magrath, "'Rags of Mortality,'" 250. See also the work of Heather Meek, which explores the complex relationships between women and physicians during this period.

29  Withey, *Physick and the Family*, 132.

30  For more on this, among others, see Boon, *The Life of Madame Necker*. See also Sturzer, "Love and Disease."

31  Lavergne l'aîné, 19 May 1772, BCU, Fonds Tissot, IS784/II/144.01.07.20.

32  Jean Frédéric Borel, 4 May 1767, BCU, Fonds Tissot, IS3784/II/149.01.01.06.

33  Cherot du Marois, 16 January 1786, BCU, Fonds Tissot, IS3784/II/144.04.01.02.

34  Madame Rigoley, Marquise d'Agrain, 4 July 1785, BCU, Fonds Tissot, IS3784/II/144.03.06.02.

35  Madame Gounon Laborde, 20 May 1773, BCU, Fonds Tissot, IS3784/II/144.02.02.07.

36  Qtd in Magrath, "'Rags of Mortality,'" 239.

37  Boon, *The Life of Madame Necker*, especially Chapter 5. See also Bérenguier, *Conduct Books for Girls*, and Bérenguier, "Lettres de Suzanne
Necker."

38  Magrath, "'Rags of Mortality,'" 249.

39  For more insight into eighteenth-century spa culture, see Wheeler, "Jane
Austen"; Hurley, "A Conversation of their Own"; Herbert, "Gender and
the Spa"; Mansén, "An Image of Paradise."

40  Herbert, "Gender and the Spa"; Mansén, "An Image of Paradise."

41  Pilloud, *Les mots du corps*, 44.

42  Cheyne, *The English Malady*.

43  I explore this more fully in Chapter 6.

44  Pilloud and Louis-Courvoisier, "Le malade et son entourage."

45  Major et Lieutenant de Bouju, 25 September 1773, BCU, Fonds Tissot,
IS3784/II/144.02.01.12.

46  Luternau, 26 January 1773, BCU, Fonds Tissot, IS3784/II/144.02.03.02.

47  Major et Lieutenant de Bouju, 25 September 1773, BCU, Fonds Tissot,
IS3784/II/144.02.01.12.

48  Thomassin, [1775], BCU, Fonds Tissot, IS3784/II/144.02.08.13.

49  Magrath, "'Rags of Mortality,'" 247.

50  Thomassin, [1775], BCU, Fonds Tissot, IS3784/II/144.02.08.13.

51  Lavergne l'aîné, October 1772, BCU, Fonds Tissot, IS784/II/144.01.07.24.

52  Ibid.

53  Lavergne l'aîné, [October 1772], BCU, Fonds Tissot, IS3784/II/144.01.
07.25.

54  Ibid.

55  Ibid.

56  Lieutenant Barbazan, 22 February 1772, undated [1772], 5 October 1772,
undated [1772], 20 May 1773, undated [1773], 12 December 1773, BCU,
Fonds Tissot, IS3784/II/149.01.04.16–149.01.04.22.

57  Lieutenant Barbazan, undated [1772], BCU, Fonds Tissot. IS3784/II/149.
01.04.17.

58  For more on sensibility, see Mullan, *Sentiment and Sociability*; Barker-
Benfield, *The Culture of Sensibility*.

59  Withey, *Physick and the Family*, 133. See also Wild, "Doctor–Patient Correspondence," 60.

60  Smith and Watson, *Reading Autobiography*, 274.

61  B. Poliansky, [1784], BCU, Fonds Tissot, IS3874/II/144.03.04.38.

62  Ibid.

63  Ibid.

64  Galliotte, 4 September 1773, BCU, IS3784/II/144.02.02.03.

65  Smith, "'An Account of Unaccountable Distemper.'"

66  A. Alvard, 30 October 1767, BCU, IS3784/II/149.01.06.07.

67  Ibid.

68  Ibid.

69 Wild, "Doctor–Patient Correspondence," 58.

70 Jaucourt, "Sensibilité (morale)" in *Encyclopédie*; Grouchy, *Lettres sur la sympathie*.

71 Williams, "'The Luxury of Doing Good,'" 77.

72 Börking, 30 November 1770, BCU, IS3784/II/149.01.05.17.

73 Dupuy *fils*, 19 November 1775, BCU, IS3784/II/149.01.03.01.

74 Ibid.

75 Roper, "Slipping out of View," 66.

76 Maillard, 12 April 1773. BCU, IS3784/II/149.01.02.07. I return to this letter in Chapter 4.

77 Thus, for example, Michael Stolberg reads the onanism letters through the lens of Foucauldian confessional culture ("An Unmanly Vice").

78 Gringet, 4 January 1784, BCU, Fonds Tissot, IS3784/II/144.03.04.21.

79 Olivier, 2 March 1774, BCU, Fonds Tissot, IS3784/II/144.02.04.10.

80 Thomassin, 28 May 1776, BCU, Fonds Tissot, IS3784/II/144.02.08.14.

81 Rossary, 13 June 1774, BCU, Fonds Tissot, IS3784/II/144.02.04.11.

82 Lanjuinais, 25 January 1790, BCU, Fonds Tissot, IS3784/II/144.05.02.12.

83 Unsigned, [1773], BCU, Fonds Tissot, IS3784/II/149.01.04.09.

84 Ibid.

85 Olivier, 2 March 1774, BCU, Fonds Tissot, IS3784/II/144.02.04.10.

86 Ibid.

87 Ibid.

88 Martin, undated, BCU, Fonds Tissot, IS3784/II/144.04.06.03.

89 Unsigned, [1773?], BCU, Fonds Tissot, IS3784/II/149.01.07.14.

90 For more on this topic, see in particular the major studies by Dena Goodman (*Becoming a Woman*) and Marie-Claire Grassi (*L'Art de la lettre*).

91 Madame Carbounié de Castelgaillard, [1775], BCU, Fonds Tissot, IS3784/II/146.01.04.19.

92 Grassi, "Epistolières au XVIIIe siècle," 103, translation mine. It is also worth noting that epistolarity, as a social practice, was a well-established site for the performance of femininity. For more on this, see Gilbert, "Deconstructing Gender," and Jensen, *Writing Love*.

93 Bernier, 25 January 1773, BCU, Fonds Tissot, IS3784/II/144.02.03.01; Luternau, 26 January 1773, BCU, Fonds Tissot, IS3784/II/144.02.03.02; A.C. Konauw (née Smith), 26 January 1773, BCU, Fonds Tissot, IS3784/II/144.02.03.03.

94 A.C. Konauw (née Smith), 26 January 1773, BCU, Fonds Tissot, IS3784/II/144.02.03.03.


## CHAPTER THREE

1 BCU, Fonds Tissot, IS3784/II/144.01.07.01.

2 Keung, "Family Ripped Apart."

3 Reynolds, *Vulnerable Communion*, 24.

4 Ibid.

5   Puar, "Coda: The Cost of Getting Better," 151.

6   Butler, *Bodies That Matter*, 2.

7   Porter, "Bodies of Thought," 99.

8   Boon, *The Life of Madame Necker*; Stolberg, *Experiencing Illness*.

9   Henke, *Shattered Subjects*, xix.

10  Pocock, "The Ideal of Citizenship," 34.

11  Shildrick, *Dangerous Discourses*, 19.

12  Pocock, "The Ideal of Citizenship," 33.

13  Isin and Wood, *Citizenship and Identity*, 4.

14  Faulks, *Citizenship*, 1.

15  Isin and Wood, *Citizenship and Identity*, 4.

16  Canning and Rose, "Gender, Citizenship and Subjectivity," 429.

17  Faulks, *Citizenship*, 6.

18  *Dictionnaire de l'Académie française*. 4th ed., s.v. "Citoyen," translation mine.

19  Féraud, "Citoyen." This concept also appears in the fifth edition of the *Dictionnaire de l'Academie françoise* (1798), translation mine.

20  *The Encyclopedia of Diderot & d'Alembert: Collaborative Translation Project*, s.v. "Citizen," trans. Sujava Dhanvantari, http://creativecommons.org/licenses/by-nc-nd/3.0/.

21  Beiner, "Introduction," 1.

22  Anderson, *Imagined Communities*, 6.

23  Revill, "Reading *Rosehill*," 119.

24  Yuval-Davis, "Women, Citizenship, and Difference," 8.

25  Gatens, *Imaginary Bodies*, 23.

26  It is worth considering, here, the words of Lauren Berlant: "health itself … can be seen as a side effect of successful normativity" (qtd in Puar, "Coda: The Cost of Getting Better," 152).

27  Hohle, "The Body and Citizenship."

28  Ibid., 286.

29  Bacchi and Beasley, "Citizen Bodies," 338.

30  Murray, "(Un/Be)Coming Out?" See also Gofmann's notion of "discredited" personhood (*Asylums*, 95) and LeBesco's "revolting bodies" (LeBesco, *Revolting Bodies?*; Braziel and LeBesco, *Bodies out of Bounds*).

31  Murray, "Normative Imperatives," 216.

32  Ibid., 213.

33  Murray, "Pathologizing 'Fatness,'" 7.

34  Murray, "Normative Imperatives," 214, italics original.

35  Murray, "(Un/Be)Coming Out?" 214.

36  For insight into some of these arguments, see, for example, Rohrer, "Toward a Full-Inclusion Feminism"; Kittay, "Forever Small"; Butler, *Precarious Life*; Butler, *Undoing Gender*, particularly Chapters 1 and 3; Wendell, *The Rejected Body*; Clare, *Exile and Pride*; Wendell, "Toward a Feminist Theory of Disability"; Garland-Thomson, "Integrating Disability."

37  BCU, Fonds Tissot, IS3784/II/144.05.02.28.

38 Rousseau, *The Social Contract*.

39 Colebrook, "On Not Becoming Man," 57. For a related view of the relationship between mind and body, see Simone de Beauvoir's *The Second Sex*, in which she contrasts the transcendent striving of man with the mute, brute immanence of the beast.

40 Bacchi and Beasley, "Citizen Bodies," 344.

41 Kirby, *Telling Flesh*, 73.

42 Kristeva, *Powers of Horror*, 3, italics original.

43 Grosz, *Volatile Bodies*; Shildrick, *Leaky Bodies and Boundaries*.

44 See, for example, Irigaray, *This Sex Which Is Not One* and Cixous, "The Laugh of the Medusa."

45 Grosz, *Volatile Bodies*, 203.

46 Beasley and Bacchi, "Citizen Bodies: Embodying Citizens," 337. See also Beasley and Bacchi, "Envisaging New Politics"; Bacchi and Beasley, "Citizen Bodies."

47 Beasley and Bacchi, "Citizen Bodies: Embodying Citizens," 344.

48 Ibid., 349.

49 Irigaray, *This Sex Which Is Not One*; Irigaray, "The Bodily Encounter with the Mother."

50 Cixous, "The Laugh of the Medusa," 275.

51 Longhurst, "Breaking Corporeal Boundaries," 84.

52 Bacchi and Beasley, "Citizen Bodies," 344.

53 Quinlan, *The Great Nation in Decline*, 6, 4.

54 Vila, "Sensible Diagnostics," 777.

55 Wellman, "Physicians and *Philosophes*," 274.

56 Vila, "Sex and Sensibility," 83.

57 Wellman, "Physicians and *Philosophes*," 273.

58 Quinlan, *The Great Nation in Decline*, 20.

59 *The Encyclopedia of Diderot & d'Alembert: Collaborative Translation Project*, s.v. "State of Nature," trans. Thomas Zemanek, http://creativecommons.org/licenses/by-nc-nd/3.0/, italics original.

60 Ibid.

61 Winston, "Medicine, Marriage, and Human Degeneration," 269.

62 Emch-Dériaz, *Tissot: Physician of the Enlightenment*, 235–6.

63 Ibid., 72.

64 Ibid., 57.

65 Necker, *Nouveaux Mélanges*, 2:135.

66 Emch-Dériaz, *Tissot: Physician of the Enlightenment*, 64.

67 Ibid., 74.

68 Ibid.

69 Fermon, *Domesticating Passions*, 26–32.

70 Tissot, *An Essay on the Disorders of People of Fashion*, 40.

71 Ibid., 7–9.

72 Ibid., 21–2.

73 Ibid., 38.

74 Unsigned, [1796], BCU, Fonds Tissot, IS3784/II/146.01.05.01.

75 Ibid.

76 Tissot, *An Essay on the Disorders of People of Fashion*, 162–3, italics original.

77 Tissot, *De la santé des gens de lettres*. Published in English as *An Essay on Diseases Incidental to Literary and Sedentary Persons*.

78 Tissot, *Essay on Diseases Incidental to Literary and Sedentary Persons*, 12.

79 Ibid., 13.

80 Ibid., 17.

81 See, for example, the Author's Preface that accompanies the 1765 English edition of the *Avis*, where Tissot writes that he was "unfeignedly affected with the Situation of the poor Sick in Country Places in Switzerland, where they are lost from a Scarcity of the best Assistance, and from a fatal Superfluity of the worst, my sole Purpose in writing this Treatise has been to serve, and to comfort them" (Tissot, *Advice to the People in General*, xix–xx).

82 Emch-Dériaz, *Tissot: Physician of the Enlightenment*, 71.

83 Major et Lieutenant de Bouju, 25 September 1773, BCU, Fonds Tissot, IS3784/II/144.02.01.12.

84 Marianne Grand, undated, BCU, Fonds Tissot, IS3784/II/149.01.05.26. See also Marquis d'Albarey [writing about la Comtesse de Mouroux], 6 September 1783, BCU, Fonds Tissot, IS3784/II/144.03.03.13.

85 BCU, Fonds Tissot, IS3784/II/144.05.05.38.

86 Martin, 16 August 1792, BCU, Fonds Tissot, IS3784/II/144.05.05.39. The Latin text is from Virgil's *First Eclogue*. In line 4, a dispossessed shepherd meets a fellow shepherd on the road and says: "Nos patriam fugimus" ["We are leaving our homeland in exile"]. My thanks to Craig Maynes for this insight.

87 Elliott, "Big Persons, Small Voices," 140.

88 Ibid.

89 G. Roche, Letter to Samuel Auguste Tissot, 17 March 1785, BCU, Fonds Tissot, IS3784/II/144.03.05.21.

90 Marquise de Cérarge de Meffray, 28 February 1777, BCU, Fonds Tissot, IS3784/II/144.03.01.01.

91 Mathis, 10 July 1773, BCU, Fonds Tissot, IS3784/II/149.01.07.11.

92 Mathis, 1 October 1773, BCU, Fonds Tissot, IS3784/II/149.01.07.12.

93 Marquis de Choisy, 22 July 1774, BCU, Fonds Tissot, IS3784/II/144.02.05.01.

94 Ibid.

95 D. Macuson [?], undated [1774], BCU, Fonds Tissot, IS3784/II/144.02.05.02.

96 Ibid.

97 Marquis de Lenoncourt, 20 July 1774, BCU, Fonds Tissot, IS3784/II/144.02.05.05.

98 Ibid.

99   Dr Kenenz, undated [1774], BCU, Fonds Tissot, IS3784/II/144.02.05.06.
100  Ibid.
101  Tissot, *An Essay on the Disorders of People of Fashion*, 38.
102  Fegely, undated, BCU, Fonds Tissot, IS3784/II/144.05.01.05.
103  Galliotte, 4 September 1773, BCU, Fonds Tissot, IS3784/II/144.02.02.03.
104  Gatens, *Imaginary Bodies*, 23.
105  Baron de Beaucouse, 25 September 1783, BCU, Fonds Tissot, IS3784/II/144.03.03.17.
106  Unsigned, undated, BCU, Fonds Tissot, IS3784/II/144.04.08.21.
107  Emily Martin, in her article, "Toward an Anthropology of Immunology: The Body as Nation State," offers a provocative reading of the suffering body itself as a nation-state under siege.
108  BCU, Fonds Tissot, IS3784/II/144.03.05.21.
109  BCU, Fonds Tissot, IS3784/II/144.05.03.02.
110  Unsigned, 15 November 1784, BCU, Fonds Tissot, IS3784/II/144.03.04.28.
111  Pictet, 17 July 1767, BCU, Fonds Tissot, IS3784/II/149.01.05.25.
112  Bouteille and Mauris, médecins, 25 March 1782, BCU, Tissot, IS3784/II/144.03.03.03.
113  Ibid.
114  Marquise de Cérarge de Meffray, 28 February 1777, BCU, Fonds Tissot, IS3784/II/144.03.01.01.
115  Robinson and Mills, "Being Observant and Observed," 423.
116  Unsigned, undated, BCU, Fonds Tissot, IS3784/II/144.04.04.23.
117  Unsigned, 30 July 1766, BCU, Fonds Tissot, IS3784/II/144.01.03.05.
118  Unsigned, undated, BCU, Fonds Tissot, IS3784/II/146.01.04.08.
119  Benoit Cattaneo, 28 March 1777, BCU, Fonds Tissot, IS3784/II/144.03.01.08.
120  Murray, "Normative Imperatives," 222.
121  Berlant, *The Queen of America*, 20.
122  Gabrielson and Parady, "Corporeal Citizenship," 380.
123  Kirmayer, "The Body's Insistence on Meaning," 323.
124  Ibid., 329.
125  See, for example, the work of Margaret Lock who considers the potential of bodily dissent ("Cultivating the Body," 141).

CHAPTER FOUR

1  Abbé de St-Véran, [1772], BCU, Fonds Tissot, IS3784/II/144.01.07.35.
2  Ibid.
3  Ibid.
4  Ibid.
5  Jacobus, "Incorruptible Milk."
6  See, for example, Cody, *Birthing the Nation*.
7  Sherman, *The Family Crucible*, 1.
8  Traer, *Marriage and the Family*, 15.

9 Sgard, "Femmes mariées chez Crebillon," 195.

10 See, for example, Darrow, "French Noblewomen"; Duncan, "Happy Mothers"; Rand, "Love, Domesticity, and the Evolution of Genre Painting"; Maza, "The 'Bourgeois' Family Revisited"; Merrick, "The Family Politics of the Marquis De Bombelles"; Bailey, "The 'Afterlife' of Parenting."

11 Winston, *From Perfectibility to Perversion*; Winston, "Medicine, Marriage, and Human Degeneration"; Quinlan, *The Great Nation in Decline*.

12 Winston, *From Perfectibility to Perversion*; Winston, "Medicine, Marriage, and Human Degeneration." See also McAlpin, *Female Sexuality and Cultural Degradation*. For more on literary and textual representations of marriage, see Roulston, *Narrating Marriage*.

13 Constant, *Un monde à l'usage des demoiselles*; Sonnet, *L'Éducation des filles*; Popiel, "Making Mothers"; Popiel, *Rousseau's Daughters*; Bérenguier, *Conduct Books for Girls*; Roulston, "Choix et accomplissement"; Roulston, *Narrating Marriage*.

14 Went-Daoust, "Madame de Charrière," 175.

15 Quinlan, *The Great Nation in Decline*; Quinlan, "Inheriting Vice."

16 Ariès, *Centuries of Childhood*.

17 Edelman, *No Future*.

18 Traer, *Marriage and the Family*, 19.

19 L. Pion, undated, BCU, Fonds Tissot, IS3784/II/144.04.05.20.

20 Madame Rigoley, Marquise d'Agrain, 4 July 1785, BCU, Fonds Tissot, IS3784/II/144.03.06.02.

21 Ibid.

22 Dupuy *fils*, 19 November 1775, BCU, Fonds Tissot, IS3784/II/149.01.03.01.

23 Ibid.

24 Traer, *Marriage and the Family*, 22–3. See also Hanley, "The Family, the State, and the Law"; Desan, *The Family on Trial*; Desan, "The Social Revolution"; Desan, "'War between Brothers and Sisters.'"

25 Unsigned, 4 June 1771, BCU, Fonds Tissot, IS3784/II/149.01.02.19.

26 Ibid.

27 Marquis de Romira, 28 March 1775, BCU, Fonds Tissot, IS3784/II/144.02.06.24.

28 Gerber, "On the Contested Margins of the Family"; Jenkins, *The Life of Property*; Lanza, *From Wives to Widows*; Hanley, "Engendering the State"; Desan, "'War between Brothers and Sisters'"; Hanley, "The Family, the State, and the Law"; Hanley, "Social Sites of Political Practice"; Locklin, *Women's Work and Identity*; Schneider, "Women before the Bench"; Corley, "Gender, Kin, and Guardianship"; Gager, *Blood Ties and Fictive Ties*.

29 Burlamaqui, *Principes du droit naturel*.

30 Fermon, *Domesticating Passions*, 19.

31 Blum, *Strength in Numbers*; McCrea, *Impotent Fathers*.

32 Marquise d'Hervilly, 25 February [1770], BCU, Fonds Tissot, IS3784/II/ 144.02.02.16.

33 Ibid.

34 [Marquise d'Hervilly and husband], undated, BCU, Fonds Tissot, IS3784/ II/144.02.02.17. These considerations, too, mark a consultation about a four-year-old boy suffering from convulsions. Here familial corporeal virtue is enacted through actions: education plans, tears and affective bonds, medical treatments such as inoculation, and other healthful behaviours all signal the family's overt commitment to their child's development. Like the d'Hervilly family, this family cocoons their child in a web of corporeal virtue (Unsigned, undated, BCU, Fonds Tissot, IS3784/II/149.01. 04.07).

35 Bon, [1790], BCU, Fonds Tissot, IS3784/II/144.05.02.36.

36 Ibid.

37 Madame Gounon Laborde, 20 May 1773, BCU, Fonds Tissot, IS3784/II/ 144.02.02.07.

38 BCU, Fonds Tissot, IS3784/II/146.01.05.03.

39 Hanafi, "'Le fruit de nos entrailles,'"48.

40 Badinter, *The Myth of Motherhood*; Brouard-Arends, *Vies et images maternelles*; Brouard-Arends, "Entre nature et histoire"; Popiel, "Making Mothers"; Duncan, "Happy Mothers"; Darrow, "French Noblewomen and the New Domesticity"; Jacobus, "Incorruptible Milk"; Cody, *Birthing the Nation*; Bowers, *The Politics of Motherhood*; Senior, "Aspects of Infant Feeding"; Bergmann, "Language and 'Mother's Milk'"; Bloch, "Women and the Reform of the Nation."

41 For more on the longer-term influence of Rousseau's thought, see Popiel, *Rousseau's Daughters*.

42 McGrath, "The Other Body," 27–58.

43 Churchill, "The Medical Practice of the Sexed Body," 3.

44 See, for example, the case of an eleven-year-old girl who was "born during a time of grief for her mother, who is of a nervous disposition very susceptible to irritation" (Unsigned, 10 November 1770, BCU, Fonds Tissot, IS3784/II/149.01.06.19). See also the work of Nahema Hanafi. Hanafi observes that the requirement of feminine modesty was to assure a child's paternity. Given this, she suggests that there is "an evident link between representations of feminine modesty and the sexual prohibitions leveled against the 'beau sexe.' Woman finds herself linked to the honour of the group, [and] to that of paternity" ("Pudeurs des souffrants," 10).

45 Primary literature in this area includes such works as Roze de l'Epinoy, *Avis aux mères*; Le Rebours, *Avis aux mères*. There is also extensive secondary literature on this subject. See, for example, Sherwood, "Treating Syphilis: The Wetnurse as Technology"; Sherwood, *Infection of the Innocents*; McClive, "Blood and Expertise."

46 Douthwaite, "Le paradoxe," 160. Cathy McClive draws on the notion of "corporeal uncertainty" in her discussion of women's reproductive bodies.

For McClive, the bodily signs and language associated with reproductive experience (from pregnancy through birth, but also in relation to questions of abortion and infanticide) were fundamentally ambiguous ("The Hidden Truths of the Belly").

47 Fermon, *Domesticating Passions*, 162.

48 Brouard-Arends, "Entre nature et histoire," 234, translation mine.

49 Popiel, "Making Mothers"; Popiel, *Rousseau's Daughters*; Bloch, "Woman and the Reform of the Nation"; Algazi, "Martyred Mothers"; Sherwood, "The Milk Factor"; Fairchilds, "Women and the Family"; Trouille, "The Failings of Rousseau's Ideals"; Richter, *Missing the Breast*; Brouard-Arends, "Entre nature et histoire"; Brouard-Arends, *Vie et images maternelles*; Richter, "Wet-Nursing, Onanism, and the Sexuality of the Breast"; Badinter, *The Myth of Motherhood*.

50 McGrath, "The Other Body"; Wilson, "Eighteenth-Century Monsters"; Golightly, "Reproduction in British Women's Novels"; Algazi, "Martyred Mothers"; Cowles, "The Economy of Maternal Loss"; DePree, *"Filles perdues?"*; DePree, *"La Fausse Couche"*; Duncan, "Happy Mothers"; Ohayon, "Rousseau's Julie"; Steinberger, "Difficult Birth of the Good Mother."

51 Azouvi, "Woman as a Model of Pathology"; Peakman and Watkins, "Making Babies"; Williams, "The Experience of Pregnancy and Childbirth"; Smith, "'La raillerie' des femmes."

52 Perry, "Colonizing the Breast"; Senior, "Aspects of Infant Feeding"; Hedenborg, "To Breastfeed Another Woman's Child"; Lastinger, "Re-Defining Motherhood"; Richter, "Wet-Nursing, Onanism, and the Sexuality of the Breast."

53 Popiel, "Making Mothers," 343.

54 Brouard-Arends, "Entre nature et histoire," 234. See also Hanafi, "'Le fruit de nos entrailles.'"

55 Rousseau, *Emile*, 325.

56 Beauvoir, *The Second Sex*.

57 For more on this, see Farrell, *Performing Motherhood*.

58 Badinter, *The Myth of Motherhood*.

59 See, for example, Epinay, *Les contre-confessions*; Charrière, *Lettres de Mistriss Henley*.

60 "Biological Data" is the title of the first chapter in Simone de Beauvoir's *The Second Sex*.

61 Hanafi, "'Le fruit de nos entrailles,'" 47–8.

62 Roy Porter and Dorothy Porter qtd in Magrath, "'Rags of Mortality,'" 239.

63 See, for example, Baronne de Vrintz (née Gugornos) whose third pregnancy and delivery almost "put [her] in the tomb" (8 April 1771, BCU, Fonds Tissot, IS3784/II/149.01.01.23).

64 For more on this, see Evans, "'Unfortunate Objects'"; Meek, "Of Wandering Wombs"; Porter, *Patient's Progress*, 178.

65 See, for example, a letter from Lasseire, which recounts his wife's troubled
reproductive history and later death, the loss of numerous children to
convulsions, and the precarious health of his last child (22 April 1778,
BCU, Fonds Tissot, IS3784/II/149.01.01.25). See also Boucé, "Imagination, Pregnant Women, and Monsters"; Vila, "Sex and Sensibility"; Peter,
"Entre femmes et médecins"; Azouvi, "Woman as a Model of Pathology";
and Huet, *Monstrous Imagination*.

66 Beauvoir, *The Second Sex*, 42, italics original.

67 McGrath, "The Other Body," 36.

68 See, for example, the stillbirths and reproductive problems experienced
by Madame Puybabillier-Mainard (Unsigned, 20 December 1792, BCU,
Fonds Tissot, IS3784/II/144.05.05.41); the miscarriage, false pregnancy,
and madness of an unidentified Portuguese woman (Costa, undated, BCU,
Fonds Tissot, IS3784/II/149.01.05.09); the death of a beloved daughter
(Unsigned, undated, BCU, Fonds Tissot, IS3784/II/138.04); miscarriage
(Unsigned, [1796], BCU, Fonds Tissot, IS3784/II/139.01.09); and the
three miscarriages experienced by Madame C. Neider Doria Cassa (30
September 1780, BCU, Fonds Tissot, IS3784/II/144.03.02.02). For more
on the representational power of miscarriage and infertility, see DePree,
"*La Fausse Couche*"; Smith, "'La raillerie' des femmes."

69 Unsigned, undated, BCU, Fonds Tissot, IS3784/II/149.01.05.27.

70 Ibid.

71 Madame de Launay, undated, BCU, Fonds Tissot, IS3784/II/144.05.02.14.
For more on this particular case, see my articles, "Epistolary Labours,"
and "Gender, Class and Epistolary Suffering."

72 Dupuy *fils*, 19 November 1775, BCU, Fonds Tissot, IS3784/II/149.01.03.
01.

73 McGrath, "The Other Body," 34–5. It is worth noting that this idea of territorial expansion was not always positively received; debates around both
wet-nursing and maternal imaginations were premised on notions of the
maternal body as threat, rather than potential.

74 Madame Necker, born and raised in Coppet and Lausanne, was one of
Tissot's compatriots. Late in her life, she was also one of his patients.

75 Golowkin, *Lettres diverses*.

76 Unsigned, undated, BCU, Fonds Tissot, IS3784/II/138.04.

77 Ibid.

78 Unsigned, undated, BCU, Fonds Tissot, IS3784/II/146.01.05.02.

79 Diderot and d'Alembert, *Encyclopédie*, s.v. "Patrie (gouvernement poli-
tique)," translation mine.

80 Rousseau, *Emile*, 13.

81 Badinter, *The Myth of Motherhood*; Boon, "Maternalising the (Female)
Breast"; Bowers, *The Politics of Motherhood*; Bowers, "'A Point of Con-
science'"; Brouard-Arends, "Entre nature et histoire"; Brouard-Arends,
*Vies et images maternelles*; Charrière, *Lettres de Mistriss Henley*; Edgren,

"Colonizing Women's Bodies"; Epinay, *Les contre-confessions*; Epinoy, *Avis aux mères*; Fildes, *Wet-Nursing: A History*; Gutwirth, "Suzanne Necker's Legacy"; Jacobus, "Incorruptible Milk"; Klimaszewski, "Examining the Wet Nurse"; Lastinger, "Re-Defining Motherhood"; Lastinger, "To Nurse and to Die"; Le Rebours, *Avis aux mères*; Ohayon, "Rousseau's Julie"; Perry, "Colonizing the Breast"; Richter, "Wet-Nursing, Onanism, and the Breast"; Senior, "Aspects of Infant Feeding"; Sherwood, "Treating Syphilis: The Wetnurse as Technology"; Sherwood, *Infection of the Innocents*; Sussman, *Selling Mothers' Milk*; *Encyclopedia of Diderot & d'Alembert: Collaborative Translation Project*, s.v. "Wet-Nurse," trans. Sonja Boon, http://creativecommons.org/licenses/by-nc-nd/3.0/; Yalom, *A History of the Breast*.

82  Epinoy, *Avis aux mères*; Le Rebours, *Avis aux mères*.

83  Some work on this topic does exist. See, for example, Gutwirth, "Suzanne Necker's Legacy"; Boon, *The Life of Madame Necker*.

84  See, for example, Roze de l'Epinoy, *Avis au meres* and the *Encyclopédie* entry on the wet nurse.

85  Boon, "Mothers and Others."

86  Hird, "The Corporeal Generosity of Maternity."

87  Madame de Bombelles, Marquise de Louvois, 29 October 1784, BCU, Fonds Tissot, IS3784/II/144.03.04.18.

88  Senior, "Aspects of Infant Feeding."

89  See, for example, Badinter, *The Myth of Motherhood*; Senior, "Aspects of Infant Feeding"; Sussman, *Selling Mothers' Milk*.

90  Senior, "Aspects of Infant Feeding," 371.

91  *The Encyclopedia of Diderot & d'Alembert: Collaborative Translation Project*, s.v. "Wet-Nurse." trans. Sonja Boon, http://creativecommons.org/licenses/by-nc-nd/3.0/.

92  For more on this, see Boon, "Mothers and Others."

93  Unsigned, undated, BCU, Fonds Tissot, IS3784/II/146.01.05.09.

94  Bonnel de La Bragrousse, *fils*, 16 January 1784, BCU, Fonds Tissot, IS3784/II/144.03.04.22.

95  Unsigned, undated, BCU, Fonds Tissot, IS3784/II/144.05.04.32.

96  Perot, 14 September 1773, BCU, Fonds Tissot, IS3784/II/144.02.03.15.

97  Negroni, 30 March 1785, BCU, Fonds Tissot, IS3784//II/144.03.06.08.

98  Unsigned, undated, BCU, Fonds Tissot, IS3784/II/144.04.04.32.

99  Madame Cagnart Briod, 18 November 1791, BCU, Fonds Tissot, IS3784/II/144.04.02.01.

100  Madame Briaux (?), undated, BCU, Fonds Tissot, IS3784/II/144.04.03.02.

101  Dollffuss, 23 February 1790, BCU, Fonds Tissot, IS3784/II/144.05.01.32.

102  Ibid.

103  Madame Moreau de La Villegille, 3 October 1773, BCU, Fonds Tissot, IS3784/II/144.02.03.25; 28 December 1773, BCU, Fonds Tissot, IS3784/II/144.01.08.18; undated [1773], BCU, Fonds Tissot, IS3784/II/144.02.

03.24. For more on the politics of breastfeeding in the letters to Tissot, see Boon, "Mothers and Others."

104 Madame Moreau de La Villegille, [1773], BCU, Fonds Tissot, IS3784/II/144.02.03.24.

105 Ibid.

106 Ibid.

107 Madame Moreau de La Villegille, 3 October 1773, BCU, Fonds Tissot, IS3784/II/144.02.03.25.

108 In her final letter, Madame Moreau de La Villegille informs Tissot that she gave birth to a healthy son on 21 October 1773. Unfortunately, her attempts to breastfeed were ultimately unsuccessful and, to her sorrow, her child was sent out to nurse (28 December 1773, BCU, Fonds Tissot, IS3784/II/144.01.08.18).

109 Madame Guillemardet, 31 January 1770, BCU, Fonds Tissot, IS3784/II/144.01.05.02.

110 Ibid.

111 Sherwood, "Treating Syphilis: The Wetnurse as Technology"; Sherwood, *Infection of the Innocents*.

112 Madame Guillemardet, 31 January 1770, BCU, Fonds Tissot, IS3784/II/144.01.05.02.

113 Hunt, *Family Romance*; Sherman, *The Family Crucible*; Germann, "Fecund Fathers and Missing Mothers"; Barker, "Painting and Reform"; Smith, "The Relative Duties of a Man"; Tuttle, "Celebrating the *père de famille*"; Merrick, "The Family Politics of the Marquise De Bombelles"; McCrea, *Impotent Fathers*.

114 Sherman, *The Family Crucible*, 18. See also Germann, "Fecund Fathers and Missing Mothers."

115 Hanley, "Engendering the State."

116 See Epinay, *Les contre-confessions* and Charrière, *Lettres de Mistriss Henley*, in particular pages 38–41. See also Bowers, "'A Point of Conscience.'"

117 Tuttle, "Celebrating the *père de famille*," 367.

118 Barker, "Painting and Reform," 46. See also Smith, "The Relative Duties of a Man"; Tuttle, "Celebrating the *père de famille*."

119 Hunt, *Family Romance*, 21.

120 Barker, "Painting and Reform," 45.

121 McClive, "Masculinity on Trial." See also McCrea, *Impotent Fathers*, which considers the literary representation of demographic decline in the UK.

122 Smith, "The Body Embarrassed?" 39.

123 See also Jennifer Grant Germann, who observes that the physical virility of the king, as embodied in his reproductive prowess, was directly linked to "the prosperity of the state" ("Fecund Fathers and Missing Mothers," 109).

124 Benoit Cattaneo, 28 March 1777, BCU, Fonds Tissot, IS3784/II/144.03.
01.08.

125 Ibid.

126 Ibid.

127 Comte de Ferray de Romans, 29 September 1779, BCU, Fonds Tissot,
IS3784/II/149.01.05.05.

128 Reydellet, 29 July 1774, BCU, Fonds Tissot, IS3784/II/144.02.05.17.

129 Marquis de Romira, 28 March 1785, BCU, Fonds Tissot, IS3784/II/144.
02.06.24.

130 Unsigned, 15 May 1792, BCU, Fonds Tissot, IS3784.II.144.05.05.59.

131 Pasteur Cart, 5 May, 8 May, 25 May, 21 June, 22–23 June 1785, BCU,
Fonds Tissot, IS3784/II/144.03.06.13–144.03.06.17. Séverine Pilloud
treats this case in *Les mots du corps*.

132 Cart, 5 May 1785, BCU, Fonds Tissot, IS3784/II/144.03.06.13.

133 Cart, 5 May, 8 May, 25 May, 21 June, 22–23 June 1785, BCU, Fonds
Tissot, IS3784/II/144.03.06.13–144.03.06.17.

134 Steinberg, undated, BCU, Fonds Tissot, IS3784/II/144.04.05.26.

135 Ibid.

136 Maillard, Letter to Samuel Auguste Tissot, 12 April 1773, BCU, Fonds
Tissot, IS3784/II/149.01.02.07. Interestingly, this letter is not about his
daughter at all, but about a countess, which suggests that the paternal
performance of tenderness may have been more strategic than authentic.
Pilloud makes a similar point about a letter written by the Chevalier de
Marmont (*Les mots du corps*, 82).

137 See also Lasseire, who writes about the illnesses of his son and wife (Lasseire, 22 April 1778, BCU, Fonds Tissot, IS3784/II/149.01.01.25), and the
Baron de Monster de Landegge, who positions himself as ideal witness
to his wife's condition (Baron de Monster de Landegge, 24 March 1779,
BCU, Fonds Tissot, IS3784/II/149.01.05.06).

138 Torchon de Lihû, 26 April 1785, BCU, Fonds Tissot, IS3784.II.144.03.
06.18.

139 For more on men's involvement in famly medicine, see Smith, "The Relative Duties of a Man."

140 Radaz chirurgien, 24 September 1786, BCU, Fonds Tissot, IS3784/II/144.
04.01.03.

141 Ibid.

142 Madame Reverdil, 17 July 1791, BCU, Fonds Tissot, IS3784/II/144.04.02.
16.

143 Ibid.

144 Marriage was understood as a way of regulating women's capricious reproductive systems. See also Hanafi, "'Le fruit de nos entrailles.'"

145 Comte de Non, 23 April 1775, BCU, Fonds Tissot, IS3784/II/144.03.06.09.

146 Ibid.

147 Comte de Ferray de Romans, 29 September 1779, BCU, Fonds Tissot,
IS3784/II/149.01.05.05.

148 Ibid.
149 Ibid.
150 Ibid.

## CHAPTER FIVE

1 BCU, Fonds Tissot, IS3784/II/144.02.05.23.
2 François Louis Gauteron, 10 July 1792, BCU, Fonds Tissot, IS3784/II/ 144.05.05.19.
3 Ibid., underlining original.
4 Ibid.
5 François Louis Gauteron, 25 September 1792, BCU, Fonds Tissot, IS3784/ II/144.05.05.21.
6 See, for example, Unsigned, 27 May 1768, BCU, Fonds Tissot, IS3784/II/ 144.01.03.07.
7 Otto, "James Graham as Spiritual Libertine," 204. See also, Porter and Hall, *The Facts of Life*, 108–18.
8 Wagner, "The Discourse on Sex," 47. For more on the Marquis de Sade, see, for example, Wyngaard, "Rétif, Sade, and the Origins of Pornography"; Ferguson, "Sade and the Pornographic Legacy"; Hénaff, *Sade, the Invention of the Libertine Body*; Hekma, "Sade, Masculinity, and Sexual Humiliation"; Phillips, "Obscenity off the Scene"; Parker, "Communal Sexuality"; Quinlan, "Shocked Sensibility"; Silver, "Libertinage et révolution"; Weiss, *Marquis de Sade's Veiled Social Criticism*. For more on Marie Antoinette, see Burrows, *Blackmail, Scandal, and Revolution*; Goodman, *Marie-Antoinette*; Thomas, *The Wicked Queen*. For more on the book trade in clandestine literature, see Darnton, *The Corpus of Clandestine Literature in France*; Darnton, *The Forbidden Best-Sellers*; and others. See also Porter and Hall, *The Facts of Life*, 21, 26; Crawford, "Sexual Knowledge"; Porter, "The Literature of Sexual Advice."
9 Crawford, "Sexual Knowledge in England," 82.
10 For more on the role of marriage as a site of bodily health, see Crawford, "Sexual Knowledge in England."
11 Ibid., 84.
12 McKeon, "The Seventeenth- and Eighteenth-Century Sexuality Hypothesis"; Pilloud, "Les mots du corps."
13 For more on this, see Pilloud, "Les mots du corps."
14 Stolberg, "Self-Pollution, Moral Reform, and the Venereal Trade," 40. See also Cook, "The Politics of Pleasure Talk."
15 For more on both works, see Stolberg, "Self-Pollution, Moral Reform and the Venereal Trade"; Stolberg, "An Unmanly Vice"; Singy, "Friction of the Genitals"; Singy, "Le pouvoir de la science."
16 *Onania*, 1.
17 Ibid., 9.
18 Ibid., 11.

19 Ibid., 20.
20 For more on the notions of reproduction and penile performativity, see Chapter 4.
21 Pilloud, "Les mots du corps."
22 While he states this as his goal, his language betrays him. His book is certainly not in the realm of the *Onania*; however, it still rests on a moral foundation.
23 Stolberg, "An Unmanly Vice," 21.
24 Tissot, *Onanism*, 2.
25 *Onania*, 25.
26 Ibid., 23.
27 Tissot, *Onanism*, 74.
28 Ibid., 73.
29 Ibid., 18–19.
30 Martin, undated, BCU, Fonds Tissot, IS3784/II/144.04.06.03.
31 Tissot, *Onanism*, 24–5.
32 Consider, for example, Rousseau's oft-cited remarks about Parisian salon women.
33 Wilson, "The Female Rake," 97.
34 See, for example, Burrows, *Blackmail, Scandal, and Revolution*; Crowston, "The Queen and Her 'Minister of Fashion'"; Goodman, *Marie-Antoinette*; Hunt, "The Many Bodies"; Thomas, *The Wicked Queen*; Weber, *Queen of Fashion*.
35 Porter and Roberts, Preface, xi.
36 Porter, "Enlightenment and Pleasure," 7.
37 See, for example, Paradis de Moncrif, *Essais sur la nécessité et sur les moyens de plaire*.
38 Roberts, "Pleasures Engendered by Gender," 49. Roberts observes, however, that not all club culture contributed to the broader social good, even as they offered spaces and sites of group identification. The notorious *Hell-Fire* clubs, for example, dedicated to the pleasures of debauchery, were condemned by royal edict (61).
39 Porter, "Enlightenment and Pleasure," 10.
40 Grouchy, *Lettres sur la sympathie*.
41 See also Williams, "'The Luxury of Doing Good.'"
42 *Dictionnaire de l'Académie française*, s.v. "Jouissance."
43 *The Encyclopedia of Diderot & d'Alembert: Collaborative Translation Project*, s.v. "Enjoyment," trans. Anoush Terjanian, http://creativecommons.org/licenses/by-nc-nd/3.0/. Terjanian makes the point that the French word *jouissance* carries numerous meanings and that "the term 'enjoyment' fails to fully capture this range of meanings."
44 Ibid.
45 Porter and Roberts, Preface, xiv.
46 *The Encyclopedia of Diderot & d'Alembert: Collaborative Translation Project*, s.v. "Enjoyment," trans. Anoush Terjanian, http://creativecommons.org/licenses/by-nc-nd/3.0/.

47  Jordanova, "Sex and Gender," 152.

48  Comte d'Adhémar and Dr de Vergennez, undated, BCU, Fonds Tissot, IS3784/II/144.03.01.11.

49  Porter, "Enlightenment and Pleasure," 3. See also Crawford, "Sexual Knowledge," 82.

50  Dawson, "Voltaire's Complaint."

51  Sturzer, "Love and Disease."

52  Young, "'Ce lieu au délices,'" 338.

53  Stolberg, "An Unmanly Vice."

54  BCU, Fonds Tissot, IS3784/II/144.02.04.32.

55  Laqueur, *Solitary Sex*, 13.

56  Grosz, *Volatile Bodies*, xii.

57  Barad, *Meeting the Universe Halfway*, ix.

58  Grosz, *Volatile Bodies*, 19.

59  Not all incidences of gonorrhea were venereal in nature. Weston, "Epistolary Consultations," 71.

60  Gounon [in the hand of Madame Gounon Laborde], [1773], BCU, Fonds Tissot, IS3784/II/144.02.02.08.

61  Ibid.

62  BCU, Fonds Tissot, IS3784/II/144.05.03.08.

63  Rousseau, *The Confessions*, 14.

64  Agin, "'*Comment se font les enfans?*'" 725.

65  Ousrard de Linière, 12 August 1772, BCU, Fonds Tissot, IS3784/II/144.01.07.26.

66  Ibid.

67  Ibid.

68  Ibid.

69  Krizler, 12 November 1791, BCU, Fonds Tissot, IS3784/II/144.05.03.08.

70  Thomas Cranfurd, 28 October 1774, BCU, Fonds Tissot, IS3784/II/144.02.05.09.

71  Chevalier de Peyrelongue, 7 September 1785, BCU, Fonds Tissot, IS3784/II/144.03.06.06.

72  Rossary, 13 June 1774, BCU, Fonds Tissot, IS3784/II/144.02.04.11.

73  Ibid.

74  Ibid.

75  *Dictionnaire de l'académie française*, 4th ed., s.v. "Chatouiller," italics original, translation mine.

76  Ibid. The same principles hold true in the 5th edition (1798).

77  Comte d'Adhémar and Dr de Vergennez, [1777], BCU, Fonds Tissot, IS3784/II/144.03.01.11.

78  Ibid.

79  Chevalier de Valpergue, 24 July 1776, BCU, Fonds Tissot, IS3784/II/144.02.08.17.

80  Ibid.

81  Ibid.

82  Ibid.

83 Weston, "Epistolary Consultations," 70. For more on understandings of syphilis in the eighteenth century, see McAllister, "Stories of the Origin of Syphilis."

84 BCU, Fonds Tissot, IS3784/II/144.02.04.11.

85 Martin, letter to Samuel Auguste Tissot, undated, BCU, Fonds Tissot, IS3784/II/144.04.06.03.

86 Ibid.

87 Ibid.

88 Ibid.

89 I return to the ideas of sight, specularity, and horror in Chapter 6.

90 Martin, undated, BCU, Fonds Tissot, IS3784/II/144.04.06.03.

91 Ibid.

92 Ibid.

93 Ibid.

94 BCU, Fonds Tissot, IS3784/II/144.02.05.23.

95 Thomassin, [1775], BCU, Fonds Tissot, IS3784/II/144.02.08.13.

96 Ibid.

97 Ibid.

98 Ibid.

99 Ibid.

100 Ibid.

101 Ibid.

102 See, for example, Madame Contrisson de Villie, 25 October 1783, BCU, Fonds Tissot, IS3784/II/146.01.01.02; Unsigned, undated, BCU, Fonds Tissot, IS3784/II/131.01; and the letters of Madame de Chastenay, 9 September 1784, 8 November 1784, 15 December 1784, and 21 February 1785, BCU, Fonds Tissot, IS3784/II/144.03.05.03-144.03.05.06. For more on this, see Pilloud, *Les mots du corps*, 274–5.

103 Unsigned, 27 May 1768, BCU, Fonds Tissot, IS3784/II/144.01.03.07. Another correspondent, the Marquis de St-Gilles, indicates that he purposely chose an alias, Gerbaut, in order to evade detection. For more on questions of confidentiality, see Louis-Courvoisier, "Que faut-il ne pas dire à qui?"

104 For more on this, see, for example, Landes, *Women and the Public*; Steinbrügge, *The Moral Sex*; and Spencer, *French Women and the Age of Enlightenment*.

105 Hanafi, "Pudeurs des souffrants," 100.

106 There is an extensive (and still growing) body of literature about domestic servants. Of interest in relation to this study are works such as Fairchilds, "Masters and Servants"; Hill, *Servants*; Kent, "Ubiquitous but Invisible"; Maza, *Servants and Masters*; Meldrum, "Domestic Service"; Morgan and Rushton, "Visible Bodies"; Steedman, "A Boiling Copper and Some Arsenic"; Steedman, *Master and Servant*; Straub, *Domestic Affairs*; Tadmor, "The Concept of the Household-Family"; Tronto, "'The Servant Problem'"; Vickery, "An Englishman's Home Is His Castle?"

107 For more on the political and personal representations of Madame de Pompadour, see Goodman, *The Portraits of Madame de Pompadour*; Hyde, "The 'Makeup' of the Marquise"; Kaiser, "Madame de Pompadour"; Lajer-Burcharth, "Pompadour's Touch"; Jones, "The Fabrication of Madame de Pompadour"; Jones, *Madame de Pompadour*; Scott, "Framing Ambition."

108 Klimaszewski, "Examining the Wet Nurse." See also Bergmann, "Language and 'Mother's Milk.'"

109 As a widower, Desbordes, for example, took up with a slave woman "who had always appeared healthy to me" (10 August 1775, BCU, Fonds Tissot, IS3784/II/149.01.03.05).

110 For more on Olympe de Gouges, see, for example, Beckstrand, *Deviant Women*; Brown, "The Self-Fashionings"; Cole, *Between the Queen and the Cabby*; Diamond, "The Revolutionary Rhetoric."

111 See, for example, McAlpin, "The Virtues of Childhood Sexual Abuse"; May, *Madame Roland and the Age of Revolution*; Goodman, *Becoming a Woman*; and Reynolds, *Marriage and Revolution*.

112 Shuckburgh, *The Memoirs of Madame Roland*, 168–9.

113 Outram, *The Body and the French Revolution*, 132.

114 Ibid. For an alternative reading, see McAlpin, *Female Sexuality and Cultural Degradation*, Chapter 5.

115 Lyons, *Before Imagination*, 77.

116 It is worth considering Rousseau's complicated relationship with Madame de Warens in this regard.

117 Chastenay-Lanty, *Mémoires de Madame de Chastenay*, 10.

118 Ibid., 12.

119 Ibid., 16.

120 See, for example, ibid., 26, 42, 51.

121 Ibid., 42.

122 Ibid.

123 Madame de Chastenay, 9 September 1784, 8 November 1784, 15 December 1784, and 21 February 1785, BCU, Fonds Tissot, IS3784/II/144.03.05.03–144.03.05.06.

124 Madame de Chastenay, 8 November 1784, BCU, Fonds Tissot, IS3784/II/144.03.05.04.

125 Chastenay-Lanty, *Mémoires de Madame de Chastenay*, 51.

126 Madame de Chastenay, 8 November 1784, BCU, Fonds Tissot, IS3784/II/144.03.05.04.

127 McAlpin, "The Virtues of Childhood Sexual Abuse," 27.

128 Irigaray, *This Sex Which Is Not One*, 24.

129 Madame de Chastenay, 8 November 1784, BCU, Fonds Tissot, IS3784/II/144.03.05.04.

130 Ibid.

131 Ibid.

132 Ibid.

133 Qtd in McAlpin, "The Virtues of Childhood Sexual Abuse," 28.

134 Madame de Chastenay, 15 December 1784, BCU, Fonds Tissot, IS3784/II/144.03.05.05.

135 Madame de Chastenay, 8 November 1784, BCU, Fonds Tissot, IS3784/II/144.03.05.04.

136 Anonymous, *Album*, 17.

137 Gonthier, Gauteron, and Iéville, *Etrennes sentimentales*.

138 Pollin, *Le hameau de l'Agnelas*.

139 Gauteron, *Lettre de Mr Gauteron*.

140 François Louis Gauteron to Philippe-Sirice Bridel, 3 October 1795, BCU, Collection Doyen Bridel, IS4177/46; François Louis Gauteron to Phlippe-Sirice Bridel, 2 April 1807, BCU, Collection Doyen Bridel, IS4177/59.

141 François Louis Gauteron, Letter to Philippe Sirice Bridel, 3 October 1795. BCU, Collection Doyen Bridel, IS4177/46.

142 François Louis Gauteron to Philippe-Sirice Bridel, 2 April 1807, BCU, Collection Doyen Bridel, IS4177/59.

143 Ibid., capitalization original.

144 Ibid.

145 Ibid., underlining original.

**CHAPTER SIX**

1 BCU, Fonds Tissot, IS3784/II/144.02.04.27.

2 BCU, Fonds Tissot, IS3784/II/144.02.08.16.

3 Vauvilliers, 14 May 1774, BCU, Fonds Tissot, IS3784/II/144.02.04.26.

4 Ibid.

5 Ibid.

6 Ibid.

7 Ibid.

8 Lawlor, "Fashionable Melancholy," 25.

9 *The Encyclopedia of Diderot & d'Alembert: Collaborative Translation Project*, s.v. "Sensibility," trans. Christelle Gonthier, http://creativecommons.org/licenses/by-nc-nd/3.0/.

10 Ahmed and Stacey, "Introduction: Dermographies," 1, italics original.

11 Ibid., 15. For more on the conceptual potential of "skinning," see Duden, *Disembodying Women*.

12 Boon, *The Life of Madame Necker*. See also the work of Michael Stolberg, *Experiencing Illness and the Sick Body*.

13 Stolberg, *Experiencing Illness and the Sick Body*, 161.

14 Doidge, *The Brain That Changes Itself*; Sacks, *The Mind's Eye*; Sacks, *The Man Who Mistook His Wife for a Hat*; Damasio, *Descartes' Error*; Hustvedt, *The Shaking Woman*; Slater, *Lying*.

15 See, for example, Bluhm, Jacobson, and Maibom, *Neurofeminism*.

16 Boon, *The Life of Madame Necker*, Chapter 5.

17 See also Peter ("Entre femmes et médecins"), who argues that the suffering body is an inherently theatrical space, and Götz, "La maladie comme effet."

18 For more on the *Convulsionnaires de St Médard*, see Kreiser, "Religious Enthusiasm in Early Eighteenth-Century Paris"; Strayer, *Suffering Saints*; Wilson, *Women and Medicine*.

19 For more on the notion of elite sociability as specular, see Stanton, *The Aristocrat as Art*; Pekacz, "The French Salon of the Old Regime as a Spectacle."

20 Porter, *Bodies Politic*, 93.

21 Wetherall-Dickson, "Melancholy, Medicine, Mad Moon and Marriage," 145.

22 The work of Heather Meek, on women's experiences of hysteria, stresses this very point.

23 See, for example, Porter, "Consumption"; Porter, "Material Pleasures." Heather Meek makes the point that "the title of George Cheyne's *The English Malady*, hints at the possible relationship between disease and culture in this period" (Meek, "[W]hat Fatigues," 379).

24 Wetherall-Dickson, "Melancholy, Medicine, Mad Moon and Marriage," 144.

25 For menstrual disorders see Williams, "Hysteria and the Court Physician," 247. Generally, I will employ the terms *nervous disorder*, *vapours*, or *convulsive disorders*. Given my understanding of the idea of nervous disorder as an umbrella term, I incorporate other secondary work, whether it be on vapours, hysteria, or hypochondria, within the broad rubric of "nervous disorder" as it was understood during this period. There was slippage in the term. Within the broad scope of nervous disorders, I have chosen to break nervous disorder down into two categories: vaporous maladies, which could be marshalled in the service of the self, and convulsive disorders (including epilepsy), which, at a fundamental level, challenged notions of the self.

26 Williams, "Hysteria and the Court Physician," 247.

27 Stolberg, *Experiencing Illness and the Sick Body*, 171.

28 See also Vauvilliers's letter, cited earlier (BCU, Fonds Tissot, IS3784/II/144.02.04.26), as well as (among others) an undated consultation written by a twenty-year-old woman (BCU, Fonds Tissot, IS3784/II/144.02.08.18), and the case of four trembling siblings, which I cite later in this chapter (BCU, Fonds Tissot, IS3784/II/144.03.04.04). For more on the role of fear in medical consultations, see Smith, "'An Account of Unaccountable Distemper.'"

29 Chevalier de Valpergue, 24 July 1776, BCU, Fonds Tissot, IS3784/II/144.02.08.17.

30 Wetherall-Dickson, "Melancholy, Medicine, Mad Moon and Marriage," 144.

31 Gaspary, 18 May 1773, BCU, Fonds Tissot, IS3784/II/144.02.02.05.

32 Stolberg, *Experiencing Illness and the Sick* Body, 178.

33 Quinlan, *The Great Nation in Decline*, 23.

34 Jonsson, "The Physiology of Hypochondria in Eighteenth-Century Britain," 18.

35 For more on this, see Jonsson, "The Physiology of Hypochondria in Eighteenth-Century Britain."

36 Lawlor, "Fashionable Melancholy," 30.

37 Diderot and d'Alembert, *Encyclopédie*, s.v. "Vapeurs (en médecine)," translation mine.

38 Emch-Dériaz, *Tissot: Physician of the Enlightenment*, 117.

39 Ibid., 118.

40 Jonsson, "The Physiology of Hypochondria."

41 Ibid., 17.

42 For more on the notion of consumption and its links with nervous disorder, see, for example, Roy Porter, "Consumption: Disease of the Consumer Society?" and "Material Pleasures."

43 Vila, "The *Philosophe*'s Stomach," 92.

44 Weyland, undated, BCU, Fonds Tissot, IS3784/II/149.02.02.05. Others, too, overtly lamented a diagnosis of epilepsy. See, for example, Madame Chevallier de Bouchet, 12 December 1769, BCU, Fonds Tissot, IS3784/II/149.01.07.04; Börking, 30 November 1770, BCU, Fonds Tissot, IS3784/II/149.01.05.17.

45 Vila, "The *Philosophe*'s Stomach," 89.

46 Jonsson, "The Physiology of Hypochondria," 15. See also Lawlor, "Fashionable Melancholy."

47 Dawson, "Voltaire's Complaint"; Vila, "The *Philosophe*'s Stomach," 97.

48 Vila, "The *Philosophe*'s Stomach," 96.

49 Williams, "Stomach and Psyche," 358.

50 Ibid., 365.

51 Jonsson, "The Physiology of Hypochondria," 15–16.

52 Stolberg, *Experiencing Illness and the Sick Body*, 187. This reading would accord with Heather Meek's assertion that, for women, hysteria was a response to their social subordination (Meek, "Of Wandering Wombs").

53 Emch-Dériaz, *Tissot: Physician of the Enlightenment*, 125.

54 Probyn, *Blush*, 38.

55 Qtd in Smith, "Brain and Mind in the 'Long' Eighteenth Century," 22.

56 La Mettrie, *L'homme machine*. Tissot's correspondent, Hartmann, describes his body as a watch (Hartmann, 19 June 1792, BCU, Fonds Tissot, IS3784/II/144.05.05.32).

57 See, for example, Fausto-Sterling, *Sex/Gender*; Barad, *Meeting the Universe Halfway*.

58 Diderot, *Rameau's Nephew and d'Alembert's Dream*, 214.

59 For more on this, see Vila, "Beyond Sympathy"; Mullan, "Hypochondria and Hysteria."

60 Diderot, *Rameau's Nephew and d'Alembert's Dream*, 183.

61 Lawlor, "Fashionable Melancholy," 47.

62 Vila, "Beyond Sympathy," 93.

63 Ingram, "Steering toward Sanity," 6.

64 Jonsson, "The Physiology of Hypochondria," 17.

65 Unsigned, undated, BCU, Fonds Tissot, IS3784/II/144.04.04.23.

66 See the work of Heather Meek for more on this. See also Mullan, "Hypochondria and Hysteria"; Barker-Benfield, *The Culture of Sensibility*.

67 Emch-Dériaz, *Tissot: Physician of the Enlightenment*, 130.

68 Heather Meek makes this point in her chapter, "[W]hat Fatigues," 376.

69 For more on the notion of inheritance, legacy, and autobiographical self-fashioning, see Boon, "Recuperative Autobiography."

70 BCU, Fonds Tissot, IS3784/II/144.03.06.24.

71 Foucault qtd in Vila, "Beyond Sympathy," 90.

72 Arnaud, "Ruse and Reappropriation"; Stolberg, *Experiencing Illness and the Sick Body*; Lawlor, "Fashionable Melancholy"; Le Menthéour, "Melancholy Vaporised."

73 Arnaud, "Ruse and Reappropriation," 177.

74 Comte Petitti de Mont[?], 1785, BCU, Fonds Tissot, IS3784/II/144.03.06.04.

75 Ibid., 179.

76 Lawlor, "Fashionable Melancholy," 27.

77 See, too, the work of Magrath ("'Rags of Mortality'") and Sturzer ("Love and Disease") for more on this.

78 Lawlor, "Fashionable Melancholy," 39–40.

79 Ibid., 38.

80 Puihabilié, 21 August 1770, BCU, Fonds Tissot, IS3784/II/149.01.05.18.

81 Ibid.

82 Unsigned, undated, BCU, Fonds Tissot, IS3784/II/146.01.05.02.

83 Unsigned, undated, BCU, Fonds Tissot, IS3784/II/146.01.05.02.

84 Meek, "Of Wandering Wombs," 107. Margaret Lock makes a similar point (Lock, "Cultivating the Body," 142). In relation to this, it is also worth considering the decidedly ambiguous and ambivalent ending of Isabelle de Charrière's *Lettres de Mistriss Henley*.

85 Berlant, "Slow Death," 754.

86 Unsigned, undated, BCU, Fonds Tissot, IS3784/II/149.01.03.08.

87 Ibid.

88 Ibid.

89 Madame Chevallier de Bouchet, 12 December 1769, BCU, Fonds Tissot, IS3784/II/149.01.07.04.

90 Ibid.

91 Ibid.

92 Ibid.

93 Ibid.

94 Comte Piossasque de Non, 23 April 1785, BCU, Fonds Tissot, IS3784/II/144.03.06.09.

95 Ibid.

96 See also the case of a nun named Soeur Lepin, also suffering from nervous disorders: "the smallest degree of heat caused her the most intense pain." Unsigned, undated, BCU, Fonds Tissot, IS3784/II/144.04.04.17.

97 Wilson, *Women and Medicine*.

98 Morel, 7 August 1784, BCU, Fonds Tissot, IS3784/II/144.03.04.04. Interestingly, Nahema Hanafi has argued that cancer, too, was understood through the lens of contagion ("Le cancer à travers").

99 Porter, *Flesh in the Age of Reason*, 316.

100 Madame Fontanes, 29 December 1774, BCU, Fonds Tissot, IS3784/II/149.01.03.09.

101 Decoppet, 29 November 1763, BCU, Fonds Tissot, IS3785/II/149.01.06.01.

102 Verdun, 6 February 1769, BCU, Fonds Tissot, IS3784/II/149.01.02.09.

103 Landsee, 11 January 1774, BCU, Fonds Tissot, IS3784/II/149.01.07.09.

104 Such arguments also lie at the heart of contemporary activisms in the area of disability.

105 Unsigned, undated, BCU, Fonds Tissot, IS3784/II/149.01.07.14.

106 Dr Sidenier, 22 May 1765, BCU, Fonds Tissot, IS3784/II/149.01.03.11.

107 Ibid.

108 Ibid.

109 Langley, 28 October 1775, BCU, Fonds Tissot, IS3784/II/149.01.07.19.

110 Colebrook, "On Not Becoming Man," 67.

### EPILOGUE

1 Rapp, *The Still Point*, 53.

2 Egan, *Burdens of Proof*, 15.

3 Cryle, "Les Choses et les Mots," 442.

4 Egan, *Burdens of Proof*, 31.

5 See, for example, Dr Cherb, 25 June 1773, BCU, Fonds Tissot, IS3784/II/149.01.05.01; Frédéric de Mulinen, 9 July 1790, BCU, Fonds Tissot, IS3784/II/144.05.01.42; Madame Possel née Fromaget, undated, BCU, Fonds Tissot, IS3784/II/144.04.06.18.

6 See, for example, Baron de Monster de Landegge, 24 March 1779, BCU, Fonds Tissot, IS3784/II/149.01.05.06; Monsieur Demandolx writing about his wife's descent into *folie* (Demandolx, undated, BCU, Fonds Tissot, IS3784/II/144.04.05.12); and the case of Madame Tollot, described by an unknown author (Unsigned, undated, BCU, Fonds Tissot, IS3784/II/149.01.05.27).

7 See, for example, Ploucquet, 24 April 1777, BCU, Fonds Tissot, IS3784/II/144.03.01.03; Unsigned, undated, BCU, Fonds Tissot, IS3784/II/144.04.06.11; Unsigned [about a Mr Jones], undated, BCU, Fonds Tissot, IS3784/II/144.04.06.11; Unsigned [about the madness of Madame Chainel], [1767], BCU, Fonds Tissot, IS3784/II/149.01.06.11.

8 Lejeune, *On Autobiography*.

9 Pomme, 12 December 1768, BCU, Fonds Tissot, IS3784/II/144.04.08.22; Cosnier, 22 December 1768, BCU, Fonds Tissot, IS3784/II/144.04.08.23; Pomme, 6 January 1769, BCU, Fonds Tissot, IS3784/II/144.04.08.24; Cosnier, 19 January 1769, BCU, Fonds Tissot, IS3784/II/144.04.08.25; Souquet, 27 May 1769, BCU, Fonds Tissot, IS3784/II/144.04.08.26; Pomme and Cosnier, 16 June 1769, BCU, Fonds Tissot, IS3784/II/144.04.08.27; Souquet, 28 July 1769, BCU, Fonds Tissot, IS3784/II/144.04.08.28; Souquet, 2 August 1769, BCU, Fonds Tissot, IS3784/II/144.04.08.29; Souquet, 3 August 1769, BCU, Fonds Tissot, IS3784/II/144.04.08.30; Cosnier, 11 September 1769, BCU, Fonds Tissot, IS3784/II/144.04.08.31; Souquet, 20 September 1769, BCU, Fonds Tissot, IS3784/II/144.04.08.32; Souquet, 29 June 1771, BCU, Fonds Tissot, IS3784/II/144.04.08.33.

10 *Archives du corps*.

11 Cosnier, 22 December 1768, BCU, Fonds Tissot, IS3784/II/144.04.08.23.

12 Souquet, 3 August 1769, BCU, Fonds Tissot, IS3784/II/13.04.03.30; Souquet, 29 June 1772, BCU, Fonds Tissot, IS3784/II/144.04.08.33.

13 Cosnier, 11 September 1769, BCU, Fonds Tissot, IS3784/II/144.04.08.31.

14 Cosnier, 22 December 1768, BCU, Fonds Tissot, IS3784/II/144.04.08.23; Souquet, 3 August 1769, BCU, Fonds Tissot, IS3784/II/144.04.08.30; Souquet, 29 June 1772, BCU, Fonds Tissot, IS3784/II/144.04.08.33.

15 Souquet, 3 August 1769, BCU, Fonds Tissot, IS3784/II/144.04.08.30.

16 Souquet, 3 August 1769, BCU, Fonds Tissot, IS3784/II/144.04.08.30; Cosnier, 22 December 1768, BCU, Fonds Tissot, IS3784/II/144.04.08.23.

17 McRuer, *Crip Theory*, 1.

18 Wendell, "Toward a Feminist Theory," 111.

19 Butler, "Violence, Mourning, Politics."

20 Ibid., 15–16.

21 Puar, "Coda: The Cost of Getting Better," 156.

22 Overboe, "Ableist Limits," 278.

23 Couser, "Paradigm's Cost," 20.

24 Smith and Watson, *Reading Autobiography*, 32.

25 Torrell, "Plural Singularities," 324.

26 Raoul et al., "Narrating the Unspeakable," 192.

27 Ibid., 193.

28 Porter, "'Expressing Yourself Ill,'" 276. See also Scarry, *The Body in Pain*.

29 Avraham, *The Invading Body*, 13.

30 Overboe, "Ableist Limits," 276.

31 Ibid., 277.

32 Diprose, "Writing in Blood," 279.

33 Egan, *Burdens of Proof*, 15.

34 Beasley and Bacchi, "Making Politics Fleshly," 112.

## { BIBLIOGRAPHY }

### MANUSCRIPT SOURCES

*Bibliothèque cantonale et universitaire de Lausanne*

Fonds Tissot
This material is also available online at *Archives du corps et de la santé au 18e siècle. Les lettres de patients au Dr. Samuel Auguste Tissot (1728–1797)*. Edited by Séverine Pilloud, Micheline Louis-Courvoisier, and Vincent Barras. http://tissot.unil.ch/fmi/iwp/cgi?-db=Tissot&-loadframes.

  IS3784/II/131
  IS3784/II/132
  IS3784/II/133
  IS3784/II/138
  IS3784/II/139
  IS3784/II/140
  IS3784/II/141
  IS3784/II/142
  IS3784/II/142bis
  IS3784/II/143
  IS3784/II/144
  IS3784/II/146
  IS3784/II/149

Collection Doyen Bridel
  IS4177/46
  IS4177/59

### PRINT SOURCES

Agin, Shane. "'*Comment se font les enfans?*' Sex Education and the Preservation of Innocence in Eighteenth-Century France." *MLN* 117, no. 4 (2002): 722–36.
Ahmed, Sara, and Jackie Stacey, eds. *Thinking through the Skin*. New York: Routledge, 2001.

Alaimo, Stacy, and Susan J. Hekman, eds. *Material Feminisms*. Bloomington: Indiana University Press, 2008.

Algazi, Lisa G. "Martyred Mothers Never Die: The Legacy of Rousseau's *Julie*." *Journal of the Association for Research on Mothering* 4, no. 1 (2002): 137–45.

Allegranti, Beatrice. *Embodied Performances: Sexuality, Gender, Bodies*. New York: Palgrave Macmillan, 2011.

Altman, Janet Gurkin. *Epistolarity: Approaches to a Form*. Columbus: Ohio State University Press, 1982.

Anderson, Benedict R. *Imagined Communities: Reflections on the Origin and Spread of Nationalism*. Rev. ed. London: Verso, 1991.

Anonymous. *Album s. sancti ministerii candidatorum collegi superioris et inferioris discipulorum in Academia Lausannensis pro anno 1789*. Lausanne: Isaac Hignou, 1789.

Anselment, Eric. "'The Want of Health': An Early Eighteenth-Century Self-Portrait of Sickness." *Literature and Medicine* 15, no. 2 (1996): 225–43.

Ariès, Philippe. *Centuries of Childhood: A Social History of Family Life*. Translated by Robert Baldick. New York: Knopf, 1962.

Armstrong, Jeannette. "Racism: Racial Exclusivity and Cultural Supremacy." In *Give Back: First Nations Perspectives on Cultural Practices*, edited by Maria Campbell, Doreen Jensen, and Joy Asham Fedorick, 73–83. North Vancouver: Gallerie, 1992.

Arnaud, Sabine. "Ruse and Reappropriation in the French Eighteenth Century: *La Philosophie des Vapeurs* by C.-J. de B. de Paumerelle." *French Studies: A Quarterly Review* 65, no. 2 (2011): 174–87.

Avrahami, Einat. *The Invading Body: Reading Illness Autobiographies*. Charlottesville: University of Virginia Press, 2007.

Azouvi, François. "Woman as a Model of Pathology in the Eighteenth Century." *Diogènes* 115 (1981): 22–36.

Bacchi, Carol, and Chris Beasley. "Citizen Bodies: Is Embodied Citizenship a Contradiction in Terms?" *Critical Social Policy* 22, no. 2 (2002): 324–52.

Badinter, Elisabeth. *The Myth of Motherhood: An Historical View of the Maternal Instinct*. Translated by Roger De Garis. London: Souvenir Press, 1981.

Baecque, Antoine de. *The Body Politic: Corporeal Metaphor in Revolutionary France, 1770–1800*. Translated by Charlotte Mandell. Stanford: Stanford University Press, 1997.

– *Glory and Terror: Seven Deaths under the French Revolution*. Translated by Charlotte Mandell. New York: Routledge, 2001.

Bailey, Joanne. "The 'Afterlife' of Parenting: Memory, Parentage, and Personal Identity in Britain, c. 1760–1830." *Journal of Family History* 35, no. 3 (2010): 249–70.

Baker, Patricia. "Hearing and Writing Women's Voices." *Resources for Feminist Research* 26, no. 1/2 (1998): 31–53.

Ballaster, Ros. "The Economics of Ethical Conversation: The Commerce of the Letter in Eliza Haywood and Lady Mary Wortley Montagu." *Eighteenth-Century Life* 35, no. 1 (2011): 119–32.

Barad, Karen. *Meeting the Universe Halfway: Quantum Physics and the Entanglement of Matter and Meaning*. Durham, NC: Duke University Press, 2007.

Barker, Emma. "Painting and Reform in Eighteenth-Century France: Greuze's 'L'Accordée de Village.'" *Oxford Art Journal* 20, no. 2 (1997): 42–52.

Barker-Benfield, G.J. *The Culture of Sensibility: Sex and Society in Eighteenth-Century Britain*. Chicago: University of Chicago Press, 1996.

Barras, Vincent, and Martin Dinges. *Maladies en lettres. 17e–21e siècles*. Lausanne: Editions BHMS, 2013.

Barras, Vincent, and Micheline Louis-Courvoisier. "Tissot et la médecine des Lumières." *Médecine et hygiène* 2369 (2001): 2341–3.

Barras, Vincent, and Micheline Louis-Courvoisier, eds. *La médecine des Lumières: Tout autour de Tissot*. Geneva and Paris: Georg Editeur, 2001.

Barras, Vincent, and Philip Rieder. "Corps et sujet à l'époque des Lumières." *Dix-huitième siècle* 37 (2005): 211–24.

Barras, Vincent, and V. Gaist. "Petit dossier Tissot." *Courrier du médecin vaudois* (1996): 3–7.

Barton, David, and Nigel Hall. Introduction to *Letter Writing as a Social Practice*, edited by David Barton and Nigel Hall, 1–14. Amsterdam and Philadelphia: John Benjamin, 2000.

Baudelaire, Charles. "L'Invitation au voyage." In *Les fleurs du mal*, 115–17. Paris: Poulet-Malassis et De Broise, 1857.

Beasley, Chris, and Carol Bacchi. "Citizen Bodies: Embodying Citizens – A Feminist Analysis." *International Feminist Journal of Politics* 2, no. 3 (2000): 337–58.

– "Envisaging a New Politics for an Ethical Future: Beyond Trust, Care and Generosity Towards an Ethic of Social Flesh." *Feminist Theory* 8, no. 3 (2007): 279–98.

– "Making Politics Fleshly: The Ethic of Social Flesh." In *Engaging with Carol Bacchi: Strategic Interventions and Exchanges*, edited by Angelique Bletsas and Chris Beasley, 99–120. Adelaide: University of Adelaide Press, 2012.

Beauvoir, Simone de. *The Second Sex*. Translated by Constance Borde and Sheila Malovany-Chevallier. London: Jonathan Cape, 2009.

Beckstrand, Lisa. *Deviant Women of the French Revolution and the Rise of Feminism*. Madison, NJ: Fairleigh Dickinson University Press, 2009.

Beiner, Ronald. "Introduction: Why Citizenship Constitutes a Theoretical Problem in the Last Decade of the Twentieth Century." In *Theorizing Citizenship*, edited by Ronald Beiner, 1–28. Albany: State University of New York Press, 1995.

Belsey, Catherine. "Textual Analysis as a Research Method." In *Research Methods for English Studies*, edited by Gabrielle Griffin, 157–74. Edinburgh: Edinburgh University Press, 2005.

Bérenguier, Nadine. *Conduct Books for Girls in Enlightenment France*. Farnham: Ashgate, 2011.

- "Lettres de Suzanne Necker à Antoine Thomas." In *Lettres de femmes: Textes inédits et oubliés du XVIe au XVIIIe siècle*, edited by Elizabeth C. Goldsmith and Colette H. Winn, 339–78. Paris: Honoré Champion, 2005.

Berg, Temma. "Truly Yours: Arranging a Letter Collection." *Eighteenth-Century Life* 35, no. 1 (2011): 29–50.

Berger, John. *Ways of Seeing*. London: Penguin Classic, 2008.

Bergmann, Emilie L. "Language and 'Mother's Milk': Maternal Roles and the Nurturing Body in Early Modern Spanish Texts." In *Maternal Measures: Figuring Caregiving in the Early Modern Period*, edited by Naomi J. Miller and Naomi Yavneh, 105–20. Aldershot: Ashgate, 2000.

Berlant, Lauren. *The Queen of America Goes to Washington City: Essays on Sex and Citizenship*. Durham, NC: Duke University Press, 1997.

- "Slow Death (Sovereignty, Obesity, Lateral Agency)." *Critical Inquiry* 33, no. 4 (2007): 754–80.

Birke, Linda. *Feminism and the Biological Body*. Edinburgh: Edinburgh University Press, 1999.

Bland, Caroline, and Máire Cross, eds. *Gender and Politics in the Age of Letter Writing, 1750–2000*. Aldershot: Ashgate, 2004.

Bloch, Jean M. "Women and the Reform of the Nation." In *Woman and Society in Eighteenth-Century France*, edited by Eva Jacobs, W.H. Barber, Jean H. Block, F.W. Leakey, and Eileen Le Breton, 3–18. London: Athlone Press, 1979.

Bluhm, Robyn, Anne Jaap Jacobson, and Heidi Lene Maibom, eds. *Neurofeminism: Issues at the Intersection of Feminist Theory and Cognitive Science*. New York: Palgrave Macmillan, 2012.

Blum, Carol. *Strength in Numbers: Population, Reproduction, and Power in Eighteenth-Century France*. Baltimore: Johns Hopkins University Press, 2002.

Boon, Sonja. "Does a Dutiful Wife Write? or, Should Suzanne Get Divorced? Reflections on Suzanne Curchod Necker, Divorce, and the Construction of the Biographical Subject." *Lumen: Selected Proceedings from the Canadian Society for Eighteenth-Century Studies/Travaux choisis de la Société canadienne d'étude du dix-huitième siècle*. Vol. 27 (2008): 59–73.

- "Epistolary Labours: Reading Childbirth and the Politics of Reproductive Medicine in Two Eigtheenth-Century Women's Letters." *Journal of the Motherhood Initiative* 5, no. 1 (2014): 160–71.

- "Gender, Class and Epistolary Suffering: Narrating the Bodily Self in Women's Medical Consultation Letters to Samuel Auguste Tissot." *Bulletin of the John Rylands University Library* 90, no. 2 (2014): 143–61.

- *The Life of Madame Necker: Sin, Redemption and the Parisian Salon*. London: Pickering & Chatto, 2011.

- "Maternalising the (Female) Breast: A Comparison of Marie-Angélique Anel Le Rebours' *Avis aux mères qui veulent nourrir leurs enfans* (1767) and La Leche League International's *The Womanly Art of Breastfeeding* (1963)." *Limina: A Journal of Historical and Cultural Studies* 15 (2009). http://www.archive.limina.arts.uwa.edu.au/past_volumes/15/boon.

- "Mothers and Others: The Politics of Lactation in Medical Consultation Letters Addressed to Samuel Auguste Tissot." In *The Secrets of Generation: Reproduction in the Long Eighteenth Century*, edited by Raymond Stephanson and Darren Wagner, 258–77. Toronto: University of Toronto Press, 2015.
- "Recuperative Autobiography and the Politics of Life Writing: Lineage, Inheritance, and Legacy in the Writings of the Marquise de La Ferté-Imbault." *Journal of Women's History* 24, no. 3 (2012): 13–38.
Bossis, Philippe. "Atelier no. 4: La Lettre Document: Approche Interdisciplinaire." In *Ecrire, publier, lire les correspondances: (problématique et économie d'un "genre littéraire"): actes du colloque international "Les correspondances,"* edited by Jean-Louis Bonnat and Mireille Bossis, 457–60. Nantes: Université de Nantes, 1983.
Boucé, Paul-Gabriel. "Imagination, Pregnant Women, and Monsters in Eighteenth-Century England and France." In *Sexual Underworlds of the Enlightenment*, edited by G.S. Rousseau and Roy Porter, 86–100. Chapel Hill: University of North Carolina Press, 1988.
Bowers, Toni. "'A Point of Conscience': Breastfeeding and Maternal Authority in Pamela, Part 2." In *Inventing Maternity: Politics, Science, and Literature, 1650–1865*, edited by Susan C. Greenfield and Carol Barash, 138–58. Lexington: University Press of Kentucky, 1999.
- *The Politics of Motherhood: British Writing and Culture, 1680–1760*. Cambridge; New York: Cambridge University Press, 1996.
Brant, Clare. *Eighteenth-Century Letters and British Culture*. New York: Palgrave Macmillan, 2006.
Braziel, Jennifer E., and Kathleen LeBesco, eds. *Bodies out of Bounds: Fatness and Transgression*. Berkeley: University of California Press, 2001.
Brouard-Arends, Isabelle. "Entre nature et histoire: Dire la maternité au siècle des Lumières." In *Sexualité, mariage et famille au XVIIIe siècle*, edited by Olga B. Cragg and Rosena Davison, 233–39. Montréal: Les presses de l'Université Laval, 1998.
- *Vies et images maternelles dans la littérature française du dix-huitième siècle*. Oxford: Voltaire Foundation, 1991.
Broomhall, Susan. *Women's Medical Work in Early Modern France*. Manchester: Manchester University Press, 2004.
Brown, Gregory S. "The Self-Fashionings of Olympe de Gouges, 1784–1789." *Eighteenth-Century Studies* 34, no. 3 (2001): 383–401.
Burke, Peter, and Roy Porter, eds. *Language, Self and Society: A Social History of Language*. London: Polity Press, 1991.
Burlamaqui, Jean-Jacques. *Principes du droit naturel*. 2 vols. Geneva: Barrillot, 1748.
Burney, Fanny. *The Journal and Letters of Fanny Burney*. Vol. 12. Edited by Joyce Hemlow, Althea Douglas, and Patricia Hawkins. Oxford: Clarendon Press.
Burrows, Simon. *Blackmail, Scandal, and Revolution: London's French Libellistes, 1758–92*. Manchester: Manchester University Press, 2006.

Burton, Antoinette. "An Assemblage/Before Me." *Journal of Women's History* 25, no. 2 (2013): 185–8.

Butler, Judith. *Bodies That Matter: On the Discursive Limits of "Sex."* New York: Routledge, 1993.

– *Gender Trouble: Feminism and the Subversion of Identity*. New York: Routledge, 1990.

– *Precarious Life: The Powers of Mourning and Violence*. London: Verso, 2006.

– *Undoing Gender*. New York: Routledge, Taylor & Francis Group, 2004.

– "Violence, Mourning, Politics." *Studies in Gender and Sexuality* 4, no. 1 (2003): 9–37.

Canning, Kathleen. "The Body as Method? Reflections on the Place of the Body in Gender History." *Gender & History* 11, no. 3 (1999): 499–513.

Canning, Kathleen, and Sonya O. Rose. "Gender, Citizenship and Subjectivity: Some Historical and Theoretical Considerations." *Gender & History* 13, no. 3 (2001): 427–43.

Charrière, Isabelle de. *Lettres de Mistriss Henley publiées par son amie*. Edited by Joan Hinde Stewart and Philip Stewart. New York: Modern Language Association, 1993.

Chastenay-Lanty, Victorine de. *Mémoires de Madame de Chastenay, 1771–1815*. Vol. 1. Edited by Alphonse Roderot. Paris: Plon, 1896.

Cheyne, George. *The English Malady, or, A Treatise of Nervous Diseases of all Kinds*. Delanco, NJ: Gryphon Editions, 2008.

Churchill, Wendy D. "Bodily Differences?: Gender, Race, and Class in Hans Sloane's Jamaican Medical Practice, 1687–1688." *Journal of the History of Medicine and Allied Sciences* 60, no. 4 (2005): 391–444.

– *Female Patients in Early Modern Britain: Gender, Diagnosis, and Treatment*. Farnham: Ashgate, 2012.

– "The Medical Practice of the Sexed Body: Women, Men, and Disease in Britain, circa 1600–1740." *Social History of Medicine* 18, no. 1 (2005): 322.

Cixous, Hélène. "The Laugh of the Medusa." In *French Feminism Reader*, edited by Kelly Oliver, 257–75. Lanham, MD: Rowman & Littlefield, 2000.

Clare, Eli. *Exile and Pride: Disability, Queerness and Liberation*. Cambridge, MA: Southend Press, 1999.

Cody, Lisa Forman. *Birthing the Nation: Sex, Science and the Conception of Eighteenth-Century Britons*. Oxford: Oxford University Press, 2005.

Cole, John R. *Between the Queen and the Cabby: Olympe De Gouges's Rights of Woman*. Montreal and Kingston: McGill-Queen's University Press, 2011.

Colebrook, Claire. "On Not Becoming Man: The Materialist Politics of Unactualized Potential." In *Material Feminisms*, edited by Stacy Alaimo and Susan Hekman, 52–84. Bloomington: Indiana University Press, 2008.

Coleman, William. "The People's Health: Medical Themes in Eighteenth-Century French Popular Literature." *Bulletin of the History of Medicine* 51 (1977): 55–74.

Constant, Paule. *Un monde à l'usage des demoiselles*. Paris: Gallimard, 1987.

Cook, Alexander. "The Politcs of Pleasure Talk in 18th-Century Europe." *Sexualities* 12, no. 4 (2009): 451–66.

Cook, Elizabeth Heckendorn. *Epistolary Bodies: Gender and Genre in the Eighteenth-Century Republic of Letters.* Stanford: Stanford University Press, 1996.

Corley, Christopher. "Gender, Kin, and Guardianship in Early Modern Burgundy." In *Family, Gender, and Law in Early Modern France,* edited by Suzanne Desan and Jeffrey Merrick, 183–222. University Park: Pennsylvania University Press, 2009.

Couser, G. Thomas. "Paradigm's Cost: Representing Vulnerable Subjects." *Literature and Medicine* 24, no. 1 (2005): 19–30.

– *Recovering Bodies: Illness, Disability, and Life Writing.* Madison: University of Wisconsin Press, 1997.

– *Signifying Bodies: Disability in Contemporary Life Writing.* Ann Arbor: University of Michigan Press, 2009.

– *Vulnerable Subjects: Ethics and Life Writing.* Ithaca, NY: Cornell University Press, 2004.

Cowles, Mary Jane. "The Economy of Maternal Loss in Rousseau's *Confessions.*" *L'Esprit Créateur* 39, no. 2 (1999): 11–19.

Cragg, Olga B., and Rosena Davison, eds. *Sexualité, mariage et famille au XVIIIe siècle.* Saint-Nicolas: Les presses de l'Université Laval, 1998.

Crawford, Patricia. "Sexual Knowledge in England, 1500–1750." In *Sexual Knowledge, Sexual Science: The History of Attitudes to Sexuality,* edited by Roy Porter and Mikulas Teich, 82–106. Cambridge: Cambridge University Press, 1994.

Crowston, Clare Haru. "The Queen and Her 'Minister of Fashion': Gender, Credit and Politics in Pre–Revolutionary France." *Gender & History* 14, no. 1 (2002): 92–116.

Cryle, Peter. "Les Choses et les Mots: Missing Words and Blurry Things in the History of Sexuality." *Sexualities* 12, no. 4 (2009): 437–50.

Cusset, Catherine. "La lettre ou l'utopie de l'amitié: Le cas de Sophie Cottin (1770–1807)." In *La lettre au XVIIIe siècle et ses avatars,* edited by Georges Bérubé and Marie-France Silver, 133–40. Toronto: Editions du Gref, 1996.

Damasio, Antonio. *Descartes' Error: Emotion, Reason and the Human Brain.* New York: Penguin, 2005.

Darnton, Robert. *The Corpus of Clandestine Literature in France, 1769–1789.* 1st ed. New York: W.W. Norton, 1995.

– *The Forbidden Best-sellers of Pre-Revolutionary France.* New York: W.W. Norton, 1995.

– *The Great Cat Massacre and Other Episodes in French Cultural History.* New York: Basic Books, 1984.

Darrow, Margaret H. "French Noblewomen and the New Domesticity." *Feminist Studies* 5, no. 1 (1979): 41–65.

Dawson, Deidre. "Voltaire's Complaint: Illness and Eroticism in *La Correspondance.*" *Literature and Medicine* 18, no. 1 (1999): 24–38.

DeJean, Joan. "(Love) Letters: Madeleine de Scudéry and the Epistolary Impulse." *Eighteenth-Century Fiction* 22, no. 3 (2010): 399–414.

DePree, Julia K. "*Filles perdues?*: French Literature in Search of the Maternal." *Intertexts* 5, no. 1 (2001): 23–31.

– "*La Fausse Couche*: Failed Potential and the Anti-Enlightenment." *Romance Quarterly* 49, no. 1 (2002): 30–5.

Desan, Suzanne. *The Family on Trial in Revolutionary France*. Berkeley: University of California Press, 2004.

– "The Social Revolution in French Revolutionary Families." *Journal of Social History* 40 (2007): 996–1003.

– "'War between Brothers and Sisters': Inheritance Law and Gender Politics in Revolutionary France." *French Historical Studies* 20, no. 4 (1997): 597–634.

Desan, Suzanne, and Jeffrey Merrick. *Family, Gender, and Law in Early Modern France*. University Park: Pennsylvania State University Press, 2009.

Diamond, Marie Josephine. "The Revolutionary Rhetoric of Olympe de Gouges." *Feminist Issues* 14, no. 1 (1994): 3–23.

*Dictionnnaire de l'Académie française*. 1st edn. 1694. ARTFL Project. Chicago: Department of Romance Languages and Literatures, University of Chicago. http://artfl-project.uchicago.edu/.

*Dictionnaire de l'Académie française*. 4th edn. 1762. ARTFL Project. Chicago: Department of Romance Languages and Literatures, University of Chicago. http://artfl-project.uchicago.edu/.

*Dictionnnaire de l'Académie française*. 5th edn. 1798. ARTFL Project. Chicago: Department of Romance Languages and Literatures, University of Chicago. http://artfl-project.uchicago.edu/.

Diderot, Denis, and Jean Le Rond d'Alembert, eds. *Encyclopédie ou Dictionnaire raisonné des sciences, des arts et des métiers*. 1751–1772. ARTFL Project. Chicago: Department of Romance Languages and Literatures, University of Chicago. http://encyclopedie.uchicago.edu.qe2a-proxy.mun.ca/.

Diderot, Denis. *Rameau's Nephew and d'Alembert's Dream*. Translated by L.W. Tancock. Harmondsworth, UK: Penguin, 1966.

Didier, Béatrice. "Ecrire pour se trouver." In *Femmes en toutes lettres: Les épistolières du XVIIIe siècle*, edited by Marie-France Silver and Marie-Laure Girou-Swiderski, 243–8. Oxford: Voltaire Foundation, 2000.

Diprose, Rosalyn. "Writing in Blood: Response to Helen Kean and Marsha Rosengarten, 'On the Biology of Sexed Subjects.'" *Australian Feminist Studies* 17, no. 39 (2002): 279–82.

Doidge, Norman. *The Brain That Changes Itself*. New York: Penguin, 2007.

Douglas, Aileen. *Uneasy Sensations: Smollett and the Body*. Chicago: University of Chicago Press, 1995.

Douthwaite, Julia. "Le paradoxe de la feminité naturelle: Marie-Angélique, Sophie et Nell." In *Sexualité, mariage et famille au XVIIIe siècle*, edited by Olga B. Cragg and Rosena Davison, 159–72. Saint-Nicolas: Les presses de l'Université Laval, 1998.

Duden, Barbara. *Disembodying Women: Perspectives on Pregnancy and the Unborn*. Translated by Lee Hoinacki. Cambridge, MA: Harvard University Press, 1993.

– *The Woman Beneath the Skin: A Doctor's Patients in Eighteenth Century Germany*. Translated by Thomas Dunlap. Cambridge, MA: Harvard University Press, 1991.

Dumonceaux, P. "Le XVIIe siècle: Aux origines de la lettre intime et du genre épistolaire." In *Ecrire, publier, lire les correspondances: Problématique et économie d'un 'genre littéraire,'* edited by Jean-Louis Bonnat and Mireille Boissis, 289–305. Nantes: Université de Nantes, 1983.

Duncan, Carol. "Happy Mothers and Other New Ideas in French Art." *Art Bulletin* 55 (1973): 570–83.

Eakin, Paul John. *The Ethics of Life Writing*. Ithaca, NY: Cornell University Press, 2004.

– *How Our Lives Become Stories: Making Selves*. Ithaca, NY: Cornell University Press, 1999.

Earle, Rebecca, ed. *Epistolary Selves: Letters and Letter Writers, 1600–1945*. Aldershot: Ashgate, 1999.

Edelman, Lee. *No Future: Queer Theory and the Death Drive*. Durham, NC: Duke University Press, 2004.

Edgren, Monika. "Colonizing Women's Bodies: Population Policies and Nationhood in Eighteenth-Century Sweden." *Journal of Women's History* 22, no. 2 (2010): 108–32.

Egan, Susanna. *Burdens of Proof: Faith, Doubt, and Identity in Autobiography*. Waterloo, ON: Wilfrid Laurier University Press, 2011.

Elliott, Charlene D. "Big Persons, Small Voices: On Governance, Obesity, and the Narrative of the Failed Citizen." *Journal of Canadian Studies/Revue d'études canadiennes* 41, no. 3 (2007): 124–49.

Emch-Dériaz, Antoinette. "L'enseignement clinique au XVIIIe siècle: L'exemple de Tissot." *Canadian Bulletin of Medical History/Bulletin canadien d'histoire de la médecine* 4 (1987): 145–64.

– *Tissot: Physician of the Enlightenment*. New York: Peter Lang, 1992.

*The Encyclopedia of Diderot & d'Alembert Collaborative Translation Project*. Ann Arbor: Michigan Publishing, University of Michigan Library, 2005. http://quod.lib.umich.edu/d/did/.

Ephron, Nora. *Heartburn*. New York: Knopf, 1983.

Epinay, Louise Florence Pétronille Tardieu d'Esclavelles, Marquise d'. *Les contre-confessions: Histoire de Madame de Montbrillant*. Edited by Elisabeth Badinter and Georges Roth. Paris: Mercure de France, 1989.

Epinoy, Roze de l'. *Avis aux mères qui veulent allaiter leurs enfans*. Paris: P.F. Didot, 1785.

Epstein, Julia L. "Writing the Unspeakable: Fanny Burney's Mastectomy and the Fictive Body." *Representations* 16 (1986): 131–66.

Evans, Tanya. "'Unfortunate Objects': London's Unmarried Mothers in the Eighteenth Century." *Gender & History* 17, no. 1 (2005): 127–53.

Faber, Diana. "Hysteria in the Eighteenth Century." In *Brain, Mind and Medicine: Essays in Eighteenth-Century Neuroscience*, edited by Harry Whitaker, C.U.M. Smith, and Stanley Finger, 321–32. New York: Springer, 2007.

Fairchilds, Cissie. "Masters and Servants in Eighteenth Century Toulouse." *Journal of Social History* 12, no. 3 (1979): 368–93.

– "Women and Family." In *French Women and the Age of Enlightenment*, edited by Samia I. Spencer, 97–110. Bloomington: Indiana University Press, 1984.

Farrell, Michèle Longino. *Performing Motherhood: The Sévigné Correspondence*. Hanover: University Press of New England, 2000.

Faulks, Keith. *Citizenship*. New York: Routledge, 2000.

Fausto-Sterling, Anne. *Sex/Gender: Biology in a Social World*. New York: Routledge, 2012.

Féraud, Jean-François. *Dictionnaire critique de la langue française*. Marseille, Mossy 1787–1788. ARTFL Project. Chicago: Department of Romance Languages and Literatures, University of Chicago. http://artfl-project.uchicago.edu/.

Ferguson, Frances. "Sade and the Pornographic Legacy." *Representations* 36, no. 36 (1991): 1–21.

Fermon, Nicole. *Domesticating Passions: Rousseau, Woman, and Nation*. Hanover, NH: Wesleyan University Press, 1997.

Fildes, Valerie. *Wet-Nursing: A History from Antiquity to the Present*. New York: Basil Blackwell, 1988.

Fleischman, Suzanne. "I Am ..., I Have ..., I Suffer from ...: A Linguist Reflects on the Language of Illness and Disease." *Journal of Medical Humanities* 20, no. 1 (1999): 3–32.

Foley, Susan. "'Your Letter is Divine, Irresistible, Infernally Seductive': Léon Gambetta, Léonie Léon, and Nineteenth-Century Epistolary Culture." *French Historical Studies* 30, no. 2 (2007): 237–67.

Fox, Christopher, Roy Porter, and Robert Wokler, eds. *Inventing Human Science: Eighteenth-Century Domains*. Berkeley: University of California Press, 1995.

Franklin, James L. "Surgery, Note by Note: Marin Marais' *Tableau de L'Opération de la Taille*," *Hektoen International* 4, no. 2 (2012). http://hektoeninternational.org/Marin-Marais.html.

Gabrielson, Teena, and Katelyn Parady. "Corporeal Citizenship: Rethinking Green Citizenship through the Body." *Environmental Politics* 19, no. 3 (2010): 374–91.

Gager, Kristin Elizabeth. *Blood Ties and Fictive Ties: Adoption and Family Life in Early Modern France*. Princeton: Princeton University Press, 1996.

Garland-Thomson, Rosemarie. "Integrating Disability, Transforming Feminist Theory." *NWSA Journal* 14, no. 3 (2002): 1–32.

Gatens, Moira. *Imaginary Bodies: Ethics, Power and Corporeality*. New York: Routledge, 1996.

Gauteron, François Louis. *Lettre de Mr. Gauteron à Mr. Ch. Pictet, de Genève, sur la fête célébrée à Hofwyl le 23 mai 1807*. Geneva: J.J. Paschoud, 1808.

Gerber, Matthew. "On the Contested Margins of the Family: Bastardy and Legitimation by Royal Rescript in Eighteenth-Century France." In *Family, Gender, and Law in Early Modern France*, edited by Suzanne Desan and Jeffrey Merrick, 225–30. University Park: Pennsylvania University Press, 2009.

Germann, Jennifer Grant. "Fecund Fathers and Missing Mothers: Louis XV, Marie Leszczinska, and the Politics of Royal Parentage in the 1720s." *Studies in Eighteenth-Century Culture* 36 (2007): 105–26.

Gilbert, Anne-Françoise. "Deconstructing Gender: Henriette's Correspondence with Rousseau." In *Gender and Politics in the Age of Letter Writing, 1750–2000*, edited by Caroline Bland and Máire Cross, 43–53. Aldershot: Ashgate, 2004.

Gilmore, Leigh. *Autobiographics: A Feminist Theory of Women's Self-Representation*. Ithaca, NY: Cornell University Press, 1994.

Gilroy, Amanda, and W.M. Verhoeven, eds. *Epistolary Histories: Letters, Fiction, Culture*. Charlottesville: University of Virginia Press, 2000.

Gofmann, Erving. *Asylums: Essays on the Social Situations of Mental Patients and Other Inmates*. New York: Anchor Books, 1961.

Goldsmith, Elizabeth C., and Colette H. Winn. *Lettres de femmes: Textes inédits et oubliés du XVIe au XVIIIe siècle*. Paris: Champion, 2005.

Golightly, Jennifer. "Reproduction in British Women's Novels of the 1790s." In *Secrets of Generation: Reproduction in the Long Eighteenth Century*, edited by Ray Stephanson and Dareen Wagner. Toronto: University of Toronto Press, 2015.

Golowkin, Fédor. *Lettres diverses, recueillies en Suisse*. Geneva and Paris: J.J. Paschoud, 1821.

Gonthier, François-Auguste-Alphonse, François Louis Gauteron, and Gabriel-Antoine Iéville. *Etrennes sentimentales et champêtres*. Lausanne: Hignou; Fischer, 1795.

Goodman, Dena. *Becoming a Woman in the Age of Letters*. Ithaca, NY: Cornell University Press, 2009.

Goodman, Dena, ed. *Marie-Antoinette: Writings on the Body of a Queen*. New York: Routledge, 2003.

Goodman, Elise. *The Portraits of Madame de Pompadour: Celebrating the Femme Savante*. Berkeley: University of California Press, 2000.

Götz, Carmen. "La maladie comme effet de constructions culturelles à l'époque des Lumières. L'exemple de l'hypocondrie." In *Maladies en lettres. 17e–21e siècles*, edited by Vincent Barras and Martin Dinges, 97–106. Lausanne: Editions BHMS, 2013.

Goubert, Jean-Pierre. "1770–1830: La première croisade médicale." *Historical Reflections/Réflexions historiques* 9, no. 1 & 2 (1982): 3–16.

Grassi, Marie-Claire. "Epistolières au XVIIIe siècle." In *La lettre au XVIIIe siècle et ses avatars*, edited by Georges Bérubé and Marie-France Silver, 91–105. Toronto: Editions du Gref, 1996.

– *L'Art de la lettre au temps de* La Nouvelle Heloïse *et du Romantisme*. Geneva: Slatkine, 1994.

Grenon, Anne-France. "'J'ai appris à souffrir, Madame; cet art dispense d'apprendre à guérir, et n'en a pas les inconvéniens.' Rousseau et le discours épistolaire de la maladie." In *Maladies en lettres. 17e–21e siècles*, edited by Vincent Barras and Martin Dinges, 107–12. Lausanne: Editions BHMS, 2013.

Grosz, Elizabeth. *Space, Time, and Perversion: Essays on the Politics of Bodies*. New York: Routledge, 1995.

– *Volatile Bodies: Toward a Corporeal Feminism*. Bloomington: Indiana University Press, 1994.

Grouchy, Sophie de. *Lettres sur la sympathie; suivies des lettres d'amour*. Montréal: Etincelle, 1994.

Gutwirth, Madelyn. "Suzanne Necker's Legacy: Breastfeeding as Metonym in Germaine de Staël's *Delphine*." *Eighteenth-Century Life* 28, no. 2 (2004): 17–40.

Haas, Christina. *Writing Technology: Studies on the Materiality of Literacy*. Mahweh, NJ: Lawrence Erlbaum Associates, 1996.

Haggarty, Sarah. "'The Ceremonial of Letter for Letter': William Cowper and the Tempo of Epistolary Exchange." *Eighteenth-Century Life* 35, no. 1 (2011): 149–67.

Hanafi, Nahema. "Des plumes singulières. Les écritures féminines du corps souffrant au XVIIIe siècle." *Clio: Femmes, Genre, Histoire* 35 (2012): 45–66.

– "Le cancer à travers les consultations épistolaires envoyées au Dr. Tissot (1728–1797)." In *Lutter contre le cancer, 1740–1960*, edited by Didier Foucault, 95–122. Toulouse: Editions Privat, 2012.

– "'Le fruit de nos entrailles': La maternité dans les écrits des nobles toulousains du siècle des Lumières." *Annales du midi* 22, no. 169 (2010): 47–74.

– "Les mères et les médecins, l'autorité médicale des mères au siècle des Lumières." In *Les mères et l'autorité, l'autorité des meres*, edited by Laure Machet, Stéphanie Ravez, and Pascale Sardin, 63–90. Bordeaux: Presses universitaires de Bordeaux, 2013.

– "Pudeurs des souffrants et pudeurs médicales." *Histoire, Médecine et Santé* 1 (2012): 9–18.

Hanisch, Carol, "The Personal is Political." In *Radical Feminism: A Documentary Reader*, edited by Barbara Crow, 113–16. New York: New York University Press, 2000.

Hanley, Sarah, "Engendering the State: Family Formation and State Building in Early Modern France." *French Historical Studies* 16, no. 1 (1989): 4–27.

– "The Family, the State, and the Law in Seventeenth and Eighteenth-Century France: The Political Ideology of Male Right versus an Early Theory of Natural Rights." *Journal of Modern History* 78 (2006): 289–332.

– "Social Sites of Political Practice in France: Lawsuits, Civil Rights, and the Separation of Powers in Domestic and State Government, 1500–1800." *American Historical Review* 102, no. 1 (1997): 27–52.

Hedenborg, Susanna. "To Breastfeed Another Woman's Child: Wet-Nursing in Stockholm, 1777–1937." *Continuity and Change* 16, no. 3 (2001): 399–422.

Hekma, Gert. "Sade, Masculinity, and Sexual Humiliation." *Men and Masculinities* 9, no. 2 (2006): 236–51.

Hénaff, Marcel. *Sade, the Invention of the Libertine Body.* Minneapolis: University of Minnesota Press, 1999.

Henke, Suzette A. *Shattered Subjects: Trauma and Testimony in Women's Life Writing.* New York: St Martin's Press, 1998.

Herbert, Amanda E. "Gender and the Spa: Space, Sociability and Self at British Health Spas, 1640–1715." *Journal of Social History* 43, no. 2 (2009): 361–83.

Hill, Bridget. *Servants: English Domestics in the Eighteenth Century.* Oxford: Clarendon Press, 1996.

Hird, Myra. "The Corporeal Generosity of Maternity." *Body and Society* 13, no. 1 (2007): 1–20.

Hohle, Randolph. "The Body and Citizenship in Social Movement Research: Embodied Performances and the Deracialized Self in the Black Civil Rights Movement 1961–1965." *The Sociological Quarterly* 50 (2009): 283–307.

How, James. *Epistolary Spaces: English Letter Writing from the Foundation of the Post Office to Richardson's Clarissa.* Aldershot: Ashgate, 2003.

Huet, Marie-Hélène. *Monstrous Imagination.* Cambridge, MA: Harvard University Press, 1993.

Hunt, Lynn. *The Family Romance of the French Revolution.* Berkeley: University of California Press, 1992.

– "The Many Bodies of Marie-Antoinette: Political Pornography and the Problem of the Feminine in the French Revolution." In *The French Revolution in Social and Political Perspective,* edited by Peter Jones, 268–84. London: Bloomsbury, 1996.

Hurley, Alison E. "A Conversation of Their Own: Watering-Place Correspondence among the Bluestockings." *Eighteenth-Century Studies* 40, no. 1 (2006): 1–21.

Hustvedt, Siri. *The Shaking Woman or A History of My Nerves.* New York: Henry Holt and Co., 2010.

Hyde, Melissa. "The 'Makeup' of the Marquise: Boucher's Portrait of Pompadour at Her Toilette." *Art Bulletin* 82, no. 3 (2000): 453–74.

Ingram, Allan. "Deciphering Difference: A Study in Medical Literacy." In *Melancholy Experience in Literature of the Long Eighteenth Century: Before Depression, 1660–1800,* edited by Allan Ingram, Stuart Sim, Clark Lawlor, Richard Terry, John Baker, and Leigh Wetherall-Dickson, 170–202. Houndmills, UK: Palgrave Macmillan, 2011.

– "Identifying the Insane: Madness and Marginality in the Eighteenth Century." *Lumen: Selected Proceedings from the Canadian Society for Eighteenth-Century Studies/Travaux choisis de la Société canadienne d'étude du dix-huitième siècle.* Vol. 21 (2002): 143–57.

– "Resisting Insanity: Language and Disorder in Eighteenth-Century Writing about Madness." *Cycnos* 19, no. 1 (2002): 3–14.

– "Steering toward Sanity: The Compass Points of Madness in Eighteenth-Century Britain." *1650–1850: Ideas, Aesthetics, and Inquiries in the Early Modern Era* 11 (2005): 3–20.

– "Time and Tense in Eighteenth-Century Narratives of Madness." *Yearbook of English Studies* 30 (2000): 60–70.

Ingram, Allan, Stuart Sim, Clark Lawlor, Richard Terry, John Baker, and Leigh Wetherall-Dickson. *Melancholy Experience in Literature of the Long Eighteenth Century: Before Depression, 1660–1800*. New York: Palgrave Macmillan, 2011.

Irigaray, Luce. "The Bodily Encounter with the Mother." In *The Irigaray Reader*, edited by Margaret Whitford and translated by David Macey, 34–46. Oxford: Basil Blackwell, 1991.

– *This Sex Which Is Not One*. Translated by Catherine Porter. Ithaca, NY: Cornell University Press, 1985.

Isin, Engin F., and Patricia K. Wood. *Citizenship and Identity*. Thousand Oaks, CA: Sage, 1999.

Jacobus, Mary. "Incorruptible Milk: Breast-Feeding and the French Revolution." In *Rebel Daughters: Women and the French Revolution*, edited by Sara E. Melzer and Leslie W. Rabine, 54–75. New York: Oxford University Press, 1992.

Jenkins, Timothy, *The Life of Property: House, Family and Inheritance in Béarn, South-West France*. New York and Oxford: Berghahn Books, 2010.

Jensen, Katharine Ann. *Writing Love: Letters, Women and the Novel in France, 1605–1776*. Carbondale and Evansville: Southern Illinois University Press, 1995.

Johnston, Lynda, and Robyn Longhurst. *Space, Place and Sex: Geographies of Sexualities*. Lanham, MD: Rowman and Littlefield, 2010.

Jones, Colin. "The Fabrication of Madame de Pompadour." *History Today* 52, no. 11 (2002): 36–43.

– *Madame de Pompadour: Images of a Mistress*. London: National Gallery of London Publications, 2002.

Jonsson, Fredrik Albritton. "The Physiology of Hypochondria in Eighteenth-Century Britain." In *Cultures of the Abdomen: Diet, Digestion, and Fat in the Modern World*, edited by Christopher E. Forth and Ana Carden-Coyne, 15–30. New York: Palgrave Macmillan, 2005.

Jordanova, Ludmilla. "Sex and Gender." In *Inventing Human Science: Eighteenth-Century Domains*, edited by Christopher Fox, Roy Porter, and Robert Wokker. 53–87. Berkeley: University of California Press, 1995.

Kadar, Marlene. *Essays on Life Writing: From Genre to Critical Practice*. Toronto: University of Toronto Press, 1992.

Kadar, Marlene, Linda Warley, Jeanne Perreault, and Susanna Egan, eds. *Tracing the Autobiographical*. Waterloo, ON: Wilfrid Laurier University Press, 2005.

Kaiser, Thomas E. "Madame de Pompadour and the Theaters of Power." *French Historical Studies* 19, no. 4 (1996): 1025–44.

Kaye, Heidi. "'This Breast – It's Me': Fanny Burney's Mastectomy and the Defining Gaze." *Journal of Gender Studies* 6, no. 1 (1997): 43–53.

Kent, D.A. "Ubiquitous but Invisible: Female Domestic Servants in Mid-Eighteenth Century London." *History Workshop Journal* 28, no. 1 (1989): 111–28.

Keung. Nicholas. "Family Ripped Apart, Immigration Says Son with Asperger's 'Inadmissible.'" *Toronto Star*, June 14, 2011. http://www.thestar.com/news/gta/2011/06/14/family_ripped_apart_immigration_says_son_with_aspergers_inadmissible.html.

King, Thomas. *The Truth about Stories*. Toronto: House of Anansi, 2003.

Kirby, Vicki. "Natural Convers(at)ions: or, What If Culture Was Really Nature All Along?" In *Material Feminisms*, edited by Stacy Alaimo and Susan J. Hekman, 214–36. Bloomington: Indiana University Press, 2008.

– *Telling Flesh: The Substance of the Corporeal*. New York: Routledge, 1997.

Kirmayer, Laurence J. "The Body's Insistence on Meaning: Metaphor as Presentation and Representation in Illness Experience." *Medical Anthropology Quarterly* 6, no. 2 (1992): 323–46.

Kittay, Eva Feder. "Forever Small: The Strange Case of Ashley X." *Hypatia* 26, no. 3 (2011): 610–31.

Klimaszewski, Melisa. "Examining the Wet Nurse: Breasts, Power, and Penetration in Victorian England." *Women's Studies* 35, no. 4 (2006): 323–46.

Kreiser, B. Robert. "Religious Enthusiasm in Early Eighteenth-Century Paris: The Convulsionaries of Saint-Médard." *Catholic Historical Review* 61, no. 3 (1975): 353–85.

Kristeva, Julia. *Powers of Horror: An Essay on Abjection*. Translated by Leon S. Roudiez. New York: Columbia University Press, 1982.

Lajer-Burcharth, Ewa. "Pompadour's Touch: Difference in Representation." *Representations* 73 (2001): 54–68.

La Mettrie, Julien Offray de. *L'homme machine*. Leiden: Elie Luzac, 1748.

Landes, Joan B. *Women and the Public Sphere in the Age of the French Revolution*. Ithaca, NY: Cornell University Press, 1988.

Lanza, Janine Marie. *From Wives to Widows in Early Modern Paris: Gender, Economy, and Law*. Aldershot and Burlington: Ashgate, 2007.

Laqueur, Thomas. *Solitary Sex: A Cultural History of Masturbation*. New York: Zone Books, 2003.

Lastinger, Valérie. "Re-Defining Motherhood: Breast-Feeding and the French Enlightenment." *Women's Studies* 25, no. 6 (1996): 603–17.

– "To Nurse and to Die: Rousseau and the Test of Fiction." *European Journal of Women's Studies* 4, no. 4 (1997): 421–33.

Lawlor, Clark. "Fashionable Melancholy." In *Melancholy Experience in Literature of the Long Eighteenth Century: Before Depression, 1660–1800*, edited by Allan Ingram, Stuart Sim, Clark Lawlor, Richard Terry, John Baker, and Leigh Wetherall-Dickson, 25–53. Houndmills, UK: Palgrave Macmillan, 2011.

LeBesco, Kathleen. *Revolting Bodies?: The Struggle to Redefine Fat Identity*. Amherst: University of Massachusetts Press, 2003.

Lejeune, Philippe. *On Autobiography*. Edited by Paul John Eakin. Translated by Katherine Leary. Minneapolis: University of Minnesota Press, 1989.

Le Menthéour, Rudy. "Melancholy Vaporised: Self-Narration and Counter-Diagnosis in Rousseau's work." In *Medicine and Narration in the Eighteenth Century*, edited by Sophie Vasset, 107–24. Oxford: Voltaire Foundation, 2013.

Le Rebours, Marie-Angélique Anel. *Avis aux mères qui veulent nourrir leurs enfans*. Utrecht and Paris: Chez Lacombe, 1767.

Lock, Margaret. "Cultivating the Body: Anthropology and Epistemologies of Bodily Practice and Knowledge." *Annual Review of Anthropology* 22 (1993): 133–55.

Locklin, Nancy. *Women's Work and Identity in Eighteenth-Century Brittany*. Aldershot: Ashgate, 2007.

Longhurst, Robyn. "Breaking Corporeal Boundaries: Pregnant Bodies in Public Places." In *Contested Bodies*, edited by Ruth Holliday and John Hassard, 81–94. New York: Routledge, 2001.

Louis-Courvoisier, Micheline. "Le malade et son médecin: Le cadre de la relation thérapeutique dans la deuxième moitié du XVIIIe siècle." *Bulletin canadien d'histoire de la médecine* 18 (2001): 277–96.

– "Qu'est-ce qu'un malade sans son corps? L'Objectivation du corps vue à travers les lettres de consultations adressées au Dr. Tissot (1728–1797)." In *Körperkonzepte = Concepts du Corps*, edited by Franziska Frei Gerlach, Annette Kreis-Schinck, Claudia Opitz, and Béatrice Ziegler, 299–310. Munich: Waxmann, 2003.

– "Que faut-il ne pas dire à qui? Le secret médical au XVIIIe siècle." *Revue médicale suisse* 2008, no. 4 (2008): 242–6.

– "Quelques traces de liens familiaux dans les consultations épistolaires envoyées au dr Tissot (1728–1797)." In *La correspondace familiale en suisse romande aux 18e et 19e siècles; affectivité, sociabilité, réseaux*, edited by Philippe Henry and Jean-Pierre Jelmini, 191–207. Neuchâtel: Alphil, 2006.

Louis-Courvoisier, Micheline, and Alexandre Mauron. "'He found me very well; for me, I was still feeling sick': The Strange World of Physicians and Patients in the 18th and 21st Centuries." *Journal of Medical Ethics* 28 (2002): 9–13.

– "'Il me trouva très bien; pour moi, je me sentois toujours malade.' La relation patient-médecin au XVIIIe et au XXe siècle." *Médecine et hygiène* 2402 (2002): 1518–22.

Louis-Courvoisier, Micheline, and Séverine Pilloud. "Consulting by Letter in the Eighteenth Century: Mediating the Patient's View?" In *Cultural Approaches to the History of Medicine*, edited by Willem Blécourt and Cornelie Usborne, 71–88. Basingstoke: Palgrave MacMillan, 2004.

– "Le malade et son entourage au XVIIIe siècle: Les médiations dans les consultations épistolaires adressées au Dr. Tissot." *Revue médicale de la Suisse Romande* 120, no. 12 (2000): 939–44.

Lyons, John D. *Before Imagination: Embodied Thought from Montaigne to Rousseau*. Stanford: Stanford University Press, 2005.

MacKenzie, Alan T., ed. *Sent As a Gift: Eight Correspondences from the Eighteenth Century*. Athens: University of Georgia Press, 1993.

Magrath, Jane. "'Rags of Mortality': Negotiating the Body in the Bluestocking Letters." *Huntington Library Quarterly* 65, no. 1/2 (2002): 235–56.

Mansén, Elisabeth. "An Image of Paradise: Swedish Spas in the Eighteenth Century." *Eighteenth-Century Studies* 31, no. 4 (1998): 511–16.

Marais, Marin. *Pièces de viole, Livre V*. Paris: Boivin, 1725.

Martin, Emily. "Toward an Anthropology of Immunology: The Body as Nation State." *Medical Anthropology Quarterly* 4, no. 4 (1990): 410–26.

May, Gita. *Madame Roland and the Age of Revolution*. New York: Columbia University Press, 1970.

Maza, Sarah C. "The 'Bourgeois' Family Revisited: Sentimentalism and Social Class in Prerevolutionary French Culture." In *Intimate Encounters: Love and Domesticity in Eighteenth-Century France*, edited by Richard Rand, 39–47. Princeton: Princeton University Press and Hood Museum of Art, 1997.

– *Servants and Masters in Eighteenth-Century France: The Uses of Loyalty*. Princeton: Princeton University Press, 1983.

McAllister, Marie E. "Stories of the Origin of Syphilis in Eighteenth-Century England: Science, Myth, and Prejudice." *Eighteenth-Century Life* 24 (2000): 22–44.

McAlpin, Mary. *Female Sexuality and Cultural Degradation in Enlightenment France*. Abingdon: Ashgate, 2012.

– "The Virtues of Childhood Sexual Abuse and Marital Infidelity in Marie-Jeanne Roland's *Mémoires particulaires* (1795)." *Journal of History of Sexuality* 21, no. 1 (2012): 16–38.

McClive, Cathy. "Blood and Expertise: The Trials of the Female Medical Expert in the Ancien-Régime Courtroom." *Bulletin of the History of Medicine* 82, no. 1 (2008): 86–108.

– "The Hidden Truths of the Belly: The Uncertainties of Pregnancy in Early Modern Europe." *Social History of Medicine* 15, no. 2 (2002): 209–227.

– "L'âge des fleurs: Le passage de l'enfance à l'adolescence dans l'imaginaire médical du XVIIe siècle." In *Regards sur l'enfance au XVIIe siècle*, edited by Anne De France, Denis Lopez, and François-Joseph Ruggiu, 171–85. Tübingen: Gunter Narr, 2007.

– "Masculinity on Trial: Penises, Hermaphrodites and the Uncertain Male Body in Early Modern France." *History Workshop Journal* 68 (2009): 45–68.

– "Menstrual Knowledge and Medical Practice in France, c. 1555–1761." In *Menstruation: A Cultural History*, edited by Andrew Shail and Gillian Howie, 76–89. Houndmills, UK: Palgrave Macmillan, 2005.

– "Quand les fleurs s'arrêtent: La ménopause et l'imaginaire médical aux XVIIe et XVIIIe siècles." In *Femmes en fleurs, femmes en corps: Sang, santé et sexualités du Moyen Âge aux Lumières*, edited by Cathy McClive and Nicole

Pellegrin, 277–99. Saint-Etienne: Publications de l'Université Saint-Etienne, 2010.

McClive, Cathy, and Nicole Pellegrin, eds. *Femmes en fleurs, femmes en corps: Sang, santé, sexualités du Moyen Âge aux Lumières*. Saint-Etienne: Publications de l'Université de Saint-Etienne, 2010.

McCrea, Brian. *Impotent Fathers: Patriarchy and Demographic Crisis in the Eighteenth-Century Novel*. Newark and London: University of Delaware Press and Associated University Press, 1998.

McGrath, Lynette. "The Other Body: Women's Inscription of their Physical Images in 16th- and 17th-Century England." *Women's Studies* 26, no. 1 (1997): 27–58.

McKeon, Michael. "The Seventeenth- and Eighteenth-Century Sexuality Hypothesis." *Signs: Journal of Women in Culture & Society* 37, no. 4 (2012): 791–801.

McRuer, Robert. *Crip Theory: Cultural Signs of Queerness and Disability*. New York: New York University Press, 2006.

Meek, Heather. "Medical Women and Hysterical Doctors: Interpreting Hysteria's Symptoms in Eighteenth-Century Britain." In *The English Malady: Enabling and Disabling Fictions*, edited by Glen Colburn, 223–47. Newcastle-upon-Tyne: Cambridge Scholars, 2008.

– "Of Wandering Wombs and Wrongs of Women: Evolving Conceptions of Hysteria in the Age of Reason." *English Studies in Canada* 35, no. 2–3 (2009): 105–28.

– "'[W]hat Fatigues We Fine Ladies Are Fated to Endure': Sociosomatic Hysteria as a Female 'English Malady.'" In *Diseases of the Imagination and Imaginary Disease in the Early Modern Period*, edited by Yasmin Haskell and German Berrios, 375–96. Turnhout: Brepols, 2011.

Meldrum, Tim. "Domestic Service, Privacy and the Eighteenth-Century Metropolitan Household." *Urban History* 26, no. 1 (1999): 27–39.

Merrick, Jeffrey. "The Family Politics of the Marquis De Bombelles." *Journal of Family History* 21, no. 4 (1996): 503–18.

Miller, Naomi J., and Naomi Yavneh, eds. *Maternal Measures: Figuring Caregiving in the Early Modern Period*. Aldershot, UK: Ashgate, 2000.

Morgan, Gwenda, and Peter Rushton. "Visible Bodies: Power, Subordination and Identity in the Eighteenth-Century Atlantic World." *Journal of Social History* 39, no. 1 (2005): 39–64.

Mukherjee, Arun, Alok Mukherjee, and Barbara Godard. "Translating Minoritized Cultures: Issues of Caste, Class and Gender." *Postcolonial Text* 2, no. 3 (2006): 1–23. http://postcolonial.org/index.php/pct/article/viewArticle/501.

Mullan, John. "Hypochondria and Hysteria: Sensibility and the Physicians." *The Eighteenth Century: Theory and Interpretation* 25, no. 2 (1984): 141–74.

– *Sentiment and Sociability: The Language of Feeling in the Eighteenth Century*. Oxford: Oxford University Press, 1988.

Murphy, Terence D. "The French Medical Profession's Perception of its Social Function between 1776 and 1830." *Medical History* 23 (1979): 259–78.

Murray, Samantha. "Normative Imperatives vs. Pathological Bodies: Constructing the 'Fat' Woman." *Australian Feminist Studies* 23, no. 56 (2008): 213–24.
– "Pathologizing 'Fatness': Medical Authority and Popular Culture." *Sociology of Sport Journal* 25 (2008): 7–21.
– "(Un/Be)Coming Out? Rethinking Fat Politics." *Social Semiotics* 15, no. 2 (2005): 153–63.
Necker, Suzanne Curchod. *Nouveaux Mélanges.* 3 vols. Paris: Pougens, 1801.
Ohayon, Ruth. "Rousseau's Julie; or, The Maternal Odyssey." CLA *Journal* 30, no. 1 (1986): 69–82.
*Onania; or, the heinous sin of self-pollution, and all its frightful consequences, in both sexes, considered, with spiritual and physical advice to Those who have already Injur'd themselves by this Abominable Practice. To which is Subjoin'd, A Letter from a Lady to the Author, (very curious) concerning the Use and Abuse of the Marriage-Bed, with the Author's Answer.* 4th ed., London, [1718?]. *Eighteenth Century Collections Online.* Gale. Memorial University of Newfoundland.
Otto, Peter. "James Graham as Spiritual Libertine." In *Libertine Enlightenment: Sex, Liberty and License in the Eighteenth Century*, edited by Peter Cryle and Lisa O'Donnell, 204–20. Houndmills, UK: Palgrave MacMillan, 2004.
Outram, Dorinda. *The Body and the French Revolution: Sex, Class and Political Culture.* New Haven, CT: Yale University Press, 1989.
Overboe, James. "Ableist Limits on Self-Narration: The Concept of Post-Personhood." In *Unfitting Stories: Narrative Approaches to Disease, Disability, and Trauma*, edited by Valerie Raoul, Connie Canam, Angela Henderson, and Carla Paterson, 275–82. Waterloo, ON: Wilfrid Laurier University Press, 2007.
Paradis de Moncrif, François-Augustin. *Essais sur la nécessité et sur les moyens de plaire.* Paris: Prault, 1738.
Pardo-Tómas, J., and A. Martínez-Vidal. "Stories of Disease Written by Patients and Lay Mediators in the Spanish Republic of Letters." *Journal of Medieval and Early Modern Studies* 38, no. 3 (2008): 467–91.
Parker, Kate. "Communal Sexuality: Mutual Pleasure in Sade's *La philosophie dans le boudoir*." *Eighteenth-Century Fiction* 25, no. 2 (2012): 407–30.
Peakman, Julie, and Sarah Watkins. "Making Babies: Eighteenth-Century Attitudes Towards Conception, Reproduction and Childbirth." In *Secrets of Generation: Reproduction in the Long Eighteenth Century*, edited by Ray Stephanson and Dareen Wagner. Toronto: University of Toronto Press, forthcoming.
Pécastaings, Annie. "Frances Burney's Mastectomy and the Female Body Politic." *Prose Studies: History, Theory, Criticism* 33, no. 3 (2011): 230–40.
Pekacz, Jolanta T. "The French Salon of the Old Regime as a Spectacle." *Lumen: Selected Proceedings from the Canadian Society for Eighteenth-Century Studies/Lumen: Travaux choisis de la Société canadienne d'étude du dix-huitième siècle.* Vol. 22 (2003): 83–102.

Perry, Ruth. "Colonizing the Breast: Sexuality and Maternity in Eighteenth-Century England." *Journal of the History of Sexuality* 22, no. 2 (1991): 204–34.

Peter, Jean-Pierre. "Entre femmes et médecins: Violence et singularités dans les discours du corps et sur le corps d'après les manuscrits médicaux de la fin du XVIIIe siècle." *Ethnologie française* 6, no. 3–4 (1976): 341–8.

Phillips, John. "Obscenity off the Scene: Sade's *La philosophie dans le boudoir*." *The Eighteenth Century* 53, no. 2 (2012): 163–74.

Pilloud, Séverine. *Documenter l'histoire de la santé et de la médecine au siècle des Lumières. Les consultations épistolaires adressées au Dr. Samuel Auguste Tissot (1728–1797)*. Lausanne: Editions BHMS, 2013.

– "Les mots du corps: L'expérience de la maladie dans les consultations épistolaires adressées au Dr Samuel Auguste Tissot (1728–1797)." PhD, Université de Lausanne, 2009.

– *Les mots du corps: Expérience de la maladie dans les lettres de patients à un médecin du 18e siècle: Samuel Auguste Tissot*. Lausanne: Editions BHMS, 2013.

– "Marges interprétatives et autorité narrative dans le récit autobiographique des maux." In *Maladies en lettres. 17e–21e siècles*, edited by Vincent Barras and Martin Dinges, 33–48. Lausanne: Editions BHMS, 2013.

– "Mettre les maux en mots, médiations dans la consultation épistolaire au XVIIIe siècle: Les malades du Dr. Tissot (1728–1797)." *Canadian Bulletin of Medical History/Bulletin canadien d'histoire de la médecine* 16 (1999): 215–45.

– "Tourisme médical à Lausanne dans la seconde moitié du XVIIIe siècle: Le réseau des patients du Dr Tissot (1728–1797)." *Revue historique vaudoise* 114 (2006): 9–23.

Pilloud, Séverine, and Micheline Louis-Courvoisier. "The Intimate Experience of the Body in the Eighteenth Century: Between Interiority and Exteriority." *Journal of Medical History* 47 (2003): 451–72.

Pilloud, Séverine, Stéphane Hächler, and Vincent Barras. "Consulter par lettre au XVIIIe siècle." *Gesnerus* 61, no. 3–4 (2004): 232–53.

Plummer, Ken. *Documents of Life 2: An Invitation to a Critical Humanism*. Thousand Oaks, CA: Sage, 2001.

Pocock, John G.A. "The Ideal of Citizenship since Classical Times." In *Theorizing Citizenship*, edited by Ronald Beiner, 29–52. Albany: State University of New York Press, 1995.

Pollin, Jean-Baptiste. *Le hameau de l'Agnelas, suivis de diverses idilles*. Vol. 1. Paris: LaVillette et cie., 1801.

Pomme, Pierre. *Traité des affections vapoureuses des deux sexes*. 2nd ed. Lyon: Benoit Duplain, 1765.

Popiel, Jennifer J. "Making Mothers: The Advice Genre and the Domestic Ideal, 1760–1830." *Journal of Family History* 29, no. 4 (2004): 339–50.

– *Rousseau's Daughters: Domesticity, Education and Autonomy in Modern France*. Durham: University of New Hampshire Press, 2008.

Portelli, Alessandro. *The Death of Luigi Trastulli, and Other Stories: Form and Meaning in Oral History*. Albany: State University of New York Press, 1991.

Porter, Dorothy, and Roy Porter. *Patient's Progress: Doctors and Doctoring in Eighteenth-Century England*. Oxford: Polity Press; Oxford: B. Blackwell, 1989.

Porter, Roy. "Bodies of Thought: Thoughts about the Body in Eighteenth-Century England." In *Interpretation and Cultural History*, edited by Joan H. Pittock and Andrew Wear, 82–108. New York: St Martin's Press, 1991.

– *Bodies Politic: Disease, Death and Doctors in Britain, 1650–1900*. London: Reaktion Books, 2001.

– "Consumption: Disease of a Consumer Society?" In *Consumption and the World of Goods*, edited by John Brewer and Roy Porter, 58–84. New York: Routledge, 1994.

– *Disease, Medicine and Society in England, 1550–1860*. 2nd ed. Cambridge: Cambridge University Press, 1993.

– "Enlightenment and Pleasure." In *Pleasure in the Eighteenth Century*, edited by Roy Porter and Marie Mulvey Roberts, 1–18. Houndmills, UK: Macmillan, 1996.

– "'Expressing Yourself Ill': The Language of Sickness in Georgian England." In *Language, Self and Society: A Social History of Language*, edited by Peter Burke and Roy Porter, 276–99. London: Polity Press, 1991.

– *Flesh in the Age of Reason*. 1st American ed. New York: W.W. Norton & Co., 2004.

– "The Literature of Sexual Advice Before 1800." In *Sexual Knowledge, Sexual Science: The History of Attitudes to Sexuality*, edited by Roy Porter and Mikulas Teich, 134–57. Cambridge: Cambridge University Press, 1994.

– "Material Pleasures in Consumer Society." In *Pleasure in the Eighteenth Century*, edited by Roy Porter and Marie Mulvey Roberts, 19–35. Houndmills, UK: Macmillan, 1996.

– "Modernité et médecine: Le dilemma de la fin des Lumières." In *La médecine des Lumières: Tout autour de Tissot*, edited by Vincent Barras and Micheline Louis-Courvoisier, 5–26. Geneva: Georg Editeur, 2001.

– "The Patient's Point of View: Doing Medical History from Below." *Theory and Society* 14, no. 2 (1985): 175–98.

Porter, Roy, ed. *The Popularization of Medicine, 1650–1850*. New York: Routledge, 1992.

Porter, Roy, and Lesley A. Hall. *The Facts of Life: The Creation of Sexual Knowledge in Britain, 1650–1950*. New Haven, CT: Yale University Press, 1995.

Porter, Roy, and Marie Mulvey Roberts. Preface to *Pleasure in the Eighteenth Century*, edited by Roy Porter and Marie Mulvey Roberts, ix–xv. Houndmills, UK: Macmillan, 1996.

Poustie, Sarah. "Re-Theorising Letters and 'Letterness.'" *Olive Schreiner Letters Project: Working Papers on Letters, Letterness & Epistolary Networks* 1 (2010): 1–50. http://www.oliveschreinerletters.ed.ac.uk/WorkingPaperSeries.html.

Probyn, Elspeth. *Blush: Faces of Shame*. Minneapolis: University of Minnesota Press, 2005.

Prosser, Jay. *Second Skins: The Body Narratives of Transsexuality*. New York: Columbia University Press, 1998.

– "Skin Memories." In *Thinking through the Skin*, edited by Sara Ahmed and Jackie Stacey, 52–68. New York: Routledge, 2001.

Puar, Jasbir. "Coda: The Cost of Getting Better." *GLQ: A Journal of Lesbian and Gay Studies* 18, no. 1 (2012): 149–58.

Quinlan, Sean M. *The Great Nation in Decline: Sex, Modernity and Health Crises in Revolutionary France, 1750–1850*. Abingdon: Ashgate, 2007.

– "Inheriting Vice, Acquiring Virtue: Hereditary Disease and Moral Hygiene in Eighteenth-Century France." *Bulletin of the History of Medicine* 80, no. 4 (2006): 649–75.

– "Shocked Sensibility: The Nerves, the Will, and Altered States in Sade's *L'Histoire de Juliette*." *Eighteenth-Century Fiction* 25, no. 3 (2013): 533–56.

Rand, Richard. "Love, Domesticity and the Evolution of Genre Painting." In *Intimate Encounters: Love and Domesticity in Eighteenth-Century France*, edited by Richard Rand, 3–19. Princeton: Princeton University Press and Hood Museum of Art, 1997.

Rankin, Alisha. "Duchess, Heal Thyself: Elisabeth of Rochlitz and the Patient's Perspective in Early Modern Germany." *Bulletin of the History of Medicine* 82, no. 1 (2008): 109–44.

Raoul, Valerie, Connie Canam, Gloria Nne Onyeoziri, James Overboe, and Carla Paterson. "Narrating the Unspeakable: Interdisciplinary Readings of Jean-Dominique Bauby's *The Diving Bell and the Butterfly*." *Literature and Medicine* 20, no 2 (2001): 183–208.

Raoul, Valerie, Connie Canam, Angela Henderson, and Carla Paterson, eds. *Unfitting Stories: Narrative Approaches to Disease, Disability, and Trauma*. Waterloo, ON: Wilfrid Laurier University Press, 2007.

Rapp, Emily. *The Still Point of the Turning World*. New York: Penguin, 2013.

Redford, Bruce. *The Converse of the Pen: Acts of Intimacy in the Eighteenth-Century Letter*. Chicago: University of Chicago Press, 1986.

Redien-Collot, Renaud. "Discours médical et pratique poétique: Les différentes figures de l'autorité, au sein de la correspondence entre Mme d'Epinay et l'abbé Galiani." In *Maladies en lettres. 17e–21e siècles*, edited by Vincent Barras and Martin Dinges, 83–96. Lausanne: Editions BHMS, 2013.

Revill, George. "Reading *Rosehill*: Community, Identity and Inner-City Derby." In *Place and the Politics of Identity*, edited by Michael Keith and Steven Pile, 115–38. London and New York: Routledge, 1993.

Reynolds, Siân. *Marriage and Revolution: Monsieur and Madame Roland*. Oxford: Oxford University Press, 2012.

Reynolds, Thomas E. *Vulnerable Communion: A Theology of Disability and Hospitality*. Grand Rapids, MI: Brazos Press, 2008.

Richardson, Laurel. "Writing: A Method of Inquiry." In *Handbook of Qualitative Research*, edited by Norman K. Denzin and Yvonna S. Lincoln, 516–29. Thousand Oaks, CA: Sage, 1994.

Richter, Simon. *Missing the Breast: Gender, Fantasy and the Body in the German Enlightenment*. Seattle: University of Washington Press, 2006.

– "Wet-Nursing, Onanism, and the Breast in Eighteenth-Century Germany." *Journal of the History of Sexuality* 7, no. 1 (1996): 1–22.

Rieder, Philip. "Correspondances historiographiques: Pour une lecture anthropologique et médicale de l'épistolarité au siècle des Lumières." In *Maladies en lettres. 17e–21e siècles*, edited by Vincent Barras and Martin Dinges, 123–34. Lausanne: Editions BHMS, 2013.

– "La Rencontre Thérapeutique au XVIIIe siècle." *L'Émoi de l'histoire* (2011): 26–39.

– "Patients and Words: A Lay Medical Culture?" In *Framing and Imagining Disease in Cultural History*, edited by George Sebastian Rousseau with Miranda Gill, David Haycock, and Malte Herwig, 215–30. London: Palgrave MacMillan, 2003.

Rieder, Philip, and Micheline Louis-Courvoisier. "Enlightened Physicians: Setting out on an Elite Academic Career in the Second Half of the Eighteenth Century." *Bulletin of the History of Medicine* 84, no. 4 (2010): 578–606.

Rieder, Philip, and Vincent Barras. "Écrire sa maladie au siècle des Lumières." In *La médecine des Lumières: Tout autour de Tissot*, edited by Vincent Barras and Micheline Louis-Courvoisier, 201–22. Geneva and Paris: Georg Editeur, 2001.

Roberts, Marie Mulvey. "Pleasures Engendered by Gender: Homosociality and the Club." In *Pleasure in the Eighteenth Century*, edited by Roy Porter and Marie Mulvey Roberts, 48–76. Houndmills, UK: Macmillan, 1996.

Robinson, James, and Sarah Mills. "Being Observant and Observed: Embodied Citizenship Training in the Home Guard and the Boy Scout Movement, 1907–1945." *Journal of Historical Geography* 38, no. 4 (2012): 412–23.

Rohrer, Judy. "Toward a Full-Inclusion Feminism: A Feminist Deployment of Disability Analysis." *Feminist Studies* 31, no. 1 (2005): 34–63.

Roper, Michael. "Slipping Out of View: Subjectivity and Emotion in Gender History." *History Workshop Journal* 59, no. 1 (2005): 57–72.

Rosario, Vernon A. *The Erotic Imagination: French Histories of Perversity*. Oxford: Oxford University Press, 1997.

Roulston, Chris. "Choix et accomplissement dans le discours sur le mariage de la fin du XVIIIe siècle." In *Sexualité, mariage et famille au XVIIIe siècle*, edited by Olga B. Cragg and Rosena Davison, 185–94. Saint-Nicolas: Les presses de l'Université Laval, 1998.

– *Narrating Marriage in Eighteenth-Century England and France*. Farnham: Ashgate, 2010.

Rousseau, G.S., and Roy Porter, eds. *Sexual Underworlds of the Enlightenment*. Chapel Hill: University of North Carolina Press, 1988.

Rousseau, Jean-Jacques. *The Confessions and Correspondence, Including the Letters to Malesherbes*. Translated by Christopher Kelly. Edited by Christopher Kelly, Roger D. Masters, and Peter G. Stillman. Hanover: University Press of New England, 1995.

– *Emile*. Translated by Barbara Foxley. London: J.M. Dent & Sons Ltd., 1974.

– *The Social Contract*. Translated by G.D.H. Cole, 1782. http://www.constitution.org/jjr/socon.htm.

Roussel, Pierre. *Système physique et moral de la femme ou Tableau philoso-phique de la constitution, des moeurs et des fonctions propres au sexe.* Paris: Vincent, 1775.

Ruberg, Willemijn. "The Letter as Medicine: Studying Health and Illness in Dutch Daily Correspondence, 1770–1850." *Social History of Medicine* 23, no. 3 (2010): 192–208.

Rublack, Ulinka. "Fluxes: The Early Modern Body and the Emotions." *History Workshop Journal* 53, no. 1 (2002): 1–16.

Russell, Penny. "Life's Illusions: The 'Art' of Critical Biography." *Journal of Women's History* 21, no. 4 (2009): 152–56.

Sacks, Oliver. *The Man Who Mistook His Wife for a Hat.* New York: Touch-stone, 1985.

– *The Mind's Eye.* New York: Alfred A. Knopf, 2010.

Scarry, Elaine. *The Body in Pain: The Making and Unmaking of the World.* New York: Oxford University Press, 1985.

Schaffer, Kay, and Sidonie Smith. *Human Rights and Narrated Lives: The Ethics of Recognition.* New York: Palgrave Macmillan, 2004.

Schneider, Gary. *The Culture of Epistolarity: Vernacular Letters and Letter Writing in Early Modern England, 1500–1700.* Newark: University of Dela-ware Press, 2005.

Schneider, Zoë A. "Women before the Bench: Female Litigants in Early Modern Normandy." *French Historical Studies* 23, no. 1 (2000): 1–32.

Scott, Katie. "Framing Ambition: The Interior Politics of Mme de Pompadour." *Art History* 28, no. 2 (2005): 248–90.

Senior, Nancy. "Aspects of Infant Feeding in Eighteenth-Century France." *Eight-eenth-Century Studies* 16, no. 4 (1983): 367–88.

Sgard, Jean. "Femmes mariées chez Crébillon." In *Sexualité, mariage et famille au XVIIIe siècle*, edited by Olga B. Cragg and Rosena Davison, 195–204. Saint-Nicolas: Les presses de l'Université Laval, 1998.

Sheller, Mimi. *Citizenship from Below: Erotic Agency and Caribbean Freedom.* Durham, NC: Duke University Press, 2012.

Sherman, Carol L. *The Family Crucible in Eighteenth-Century Literature.* Aldershot: Ashgate 2005.

Sherwood, Joan. *Infection of the Innocents: Wet Nurses, Infants, and Syphilis in France, 1780–1900.* Montreal and Kingston: McGill-Queen's University Press, 2010.

– "The Milk Factor: The Ideology of Breast-Feeding and Post-Partum Illnesses, 1750–1850." *Canadian Bulletin of Medical History* 10 (1993): 25–47.

– "Treating Syphilis: The Wetnurse as Technology in an Eighteenth-Century Parisian Hospital." *Journal of the History of Medicine and Allied Sciences* 50, no. 3 (1995): 315–39.

Shildrick, Margrit. *Dangerous Discourses of Disability, Subjectivity and Sexual-ity.* Houndmills, UK: Palgrave Macmillan, 2009.

– *Leaky Bodies and Boundaries: Feminism, Postmodernism and (Bio)Ethics.* New York: Routledge, 1997.

Shuckburgh, Evelyn. *The Memoirs of Madame Roland: A Heroine of the French Revolution*. New York: Moyer Bell, 1990.

Shuttleton, David. "'Not the meanest part of my works and experience': Dr. George Cheyne's Correspondence with Samuel Richardson." In *Medicine and Narration in the Eighteenth Century*, edited by Sophie Vasset, 65–82. Oxford: Voltaire Foundation, 2013.

Silver, Marie-France. "Libertinage et révolution: Les romans du Marquis de Sade." *Man and Nature/Homme et nature* 8 (1989): 129–36.

Singy, Patrick. "Friction of the Genitals and Secularization of Morality." *Journal of the History of Sexuality* 12, no. 3 (2003): 345–64.

– "Le pouvoir de la science dans *L'Onanisme* de Tissot." *Gesnerus: Swiss Journal of the History of Medicine and Sciences* 57 (2000): 27–41.

– "The Popularization of Medicine in the Eighteenth Century: Writing, Reading and Rewriting Samuel Auguste Tissot's *Avis au peuple sur sa santé*." *Journal of Modern History* 82 (2010): 769–800.

Slater, Lauren. *Lying: A Metaphorical Memoir*. New York: Penguin, 2001.

Smith, C.U.M. "Brain and Mind in the 'Long' Eighteenth Century." *Brain, Mind and Medicine: Essays in Eighteenth-Century Neuroscience*, edited by Harry Whitaker, C.U.M. Smith, and Stanley Finger, 15–28. New York: Springer, 2007.

Smith, Lisa Wynne. "'An Account of Unaccountable Distemper': The Experience of Pain in Early Eighteenth-Century England and France." *Eighteenth-Century Studies* 41, no. 4 (2008): 459–80.

– "The Body Embarrassed? Rethinking the Leaky Male Body in Eighteenth-Century England and France." *Gender & History* 23, no. 1 (2010): 26–46.

– "'La raillerie' des femmes? Les femmes, la stérilité et la société en France à l'époque moderne." In *Femmes en fleurs, femmes en corps: Sang, santé, sexualités du Moyen Âge aux Lumières*, edited by Cathy McClive and Nicole Pellegrin, 203–20. Saint-Etienne: Publications de l'Université de Saint-Etienne, 2010.

– "Reassessing the Role of the Family: Women's Medical Care in Eighteenth Century England." *Social History of Medicine* 16, no. 3 (2003): 327–42.

– "The Relative Duties of a Man: Domestic Medicine in England and France, ca. 1685–1740." *Journal of Family History* 31, no. 3 (2006): 237–56.

Smith, Sidonie. *A Poetics of Women's Autobiography: Marginality and the Fictions of Self-Representation*. Bloomington: Indiana University Press, 1987.

– *Subjectivity, Identity, and the Body: Women's Autobiographical Practices in the Twentieth Century*. Bloomington: Indiana University Press, 1993.

Smith, Sidonie, and Julia Watson. *Reading Autobiography: A Guide for Interpreting Life Narratives*. 2nd ed. Minneapolis: University of Minnesota Press, 2010.

Smith, Sidonie, and Julia Watson, eds. *Getting a Life: Everyday Uses of Autobiography*. Minneapolis: University of Minnesota, 1996.

– *Interfaces: Women, Autobiography, Image, Performance*. Ann Arbor: University of Michigan Press, 2002.

Sonnet, Martine. *L'Education des filles au temps des Lumières*. Paris: Le Cerf, 1987.

Sontag, Susan. *AIDS and Its Metaphors*. New York: Farrar, Straus and Giroux, 1989.

– *Illness as Metaphor*. New York: Farrar, Straus and Giroux, 1978.

– *Illness as Metaphor; and, AIDS and Its Metaphors*. New York; Toronto: Doubleday, 1990.

Spencer, Samia I., ed. *French Women and the Age of Enlightenment*. Bloomington: Indiana University Press, 1984.

Stanley, Liz. "The Epistolarium: On Theorizing Letters and Correspondences." *A/b: Auto/Biography Studies* 12, no. 3 (2004): 201–35.

– "The Epistolary Gift, the Editorial Third-Party, Counter-Epistolaria: Rethinking the Epistolarium." *Life Writing* 8, no. 2 (2011): 135–52.

Stanley, Liz, Helen Dampier, and Andrea Salter. "The Epistolary Pact, Letterness, and the Schreiner Epistolarium." *A/b: Auto/Biography Studies* 27, no. 2 (2012): 262–93.

Stanton, Domna C. *The Aristocrat as Art: A Study of the Honnête Homme and the Dandy in Seventeenth and Nineteenth-Century French Literature*. New York: Columbia University Press, 1980.

Steedman, Carolyn. "A Boiling Copper and Some Arsenic: Servants, Childcare, and Class Consciousness in Late Eighteenth-Century England." *Critical Inquiry* 34, no. 1 (2007): 36–77.

– *Dust: The Archive and Cultural History*. Manchester: Manchester University Press, 2001.

– *Master and Servant: Love and Labour in the English Industrial Age*. Cambridge: Cambridge University Press, 2007.

Steinberger, Deborah. "The Difficult Birth of the Good Mother: Donneau de Visé's *L'Embarras de Godard, ou l'Accouchée*." In *Maternal Measures: Figuring Caregiving in the Early Modern Period*, edited by Naomi J. Miller and Naomi Yavneh, 201–11. Aldershot: Ashgate, 2000.

Steinbrügge, Lieselotte. *The Moral Sex: Woman's Nature in the French Enlightenment*. Translated by Pamela E. Selwyn. New York: Oxford University Press, 1995.

Steinke, Hubert. "Maladie en contexte. Lettres familières, lettres de savants et lettres de patients au 18e siècle." In *Maladies en lettres. 17e–21e siècles*, edited by Vincent Barras and Martin Dinges, 49–58. Lausanne: Editions BHMS, 2013.

Stolberg, Michael. *Experiencing Illness and the Sick Body in Early Modern Europe*. Translated by Leonhard Unglaub and Logan Kennedy. Houndmills, UK: Palgrave Macmillan, 2011.

– "Les lettres de patients et la culture médicale pré-moderne." In *Maladies en lettres. 17e–21e siècles*, edited by Vincent Barras and Martin Dinges, 23–32. Lausanne: Editions BHMS, 2013.

– "Medical Popularization and the Patient in the Eighteenth Century." In *Cultural Approaches to the History of Medicine: Mediating Medicine in Early*

*Modern and Modern Europe*, edited by Willem de Blécourt and Cornelie Usborne, 89–107. Houndmills, UK: Palgrave Macmillan, 2004.

– "The Monthly Malady: A History of Premenstrual Suffering." *Medical History* 44 (2000): 301–22.

– "Self-Pollution, Moral Reform, and the Venereal Trade: Notes on the Sources and Historical Context of *Onania* (1716)." *Journal of the History of Sexuality* 9, no. 1/2 (2000): 37–61.

– "An Unmanly Vice: Self-Pollution, Anxiety, and the Body in the Eighteenth Century." *Social History of Medicine* 13 (2000): 1–22.

– "A Woman's Hell? Medical Perceptions of Menopause in Preindustrial Europe." *Bulletin of the History of Medicine* 73, no. 3 (1999): 404–28.

Straub, Kristina. *Domestic Affairs: Intimacy, Eroticism, and Violence between Servants and Masters in Eighteenth-Century Britain*. Baltimore: Johns Hopkins University Press, 2009.

Strayer, Brian E. *Suffering Saints: Jansenists and Convulsionnaires in France, 1640–1799*. Brighton: Sussex Academic Press, 2008.

Sturzer, Felicia B. "Love and Disease: The Contaminated Letters of Julie de Lespinasse." *Studies on Voltaire and the Eighteenth Century* 2000, no. 8 (2000): 3–16.

Sussman, George D. *Selling Mothers' Milk: The Wet-Nursing Business in France, 1715–1914*. Urbana: University of Illinois Press, 1982.

Tadmor, Naomi. "The Concept of the Household-Family in Eighteenth-Century England." *Past & Present* no. 151 (1996): 111–40.

Teysseire, Daniel. "Mort du roi et troubles féminins: Le premier valet de chambre de Louis XV consulte Tissot pour sa jeune femme (mai 1776)." In *Santé et maladie au XVIIIe siècle*, edited by Helmut Holshey and Urs Boschung, 49–56. Amsterdam: Rodopi, 1995.

Thomas, Chantal. *The Wicked Queen: The Origins of the Myth of Marie-Antoinette*. New York: Zone Books, 1999.

Tissot, Samuel Auguste. *Advice to the People in General, with Regard to Their Health*. Translated by J. Kirkpatrick. London, 1765. *Eighteenth Century Collections Online*. Gale. Memorial University of Newfoundland.

– *Avis au peuple sur sa santé*. Lausanne: François Grasset, 1761.

– *De la Médecine civile, ou de la Police de la Médecine*. Edited by Miriam Nicoli. Lausanne: Editions BHMS, 2009.

– *De la santé des gens de lettres*. Lausanne: Grasset, 1768.

– *Essai sur les maladies des gens du monde*. Laussane: Grasset, 1770.

– *An Essay on Diseases Incidental to Literary and Sedentary Persons*. Dublin: James Williams, 1769.

– *An Essay on the Disorders of People of Fashion*. Translated by Francis Bacon Lee. London: Richardson and Urquhart, 1771.

– *L'Onanisme*. Lausanne: Chapuis, 1760.

– *Onanism: Or a Treatise upon the Disorders Produced by Masturbation: Or, the Dangerous Effects of Secret and Excessive Venery*. Translated by A. Hume. London: J. Pridden, 1766.

– *Traité des nerfs et de leurs maladies*. Lausanne: Grasset, 1778–80.

Torrell, Margaret Rose. "Plural Singularities: The Disability Community in Life-Writing Texts." *Journal of Literary & Cultural Disability Studies* 5, no. 3 (2011): 321–38.

Traer, James F. *Marriage and the Family in Eighteenth-Century France*. Ithaca, NY: Cornell University Press, 1980.

Tronto, Joan. "'The Servant Problem' and Justice in Households." *Iris: European Journal of Philosophy and Public Debate* 2, no. 3 (2010): 67–86.

Trouille, Mary Seidman. "The Failings of Rousseau's Ideals of Domesticity and Sensibility." *Eighteenth-Century Studies* 24, no. 4 (1991): 451–83.

Tuttle, Leslie. "Celebrating the *père de famille*: Pronatalism and Fatherhood in Eighteenth-Century France." *Journal of Family History* 29, no. 4 (2004): 366–81.

Tyler, Imogen. "Skin-Tight: Celebrity, Pregnancy and Subjectivity." In *Thinking through the Skin*, edited by Sara Ahmed and Jackie Stacey, 69–83. New York: Routledge, 2001.

Vasset, Sophie, ed. *Medicine and Narration in the Eighteenth Century*. Oxford: Voltaire Foundation, 2013.

Venel, Jean-André. *Essai sur la santé et sur l'éducation médicinale des filles destinées au mariage*. Yverdon: Chez la Société Littéraire & Typographique, 1776.

Vess, David M. *Medical Revolution in France, 1789–1796*. Gainesville: Florida State University Press, 1975.

Vickery, Amanda. "An Englishman's Home is His Castle? Thresholds, Boundaries and Privacies in the Eighteenth-Century London House." *Past and Present* 199, no. 1 (2008): 147–73.

Vigroux, Hélène. "Marin Marais et le *Le tableau de l'opération de la taille*." *Médecine des arts: Approche médicale et scientifique des pratiques artistiques* 4 (1993): 25–7.

Vila, Anne C. "Alternative Pleasures: Sex, Sociability, and the Scholarly Imagination in Eighteenth-Century France." In *Imagination und Sexualität: Pathologien der Einbildungskraft im Medizinischen Diskurs der Frühen Neuzeit*, edited by Stefanie Zaun, Daniela Watzke, and Jörn Steigerwald, 101–18. Frankfurt: Vittorio Klostermann, 2004.

– "Beyond Sympathy: Vapors, Melancholia, and the Pathologies of Sensibility in Tissot and Rousseau." *Yale French Studies* 92 (1997): 88–101.

– "Enlightened Minds and Scholarly Bodies from Tissot to Sade." *Studies in Eighteenth-Century Culture* 23, no. 1 (1994): 207–20.

– *Enlightenment and Pathology: Sensibility in the Literature and Medicine of Eighteenth-Century France*. Baltimore: Johns Hopkins University Press, 1998.

– "Reading the 'Sensible' Body: Medicine, Philosophy, and Semiotics in Eighteenth-Century France." In *Data Made Flesh: Embodying Information*, edited by Robert Mitchell and Phillip Thurtle, 27–45. New York: Routledge, 2004.

– "The *Philosophe*'s Stomach: Hedonism, Hypochondria, and the Intellectual in Enlightenment France." In *Cultures of the Abdomen: Diet, Digestion, and Fat in the Modern World*, edited by Christopher E. Forth and Ana Carden-Coyne, 89–104. Houndmills, UK: Palgrave Macmillan, 2005.

– "Sensible Diagnostics in Diderot's *La Religieuse*," *MLN* 105, no. 4 (1990): 774–99.

– "Sex and Sensibility: Pierre Roussels *Système physique et moral de la femme*." *Representations* 52 (1995): 76–93.

Wagner, Peter. "The Discourses on Sex – or Sex as Discourse: Eighteenth-Century Medical and Paramedical Erotica." In *Sexual Underworlds of the Enlightenment*, edited by G.S. Rousseau and Roy Porter, 46–68. Chapel Hill: University of North Carolina Press, 1988.

Weber, Caroline. *Queen of Fashion: What Marie Antoinette Wore to the Revolution*. 1st ed. New York: H. Holt, 2006.

Weiss, James R. *Marquis de Sade's Veiled Social Criticism: The Depravities of Sodom as the Perversities of France*. Lewiston, NY: Edwin Mellen Press, 2008.

Wellman, Kathleen. "Physicians and *Philosophes*: Physiology and Sexual Morality in the French Enlightenment." *Eighteenth-Century Studies* 35, no. 2 (2002): 266–77.

Wendell, Susan. *The Rejected Body: Feminist Philosophical Reflections on Disability*. New York: Routledge, 1996.

– "Toward a Feminist Theory of Disability." *Hypatia* 4, no. 2 (1999): 104–24.

Went-Daoust, Yvette. "Madame de Charrière et l'impératif du mariage." In *Sexualité, mariage et famille au XVIIIe siècle*, edited by Olga B. Cragg and Rosena Davison, 173–83. Saint-Nicolas: Les presses de l'Université Laval, 1998.

Weston, Robert. "Epistolary Consultations on Venereal Disease in Eighteenth-Century France." *French History and Civilisation. Papers from the George Rudé Seminar* 3 (2009). http://www.h-france.net/rude/rudevolumeiii/ Weston Vol3.pdf.

– *Medical Consulting by Letter in France, 1665–1789*. Farnham, Surrey: Ashgate, 2013.

Wetherall-Dickson, Leigh. "Melancholy, Medicine, Mad Moon and Marriage: Autobiographical Expressions of Depression." In *Melancholy Experience in Literature of the Long Eighteenth Century: Before Depression, 1660–1800*, edited by Allan Ingram, Stuart Sim, Clark Lawlor, Richard Terry, John Baker, and Leigh Wetherall-Dickson, 142–69. Houndmills, UK: Palgrave Macmillan, 2011.

Wheeler, David. "Jane Austen and 18th-Century English Spa Culture." *English Studies: A Journal of English Language and Literature* 85, no. 2 (2004): 120–33.

Wild, Wayne. "Doctor–Patient Correspondence in Eighteenth-Century Britain: A Change in Rhetoric and Relationship." *Studies in Eighteenth-Century Culture* 29 (2000): 47–64.

– *Medicine-by-Post: The Changing Voice of Illness in Eighteenth-Century British Consultation Letters and Literature*. Amsterdam: Rodopi, 2006.

Williams, Carolyn D. "'The Luxury of Doing Good': Benevolence, Sensibility, and the Royal Humane Society." In *Pleasure in the Eighteenth Century*, edited by Roy Porter and Marie Mulvey Roberts, 77–107. Houndmills, UK: Macmillan, 1996.

Williams, Elizabeth A. "Hysteria and the Court Physician in Enlightenment France." *Eighteenth-Century Studies* 35, no. 2 (2002): 247–55.

– "Stomach and Psyche: Eating, Digestion and Mental Illness in the Medicine of Philippe Pinel." *Bulletin of the History of Medicine* 84, no. 3 (2010): 358–86.

Williams, Samantha. "The Experience of Pregnancy and Childbirth for Unmarried Mothers in London, 1760–1866." *Women's History Review* 20, no. 1 (2011): 67–86.

Wilson, Kathleen. "The Female Rake: Gender, Libertinism and Enlightenment." In *Libertine Enlightenment: Sex, Liberty and License in the Eighteenth Century*, edited by Peter Cryle and Lisa O'Donnell, 95–111. Houndmills, UK: Palgrave MacMillan, 2004.

Wilson, Lindsay B. *Women and Medicine in the French Enlightenment*. Baltimore: Johns Hopkins University Press, 1993.

Wilson, Philip K. "Eighteenth-Century 'Monsters' and Nineteenth-Century 'Freaks': Reading the Maternally-Marked Child." *Literature and Medicine* 21, no. 1 (2002): 1–25.

Winston, Michael E. *From Perfectibility to Perversion: Meliorism in Eighteenth-Century France*. New York: Peter Lang, 2005.

– "Medicine, Marriage, and Human Degeneration in the French Enlightenment." *Eighteenth-Century Studies* 38, no. 2 (2005): 263–81.

Withey, Alun. *Physick and the Family: Health, Medicine and Care in Wales, 1600–1750*. Manchester: Manchester University Press, 2011.

Wolff, Eberhard. "Perspectives on Patients' History: Methodological Considerations on the Example of Recent German-Speaking Literature." *Canadian Bulletin of Medical History* 15, no. 1 (1998): 207–28.

Woolf, Virginia. "On Being Ill." *The New Criterion* 4, no. 1 (1926): 32–45.

– *A Room of One's Own and Three Guineas*. Oxford: Oxford University Press, 1998.

Wyngaard, Amy S. "Rétif, Sade, and the Origins of Pornography: *Le Pornographe* as Anti-Text of *La philosophie dans le boudoir*." *Eighteenth-Century Fiction* 25, no. 2 (2012): 383–406.

Yalom, Marilyn. *A History of the Breast*. New York: Ballantine Books, 1997.

Young, Iris Marion. *On Female Body Experience: "Throwing Like a Girl" and Other Essays*. Studies in Feminist Philosophy. New York: Oxford University Press, 2005.

Young, Paul J. "'Ce lieu au délices': Art and Imitation in the French Libertine Cabinet." *Eighteenth-Century Fiction* 20, no. 3 (2008): 335–56.

Yuval-Davis, Nira. "Women, Citizenship, and Difference." In *Citizenship: Pushing the Boundaries*, edited by Feminist Review Collective, 4–17. Abingdon, UK: Taylor & Francis, 1997.

epilepsy, 75, 164, 214, 228, 232. *See also* convulsive disorder; nervous disorder

Epinoy, Roze de l', 139

epistolarity: and art of pleasing, 222; complexities of, 81–2; epistolary pact, 44; epistolarium, 47–8; and gender, 40, 82–3; in libertine literature, 172; medical, 10, 29–34; and narrative choice, 82; skin as metaphor, 50; as social practice, 38–9. *See also* letters

*Essai sur les maladies des gens du monde*, 102–5

état de nature. *See* Nature

excess: as basis for personal transformation, 119; and body resistance, 224; and corporeal stigmata, 187; and elite identity, 100, 103–5, 211, 213–14, 229; and failed citizens, 93, 179, 200; and libertinage, 168; luxury and, 214; and the unruly body, 96, 97; and will, 78, 80. *See also* citizenship; *jouissance*; nervous disorder; onanism; pleasure

experience: authenticity and, 24; discursive, 243–4; interpretations of, 177; as site of inquiry, 24

failed citizens, 93, 247

family: affective, 124; as basis for civic happiness, 62; and the body, 130; as business transaction, 123; eighteenth-century understandings of, 123–4, 126–7; horizontal axis, 131–2; ideologies of, 128; legal understandings of, 127; lineage and, 122–3, 124, 126, 128, 155; *mal* and *maux de famille*, 122, 130; Rousseau's understandings, 125, 128; source of the nation, 122; vertical axis, 131–2. *See also* kinship

fatherhood: in eighteenth-century family, 123; as gatekeeper of maternal performance, 148; ideologies of, 147–8; and paternal intimacy, 152, 272n136; and paternal masculinity,

150–1; and paternal subjectivity, 149; and penile performativity, 149, 153; *père de famille*, 148; as performance, 31, 152, 153; sensibility and, 149. *See also* family; kinship; motherhood

fear: and bodily disorder, 111; and compromised citizenship, 127, 167, 170, 228; and convulsive disorders, 231. *See also* shame

femininity: dissimulation, 41–2; and elite identity, 222; letters and, 40; performance of, 222, 226, 232; reproductive fecundity and, 222; and sexual pleasure, 175–6, 195, 197; and virtue, 197, 198

Fermon, Nicole, 102, 128, 133

*Fonds Tissot*: approachability of, 22–3; geographic scope, 11–12; characteristics of letters in, 15; correspondence language in, 12; lay letters, 15–18; professional letters, 16; sociological profile, 12. *See also* epistolarity; letters

Foucault, Michel, 43, 220

French Revolution, 16, 90, 108

Galliotte (Tissot correspondent), 73–4, 113

Gatens, Moira, 92, 113

Gauteron, François Louis: and body crimes, 159–60; letters to Philippe-Sirice Bridel, 203–5; letters to Tissot, 158–9; publications, 203; and social utility, 170. *See also* pleasure

Gay, J. Pierre, 12

gaze: autoerotic, 172; doubled, 6, 173; external 57; Foucauldian 160; internal 67; letters 172, 173; medical, 14, 67, 88, 242, 243; spectacle, 189; voyeurism, 20. *See also* letters

Germigny, Monsieur de, 32

Gilmore, Leigh, 36

Gounon (Tissot correspondent), 50, 177, 192–3

Grand, Marianne, 107

Grassi, Marie-Claire, 41, 82

Gringet, Monsieur, 32–4, 40, 52, 77

and intergenerational responsibility, 163–4; invisibility and, 164; and nervous disorder, 202; and performance of masculinity, 175, 181, 191, 192; and reproduction, 163; and seminal fluid, 165; and sexual excess, 164; and sexual initiation, 178–80, 183, 194; and shame, 180, 205; social effects of, 163; as spectacle, 167; and virility, 159, 183, 191, 193; women and, 193–5. *See also Onania*; *Onanisme, L'*; pleasure

*Onanisme, L'*: in letters, 33, 74–5, 173, 179; and onanytic epistolarity, 173; success of, 162; in relation to Tissot's other publications, 213; understandings of onanism in, 164–7. *See also Onania*; onanism; pleasure

"On Being Ill", 46–7

Overboe, James, 243, 245, 246

pain: onanism and, 164; pleasure and, 174, 190; in "Tableau de l'opération de la taille," 4–5

patient: as correspondent, 16–17; definition of, 30; docile, 242; doctor–patient relations, 14, 17, 177, 207, 217–20, 245; experience, 26; as medical knower, 14; methodological implications of, 30–1; as *ouvrage*, 64, 65

*patrie. See* homeland

penile performativity, 150, 151, 153, 164, 191

Peyrelongue, Chevalier de, 181

Pictet (Tissot correspondent), 116

Pilloud, Séverine: interiority and exteriority in Tissot correspondence, 51–2; mediation in Tissot correspondence, 13, 63; onanism, 164; parameters of Fonds Tissot, 250n23, 250n24, 251n26, 251n29, 251n38; and suffering in community, 31. *See also* Louis-Courvoisier, Micheline

*plaisir*: as imagined community, 169; and social discipline, 169; *l'art de plaire*, 169; citizenship and, 169; and

*jouissance*, 171, 174, 175, 176. *See also* pleasure

pleasure: autoeroticism and, 160, 199, 202, 204; and biblical fall, 170; and bodily crime, 160; class and, 194; and consumption, 214; corporeal stigmata and, 181, 183, 187; Diderot's definition, 170–1; and divine grace, 205; as earthly entitlement, 171; eighteenth-century understandings of, 161–2; and elite identity, 167–8, 169; erotic sociability and, 173; flirtation and, 161, 184; gallantry, 161, 168; illicit, 159, 174, 176, 180; imagination and, 165–6, 199–202; libertine fiction and, 161, 172, 194–5; libertinage, 168; Madame Roland and, 196–7; masculinity and, 175–6, 181, 185–6; as moral virtue, 171; and nervous disorder, 214; pleasure-seeking body, 171, 176–7, 183–5, 190–2, 200; politics of, 168, 174–5; as punishment, 160; reproduction and, 163–4; self pleasure, 170, 184; sexual initiation, 178–80, 182–3; shame, 169, 176, 180, 203–5, and social discipline, 169, 174, 180; as somatic memory, 172; Temple of Health, 161; tickling and, 183–5; voyeurism and, 172, 174, 175, 181; women and, 193–5, 197–8. *See also* gaze, imagination; *jouissance*; onanism; *plaisir*; voyeurism

Poliansky, B., 71–3

Pomme, Pierre, 240–1

Pompadour, Madame de, 194, 195

Porter, Roy: and illness and identity, 58, 62, 246; and medical history from below, 24; understanding of nervous disorder, 209, 215, 231; understanding of pleasure, 169, 171

post-personhood, 246. *See also* disability studies

Probyn, Elspeth, 216

Prosser, Jay, 50

Puar, Jasbir, 86, 243